THE HOLT INSTITUTE OF MEDICINE
PRESENTS:

A Primer of Natural Therapeutics

A CERTIFICATION PROGRAM FOR DIETARY SUPPLEMENT COUNSELORS (Dip. DSC)

Stephen Holt MD

The Holt Institute of Medicine
www.hiom.org

Cover design and layout by Jonathan Gullery.
Edited by Cecily MacConchie

Manufactured in the United States.
Library of Congress catalogue in-publication data.
Holt, Stephen 1950-

A Primer of Natural Therapeutics: A Certification Program
for Dietary Supplement Counselors

Author: Stephen Holt MD with a Forewords by Thomas V. Taylor, MD
and Charles McWilliams, ND

ISBN: 978-0-9747198-1-8

Key Words: 1. dietary supplements 2. natural medicine 3. certification program 4. alternative medicine 5. nutraceuticals 6. lifestyle 7. herbs 8. botanical medicine 9. nutrition 10. vitamins 11. minerals 12. integrative medicine

CONTENTS

PUBLISHER'S NOTES … … … … … … … … … … … … … … … … … 5

WHAT IS THIS BOOK … … … … … … … … … … … … … … … … … 6

FOREWORD 1 … … … … … … … … … … … … … … … … … 7

FOREWORD 2 … … … … … … … … … … … … … … … … 10

PREFACE … … … … … … … … … … … … … … … … … 12

HOW TO USE THIS BOOK … … … … … … … … … … … … … 15

CHAPTER 1 MULTIVITAMINS … … … … … … … … … 17

CHAPTER 2 SLEEP … … … … … … … … … … … … 25

CHAPTER 3 MENOPAUSE AND PMS: THE MENOPLAN … 31

CHAPTER 4 ANTIOXIDANTS … … … … … … … … … … 36

CHAPTER 5 ANTIAGING: PREVENTING PREMATURE
DISABILITY AND DEATH … … … … … … … 45

CHAPTER 6 OSTEOPOROSIS OR THIN BONES: THE
ANTIPOROSIS® PLAN … … … … … … … … 54

CHAPTER 7 IMMUNE FUNCTION … … … … … … … … 59

CHAPTER 8 JOINT CARE … … … … … … … … … … … 66

CHAPTER 9 DIGESTION … … … … … … … … … … … 73

CHAPTER 10 HEARTBURN … … … … … … … … … … 84

CHAPTER 11 COLON CLEANSING … … … … … … … … 91

CHAPTER 12 FIBER … … … … … … … … … … … … … 96

CHAPTER 13 ENZYMES … … … … … … … … … … … 102

CHAPTER 14 CORAL CALCIUM … … … … … … … … … … 109

CHAPTER 15 WEIGHT MANAGEMENT … … … … … … … 113

CHAPTER 16 SYNDROME X AND NUTRITIONAL FACTORS 121

CHAPTER 17 BLOOD SUGAR … … … … … … … … … 132

CHAPTER 18	FISH OIL … … … … … … … … … … … … …	144
CHAPTER 19	CHOLESTEROL: DON'T FORGET	
	HOMOCYSTEINE! … … … … … … … … …	154
CHAPTER 20	HEART … … … … … … … … … … … … … …	166
CHAPTER 21	PROSTATE … … … … … … … … … … … … …	171
CHAPTER 22	SEX NATURALLY … … … … … … … … … … …	174
CHAPTER 23	MEMORY: BRAIN FUNCTION … … … … …	178
CHAPTER 24	SKIN, NAILS AND HAIR SUPPORT … … … …	187
CHAPTER 25	EYE CARE … … … … … … … … … … … … …	190
CHAPTER 26	HIGH ENERGY … … … … … … … … … … …	192
CHAPTER 27	NATURES CALCIUM® AND CALCIUM	
	SUPPLEMENTS … … … … … … … … … … …	196
CHAPTER 28	ANTI-DEPENDENCE … … … … … … … …	199
CHAPTER 29	MOOD … … … … … … … … … … … … … …	205
CHAPTER 30	ALLERGY … … … … … … … … … … … … …	209
CHAPTER 31	SPECIFIC ANTI-AGING FACTORS	
	FOR NATURAL CLINICIANS … … … … … …	215
CHAPTER 33	PETS … … … … … … … … … … … … … … …	288
CHAPTER 34	WELLNESS EDUCATION … … … … … … …	292
APPENDIX A	VERY IMPORTANT AND SPECIAL	
	WARNINGS TO READERS … … … … … … …	295
APPENDIX B	ABOUT THE AUTHOR … … … … … … … …	299
APPENDIX C	METABOLIC SYNDROME, SYNDROME X:	
	SYNDROME X, Y, Z…? … … … … … … … …	301
CERTIFICATION EXAMINATION… … … … … … … … … …	343
INSTRUCTIONS	… … … … … … … … … … … … … … … … … …	343
QUESTIONS	… … … … … … … … … … … … … … … … … …	345
ANSWER SHEET	… … … … … … … … … … … … … … … … … …	365
INDEX	… … … … … … … … … … … … … … … … … …	369

PUBLISHER'S NOTES

THIS book describes the use of dietary supplements and their potential applications for the support of body structures and functions. The author of this book is not attempting to provide advice on the treatment or prevention of disease with dietary supplements, given the US Dietary Supplement and Health Education Act, DSHEA (1994). It is not the intention of the author to interfere with physician/client relationships. Readers are encouraged to share the information in this book with healthcare practitioners. The use of dietary supplements and health food is being incorporated increasingly into medical practice in the 21st century. This book was not written to endorse the use of any specific products or for any treatment purposes. The book describes concepts of dietary supplement formulation using combinations of nutrients, botanicals and herbs. The author uses examples of his own work on formulation and provides reference sections for individuals to make their own informed judgments. Any opinions expressed in this book represent the author's opinions on medical, scientific, folkloric and lay writings on the topics discussed. The author acknowledges that medical opinion varies on the value of nutrition or dietary supplements in standard medical practice. The author is not advising any deviation from usual and customary standards of medical care, but the author believes strongly that the healthcare recipient is the key decision maker in the management of their own disease. Many people in industrialized societies are seeking natural, medical alternatives. The author does not support disease treatment claims that accompany the sale of some dietary supplements. This book is not intended to be a product label and it should be displayed in a retail setting only with geographic separation from any health food or dietary supplement. The publisher believes that this is the first published work that summarizes information, in one short synopsis, on "how to use" dietary supplements.

www.hiom.org

WHAT IS THIS BOOK?

A Certification Program for Individuals who wish to counsel on the use of dietary supplements (nutraceuticals). This book was written primarily for health enthusiasts, retail store or office staff to improve their knowledge and skills in counseling on the use of dietary supplements. However, clinicians seeking basic knowledge on supplements may benefit from this introductory course.

This program is complemented by on-site educational resources at the Holt Institute of Medicine [NJ, USA], where training sessions can be scheduled for group learning.

At the end of the book is a Certification Examination with an answer key that can be detached and mailed to "Dietary Supplement Counselor Certification Program," Holt Institute of Medicine, 61 Stevens Ave, Little Falls, NJ 07424 (Tel (973) 890-2378).

After the answer pages for the examination are completed, and the answer key is detached and mailed to the above address, an oral examination will be held by telephone or in person with Stephen Holt MD or a member of his personal staff. The oral exam will test general knowledge and skills on dietary supplements usage.

Upon completion of these requirements, a certificate for a "Certified Dietary Supplement Counselor," the Diploma of Dietary Supplement Counseling (Dip. DSC.), will be issued by the Holt Institute of Medicine, in affiliation with the World Organization of Natural Medical Practitioners and the Pan American School of Natural Medicine, Nevis, WI.

Successful completion of this course provides credits toward a Naturopathic Degree from the Pan American School of Natural Medicine (call (973) 256-4660).

www.hiom.org

FOREWORD I

MILLIONS of Americans are using dietary supplements to promote health and wellbeing; but many healthcare consumers may lack enough scientific or "medical" knowledge to comprehend their correct use. Natural remedies or dietary supplements are valuable health interventions. Health food stores and chain stores contain a vast array of supplement product offerings. This creates frequent consumer confusion, and sometimes expressions of "uncertainty" on the part of retail staff. The retail store staff is consulted often for supplement recommendations, but training in supplement usage is not structured and it is sometimes limited to biased marketing information about nutraceuticals. Much marketing information on dietary supplements is disseminated by individuals with no biomedical training or credentials.

No institution or association in the dietary supplement industry has produced a "core program" to educate on dietary supplement usage. Industry trade publications contain editorial content that is often written by individuals with limited, if any, medical experience. Such authors may have to appease the needs of their advertisers. Trade "associations" in the US or global dietary supplement industry tend sometimes to select lecturers at national or regional meetings that have paid for a forum in which to speak; and they operate with little or no formal process of speaker credentialing. Furthermore, the government has not accepted the need to educate the public about disease treatment or prevention without a conventional medical intervention (drugs or surgery).

Positive lifestyle change with good nutrition is a first line option for wellness promotion, but these options should be exercised with a reasonable base of knowledge. Stephen Holt MD has committed himself to educate the public on more simple gentle and natural pathways to health, "without turning his back" on the appropriate application of conventional medicine. This approach constitutes the modern discipline of Integrative Medicine.

This book is a unique contribution to the dietary supplement industry. It represents new and novel descriptions of dietary supplements that have a reasonable evidence-base for nutritional support of body structures and functions. In this book, Dr. Holt describes allowable but limited claims concerning dietary supplements. These limited, wellness claims conform to the US Dietary Supplement and Health Education Act of 1994 (DSHEA). Dr. Holt has described the far reaching consequences of DSHEA for American consumers and purveyors of dietary supplements, in peer-reviewed literature. In this forum, he has attempted to offer guidelines for the ethical sale of dietary supplements with appropriate education. Dietary supplements are not to be used to prevent, diagnose or treat any disease... at law. This book reacts strongly against the description elsewhere of "Natural Cures" that do not exist.

I am proud and pleased to write a foreword to this revolutionary account of dietary supplement applications in wellness promotion. Dr. Holt proposes nutritional supplements that are made often by combining several natural substances in a synergistic manner. The term synergy is derived from the Greek word "synergia" which means "to work together." Natural ingredients in dietary supplements can take advantage of cooperative actions that are powerful modifiers of biological responses. Cooperative actions, in a combination of additive effects, can result in biological actions that may be greater than the sum of the individual components of the proposed mixture of natural substances. In other words, synergistic formulations of dietary supplements have the advantage of combined or correlated actions of two or more natural agents. This approach represents leading-edge nutraceutical technology which is beyond the ability of many marketers or sellers of supplements who "formulate" for commercial purposes.

While this book describes the use of dietary supplement formulations that are designed to operate in an additive manner for health benefits, it does not claim that supplements are "magic bullets." This book emphasizes that dietary supplements should not be used as a substitute for a poor diet; and they must be applied with positive lifestyle changes for the promotion of health and wellbeing. Dr. Holt emphasizes that dietary supplements that are accompanied by "curative claims," should be avoided and he stresses a need to inform healthcare consumers or healthcare givers about both the advantages and the limitations of self medication with supplements.

Sir Stephen Holt MD, LLD(Hon.), PhD, ND, FACP, FRCP (C), FACG, FACN, MRCP (UK), FACAM, a Knight of Grace of the Holy Order of St. John is uniquely qualified to formulate health giving, dietary supplements. He has practiced medicine for 36 years and is a double board certified physician with higher training in nutrition and clinical pharmacology. His impressive credentials are combined with his extensive background of medical research and long term involvement in pharmaceutical, food and supplement development.

The modern consumer of dietary supplements has become increasingly knowledgeable about remedies of natural origin. These educated healthcare consumers are now taking a long, hard look at **who is formulating the dietary supplements they are using?** It is quite surprising that many people may use supplements that have been formulated or recommended by individuals with very little biomedical training, no medical credentials, or no clinical experience in natural medicine. In fact, it is of great concern that some people may not educate themselves so that they can exert care or informed judgments in their choice of supplement formulations.

I can state with confidence that Stephen Holt MD has brought an unsurpassed level of excellence in the research and development of drugs, functional foods and dietary supplements over the past four decades. Stephen Holt MD works at many levels in the supplement industry including: basic science research on new supplement ingredients, manufacturing, formulation and education. With that said, Dr. Holt's formulations are among the most copied of all formulations in the modern history of the US dietary supplement industry.

Stephen Holt MD has been described as an icon and visionary in the global dietary supplement industry. He has contributed greatly to the education of consumers, retailers and professionals on the correct use of supplements for specific health purposes or conditions. With more than 20 books in international distribution, and several hundred published peer-reviewed, scientific communications, Dr. Holt is a pioneer of Integrative Medicine and he is the Chairman of a Department of Integrative Medicine in New York, where he holds the most senior of all academic ranks as a Distinguished Professor of Medicine.

Stephen Holt MD will not support illegal treatment claims about dietary supplements or foods, but he has a passion for natural medicine. Dr. Holt has worked diligently to incorporate dietary supplements into modern healthcare and his efforts have been recognized by the granting of honorary degrees. For his lifetime contributions to society, Dr. Holt was Knighted by the Holy Order of St. John. It is with great pleasure that I support the contributions of Dr. Stephen Holt MD to Integrative Medicine, or Pluralistic Medicine... as he prefers to call it!

TV Taylor MD
Clinical Professor, Baylor College of Medicine, and University of Texas. Chairman of Academic Surgery, St. Joseph's Hospital, Houston, TX. Knight of Honor, Holy Order of St. John.

FOREWORD 2

IT is a great pleasure to introduce this unique book and program that provides an ability to rapidly assimilate information on the use of "natural medicines" (dietary supplements). Dr. Holt is well known on a global basis for his pioneering work in Integrative Medicine and many honors have been bestowed upon him for his lifetime contribution to both natural and allopathic medicine. This book is written with eloquence, clarity and simplicity. It is a great feat to synthesize an enormous amount of evidence-based information into a summarized text, which Dr. Holt does so often with ease. This book permits the student to enter the intellectual thoughts of Dr. Holt and it demonstrates his ability to navigate huge amounts of information through the natural medical literature.

Most accounts of the use of dietary supplements or natural medicines talk about supplements in a phenomenological manner. Dr. Holt has gone beyond the realm of supplement description by describing the therapeutic approach with nutrients, herbs and botanicals. Dr. Holt admits that his thoughts have been stimulated most by physicians of the late Victorian era who first proposed the concept of "harmony of the body." It is not apparent to many people who know about Dr. Holt's contemporary contributions to natural medicine that he is a trained clinical pharmacologist as well as a board certified gastroenterologist and internist in the US, Canada and the EU. Dr. Holt has made meritorious contributions to drug development and he utilizes his unique background in pharmaceutical research to probe the real biopharmaceutical potential of herbs, botanicals and nutrients. Do not be fooled by the simplicity of the statements made in this book. Dr. Holt presents all material in an understandable manner, but he is armed with an encyclopedic knowledge of conventional and alternative medical literature.

Stephen Holt is the Academic President of the World Organization of Natural Medical Practitioners (www.wonmp.us) and he holds the academic rank of Distinguished Professor of Medicine. In fact, Dr. Holt's credentials are unique in the Integrative Medical community and he chairs the New York Department of Integrative Medicine. I have witnessed Dr. Holt's powerful teaching presentations at many medical conferences and he is an educator par excellence. Dr. Holt has major peer recognition and this book is an example of his skill and ability to teach others. It is clear to me that Dr. Holt's commitment is to educate the population as a way of improving health and wellbeing. He has done this in an unselfish manner and he has written for many scientific journals, lay publications and his books have achieved best seller status.

I have been so taken with this basic introduction to the rational use of dietary supplements that I presented it to the curriculum committee of the Pan American School of Natural Medicine who have embraced this teaching as a qualification for credits towards a degree in Natural (Naturopathic) Medicine. Please enjoy Dr. Holt's teachings and they should enrich your ability to help promote the health and well being of you and your loved ones.

Charles McWilliams, ND
Dean, Pan American School of Natural Medicine
Grand Master - Sovereign Medical Order of the Knights
Hospitaller (www.smokh.org)

PREFACE

THERE is a revolution in modern medicine. These days, the American public seeks safe, simple, natural and gentle options to promote their health and well-being. This explosion in the use of health food, dietary supplements and natural medicine has been prompted by several circumstances. This book was written primarily to give retail, professional or office staff in dietary supplement sales and others a basic education on dietary supplement usage. However, this work is relevant to any healthcare giver who wants to know more about supplement usage. The use of dietary supplements is part of a new treatment paradigm in medical care.

Healthcare consumers have expressed some disenchantment with standard conventional medicine; and there is an increasing trend towards self-diagnosis of illness with self-medication. The expanding elderly population and millions of "baby boomers" are seeking longevity, not just long life. Longevity must involve the maintenance of wellbeing. It is clear that people do not want to age with poor quality of life caused by chronic disease. Preventing illness, promoting health, and going to the plateau of wellness are key objectives for modern humankind.

In recent times, conventional medicine has presented an ever-increasing number of drugs and surgical procedures for disease management, but a significant proportion of patients and their families are second guessing these allopathic ("standard") treatments. The past decade has witnessed unprecedented skepticism about "drug promises." The idea that there is a "techno-fix" with a drug to treat or prevent disease is being challenged, as everyone realizes the importance of positive lifestyle in health maintenance. Consumer confidence is rocked by recurrent epidemics of adverse drug effects and their consequences of disability and death.

In this book, I present some viable natural options to help address major public health problems. Natural approaches to health, with the use of lifestyle modification, good nutrition and dietary supplements are now part of mainstream medicine. The advent of natural ways to promote health has come from a large consumer lobby. This lobby has not accepted the risks that are posed by some pharmaceutical treatments. Nowhere is this more obvious than in the management of common disorders such as arthritis, obesity, weight control, thin bones, cardiovascular health and the modern epidemics of pre-diabetes, metabolic syndrome X, and diabetes mellitus. With that said, I have not turned my back on drug treatments that have proven valuable in disease management, but I have a problem in identifying many drugs that "cure illness." The drive to use most popular drugs is "symptom relief."

Major medical institutions and important national bodies of opinion are redefining the management approach to major lifetime disorders such as obesity related disease, aging and the menopause. Menopause is not a disease, despite attempts to label it as such. The nation is presented with the frightening combination of being overweight, having abnormal blood cholesterol and/or high blood pressure, all linked by the underlying problem of resistance to the hormone insulin. This condition is called Syndrome X or the Metabolic Syndrome. This "Syndrome" affects 70 million Americans as a "hidden pandemic." Syndrome X is often mismanaged. Furthermore, Syndrome X remains a well-kept secret, perhaps because there is no alleged, drug techno-fix.

Natural interventions are becoming part of mainstream medicine, but there has been some concern expressed about unsupported claims concerning the health benefits of some dietary supplements. Indeed, I acknowledge there are many dietary supplements that have been sold with meager evidence of marginal benefit. Marketing predators have, on occasion, seriously misled the public on the benefits of some supplements, especially by the use of TV infomercials. Fortunately, the Federal Government and Dietary Supplement Industry Associations have intervened to stop this activity. This misleading activity is sometimes also present in "pharmaceutical claims." It is my intention to help people understand the positive benefits of good nutrition, dietary supplements and positive lifestyle change for the promotion of health and well-being, among their loved ones and themselves.

This book represents a number of options for natural pathways to health with an emphasis on lifestyle change. Today, medicine still follows the teaching of Hippocrates, the Father of Modern Medicine. Hippocrates would not divorce the concept of food from medicine and he was a proponent of "clean living."

Please enjoy the contents of this book which attempt to define the evidence that is available in scientific literature to define natural pathways to health. Of course, my writings reflect my own opinions. I want to avoid commercial bias. The modern health care consumer has been introduced to the absurd concept of "lifestyle drugs," but the solution to any lifestyle problem is positive lifestyle change, not a drug! In this new millennium, many people are looking towards vibrant health and anti-aging tactics that are clearly rooted in good lifestyle and the practice of Eclectic or Pluralistic Medicine or Integrative Medicine.

Stephen Holt MD, LLD (Hon.), PhD, ND, FACP, FRCP (C), FACG, FACN, MRCP (UK), FACAM, OSJ, Little Falls, NJ, 2008, Chairman, New York Department of Integrative Medicine, NYCPM, NY, Distinguished Professor of Medicine, President World Organization of Natural Medical Practioners, Knight of Grace, Holy Order of St. John. Board Member, Integrative Medicine Asia and GFIM. www.hiom.org

HOW TO USE THIS BOOK

- This book has an easy contents page that directs an individual to a specific health condition or use of a specific category of dietary supplements.
- The book contains cross-references and it attempts to show how many different nutrient or botanical or herbal ingredients can be applied as nutritional support for body structures and functions.
- This book is NOT a manual for disease prevention or treatment.
- This book provides a strong message that positive lifestyle changes must be undertaken for any dietary supplement or drug to be effective; and taking of dietary supplements is not a substitute for a lousy diet.
- Each chapter contains a keynote summary on the subject in question at the end of each chapter. This serves as a quick reference guide.
- The book will be useful to consumers or purveyors of many dietary supplements and it serves as a quick reference guide for retailers of dietary supplements or office staff of care-givers. Care-givers may benefit from this "primer" information.
- References are given at the back of the book to support the notions of "good scientific agreement." However, there is some disagreement in several areas of medicine concerning what constitutes "good scientific agreement." The author encourages dialogue.
- Self medication is becoming more common as healthcare becomes less portable. Please educate yourself before self medication or before making recommendations to others.
- Favorable statements about the use of supplements for health must be interpreted with the knowledge that many dietary supplements have not been studied in formal, controlled clinical trials. The author does not accept testimonials of benefit as evidence of the treatment potential of any drug or supplement. Studies used to assess the benefit of dietary supplements have often involved the study of only a few subjects or individuals. Repetition in this book is intentional to highlight important concepts.
- The book has an index which provides quick page references.

- Dietary supplements cannot be used to diagnose, prevent or treat any disease. This book is not a supplement label.
- At the end of this book is a multiple choice examination which is able to be used as part of the reader's revision of their acquired knowledge.
- The answer sheet (only) on the exam should be detached and mailed to the Holt Institute of Medicine, 61 Stevens Ave., Little Falls, NJ 07424 (Attention: Certified Dietary Supplement Counselor), (Dip. DSC).
- The answers to the questions in the book are given as part of an honor code. Anyone who uses the answer key inappropriately is only fooling themselves.
- Please learn and share your knowledge to "keep your nation well."

CHAPTER I

MULTIVITAMINS

"VITAMIN THERAPIES": ASSESSING VITAMIN NEEDS

T HERE are few people who doubt the benefit of supplementing the Standard American Diet (SAD) with essential vitamins and selected minerals. Vitamins are a group of naturally occurring substances that are essential for the maintenance of all body structures and functions. Vitamins cannot be made by the human body, with the notable exception of Vitamin D. There has been much recent research that shows that the correct dosages of vitamins in the diet can improve health and wellbeing in many ways. While dietary supplements have been labeled as "not to be used for the prevention or treatment of diseases," the exceptions to this "legal rule" are arguably vitamins and minerals, especially when they are prescribed by a physician. Vitamins and minerals have been shown to variably reduce the chances of developing many diseases, when used correctly; and they are known to promote health and well-being, most notably in states of deficiency.

Food scientists are correct in their assertion that vitamins and minerals are best obtained from the diet. However, much processed food in Western societies and in urban areas in third world countries, has been manipulated to a degree that it has been robbed of many vitamins and minerals. There is a new problem emerging in potential vitamin and mineral deficiencies. This problem is related to the obesity epidemic. Individuals who are trying to control their weight may often reduce the amount of food they eat. If they are reducing the intake of processed food, that may already be deficient in vitamins, they are putting themselves at risk of vitamin or mineral deficiencies.

It is known that excessive calorie intake in the diet is one major cause for being overweight, but much food that is purchased in convenient restaurants or supermarkets is manufactured to be cheap food with high calorie content. I am not suggesting that people are walking around with obvious signs or symptoms of vitamin deficiency, but it must be clearly understood that marginal deficiency of several vitamins or minerals is quite common, especially in the elderly or in the segment of the population that relies upon "fast," processed, or junk foods.

Many physicians or healthcare givers have changed their opinions about the need for vitamin or mineral supplements. There are many examples of population studies that show intakes of essential vitamins to be often below recommended daily intakes or values (RDI, RDV). Healthcare consumers must understand that the concept of the RDI was generated from assessments of vitamin intake that would prevent nutrient deficiencies. This does not necessarily mean that the RDI of a vitamin is enough for health and wellbeing. This has led to the suggestion that there may be optimal levels of intake of vitamins that are higher than the so-called RDI. In addition, there are some circumstances where physicians use vitamins in higher dosages for therapeutic (treatment) effects. High dosage vitamin therapies should not be self-administered, especially if the vitamin is known to be toxic in high dosage (e.g. Vitamins A, D or K).

I believe that it is no longer possible to rely upon the average Western diet or Standard American Diet (SAD) as a means of achieving an optimal vitamin or mineral intake. There are glaring examples of these circumstances. For example, many elderly people do not have enough vitamin D to maintain healthy bones, teeth and other body structures, even though this is a vitamin that can be synthesized by the body. Vitamin D is synthesized as a consequence of exposure to sunlight. Furthermore, there are many references concerning the inability of individuals to receive a necessary amount of vitamin E from dietary sources. Many Americans are strangers to fruit and vegetables and even daily, dietary intakes of vitamin C may be inadequate in many people. Only a limited segment of the population obtains the recommended five servings of fruit and vegetables per day (USDA, Food Pyramid Guide).

There are many circumstances in which I believe vitamin supplementation is absolutely necessary. Such circumstances include calorie-controlled dieting and acute or chronic illness, or the presence of risk factors for illness, where the need for extra vitamins may be mandatory. For example, the 20 million people in the United States with diabetes mellitus may "leak" water soluble vitamins and some minerals from their body. In fact, the word diabetes means "siphon." Excessive urination in diabetes flushes out vitamins and essential minerals (e.g. magnesium and zinc) which must be taken in the diet in greater amounts in these individuals.

Western society is constantly "on the go" and people are eating food that is often deficient in vital nutrients. This situation is made worse by the lack of time that people have to shop for well balanced food substances and prepare their own meals. This basic information about nutrition provides a compelling argument for every person to consider their daily needs of essential vitamins and minerals.

NEW HORIZONS FOR THE USE OF VITAMINS

Many scientists and healthcare givers believe in taking enough vitamins to help ensure health and wellbeing. Therefore, the modern use of vitamins has more to do with the promotion of wellness than the mere act of avoiding vitamin deficiencies. The scientists who proposed and modified recommended daily intakes of vitamins were quite frank with their opinion that it is not easy to determine what constitutes the ideal dosages of essential vitamins. There is a growing medical opinion that these dosages are likely to be much higher than the standard recommendations, or (RDI) values, that currently prevail in people's minds.

Vitamin needs change dramatically with age, disease status, environmental conditions and health status… to name a few circumstances. Adequate vitamin or mineral intake cannot be effective in promoting health without positive lifestyle changes, such as the use of a balanced, nutrient dense diet that is somewhat restricted in saturated fat, simple sugar and animal protein. Modern dietary recommendations for health must stress the importance of increasing dietary fiber intake, with a more liberal use of healthy fats, such as omega 3 fatty acids, found in fish oil (see Fish Oil, Chapter 18).

Much concern continues to be expressed about the adverse effects of taking too many vitamins. I think that this fear has been somewhat overestimated because there are relatively few reports of toxicity from the use of vitamin supplements. However, a general rule is that the fat soluble vitamins A, D, E and K are not to be taken in high dosages without medical supervision. Healthcare consumers become confused when studies are reported that allege negative outcomes from taking larger dosages of a single vitamin. In recent times, this situation has arisen with the use of vitamin E. However, many studies that focus on the single use of a nutritional substance are able to be criticized by their construction. The "construction" of a study may not result in a conclusion that can be generally applied to the population. I believe that this was the case in the recent reports of the dangers of using vitamin E in patients with heart disease. That said, vitamin E is an antioxidant vitamin and the dietary supplement industry may have been over-promoting the use of antioxidants as "single agents" which in high dosages can cause unwanted actions, such as pro-oxidant effects (see Antioxidants, Chapter 4).

Some scientists have suggested that vitamin supplementation can be tailored to a patient's individual needs. Unfortunately, this commendable approach is very difficult to achieve by self management. The background that I present for vitamin usage means that there is a compromise to be achieved between the RDI of vitamins and the avoidance of adverse effects of certain types of vitamin excess. Naturopathic physicians and practitioners of natural medicine, in general, may tailor vitamin needs to their patients, so that they can achieve wellbeing, beyond simple health. This approach is not often found in the practice of conventional medicine. Many drugs are known to deplete certain vitamins or minerals and the act of adding supplements with pharmaceutical prescriptions is often overlooked. I call upon my colleagues in pharmacy practice to be more aware of "drug-induced nutrient depletions."

AN OVERVIEW OF THE HEALTH BENEFITS OF VITAMINS

There are many accounts of the actions of individual vitamins on body structures and functions. Recent research has identified many previously ignored functions of vitamins. Vitamin A is present in the body in many different chemical forms. There are retinoids which are "formed-types" of vitamin A and a series of naturally occurring compounds called carotenoids that can be converted variably into vitamin A itself. Vitamin A plays a major role in supporting eye function, body linings, normal bone growth, immune functions and reproduction. Vitamin A or beta carotene may reduce the risk of cancer in some circumstances, but opinions are divided. Excessive amounts of vitamin A should be avoided, especially during pregnancy.

Vitamin D is probably best not referred to as a vitamin, because it can be manufactured in the body, unlike other vitamins. It occurs in chemical forms called calciferols. The natural, active form of vitamin D is vitamin D3 which has many "hormonal actions" in the body. Vitamin D is best known for its ability to increase calcium and phosphorus absorption; and it has an important role in the formation of bones and teeth. Also, Vitamin D supports the production of insulin, promotes healthy immune function and it has a role in cancer prevention. Excessive amounts of vitamin D are not recommended, because of potential toxicity; but adverse effects are only seen at high dosages, taken continuously.

Vitamin E (like Vitamin A and D) occurs in several forms that are called tocopherols and tocotrienols. There is evidence that natural origins of vitamin

E are more effective than synthetic vitamin E. Vitamin E is a class vitamin and it plays a major role in protecting cell membranes aga (antioxidant effects). Vitamin E works in concert with vitamins A classic antioxidant and it supports reproductive function. Wheth vitamin E is toxic in high dosages remains arguable, but the taking more than 400 IU of vitamin E per day, continuously, should only be used under medical supervision. Vitamin K is the classic vitamin utilized by the body in blood clotting and this vitamin is not often deficient in the diet. Vitamin K can be synthesized by bacteria in the colon.

B vitamins include niacin (vitamin B3), pyridoxine (vitamin B6), cobalamin (vitamin B12), thiamin (vitamin B1), riboflavin (vitamin B2), pantothenic acid, biotin and folic acid. All B vitamins are water soluble and they serve many basic functions, including: blood formation, support of central nervous system function, support of general body chemistry, genetic functions and other important activities. In general, B vitamins do not have a tendency to cause adverse effects, even in relatively high dosages. An exception is niacin, which can cause liver damage when used in gram amounts, over a significant period of time. Crystalline niacin is less likely to damage the liver than "sustained-release" niacin. Niacin is valuable in detoxification programs.

Vitamin C requires little introduction. This vitamin is essential for the health of supporting tissues in the body, blood vessel functions, wound healing and the production of body hormones or messenger substances. Vitamin C is a powerful antioxidant. Much evidence implies that vitamin C may protect against the common cold, prevent certain types of cancer, promote cardiovascular health, support memory, prevent cataract formation, exert anti-allergic effects and it has documented anti-aging properties.

WHAT ARE THE BEST VITAMIN SUPPLEMENTS?

Simply stated, you get what you pay for when you purchase a vitamin supplement. Cheaper types of vitamin supplements are often presented in pressed, hard tablets that are difficult to swallow; and their contents are often poorly absorbed. Some vitamin tablets are so poorly absorbed that they may be passed in the stool in an intact form. Clearly, vitamin supplements are best administered in capsules and vegetable capsules are preferred, because of concerns about bovine gelatin as a possible source of mad cow disease. Vegetable capsules are more expensive than regular gelatin capsules, but they are advantageous and used in superior supplement products.

Many people are confused about the ideal amounts of vitamins that should taken on a daily basis. The amounts of several vitamins in advanced vitamin formulae often exceed RDI, but the amounts of vitamins used will not produce toxic effects in average use. Superior vitamin supplements are distinguished by the addition of several other vital nutrients which are not able to be classified as vitamins per se, but these added nutrients have other potential health benefits by acting as co-factors. Many of the benefits of these advantageous, extra additions to vitamin supplements are discussed in other areas of this book. These value-added nutrients include green tea extract, turmeric or curcuminoids, choline, inositol, PABA, grape seed extract, lutein and lycopene. Small amounts of black pepper are added sometimes, to multivitamin formulations for anti-oxidant functions and the promotion of better vitamin absorption.

ARE MULTIVITAMINS A HEALTH RISK?

Throughout this book, you will experience statements about different "opinions" on the safety and effectiveness of dietary supplements. Airing differences of opinion can cause consumer confusion, but they are necessary in order to reach an informed decision. In May, 2006, the National Institutes of Health (NIH), held an "NIH State-of-the-Science Conference" on Multivitamin/Multimineral supplements and Chronic Disease Prevention. The members of this expert panel proposed that multivitamins may pose some theoretical health risks, especially in circumstances of self medication. Of course, anything in medicine has a theoretical risk.

Protests to the conclusions of the NIH panel emerged rapidly. For example, the National Nutritional Food Association (NNFA, a US body representing the dietary supplement industry) labeled the NIH panel as irresponsible and uninformed in their process of "theorizing" on the risks of multivitamins.

Let it please be clear that any and all medical interventions pose risks and this is why the good practice of medicine always involves an assessment of risks versus benefits. In the case of multivitamins, it is clear that only a small proportion of the estimated 100 million users of vitamins have adverse reactions. Such reactions are infrequent and in many cases, minor or rapidly reversible. Data produced by the American Association of Poison Control imply that only 4% of all adverse reactions to prescription or over the counter "drugs" can be linked to vitamin usage (cited by NNFA).

The NIH panel expressed concerns about lack of regulatory authority on supplement sales and the need for more research to assess supplement benefits, or lack thereof. One major problem is the unwillingness of some scientists to accept benefits of nutritional factors described in observational or population studies. If one waited for "conclusive," clinical data on supplement usage, one may wait forever! Economic rewards rest most often with drugs.

Dietary supplements do not fit the economic models of patented drugs, and there is little incentive and limited financial backing for supplement research. I trust that readers of this book will consider benefits and risks of dietary supplement usage. The circumstances are confounded by the questionable legalities of comparing drugs with dietary supplements.

KEYNOTE SUMMARY: MULTIVITAMIN INTAKE

Almost every medical practitioner believes in the benefits of vitamin supplementation of the diet. Vitamins are essential substances in the diet that exert major controls over the chemistry of life. Modern research demonstrates that certain vitamins have disease prevention and even treatment capabilities when taken in the correct amounts or forms. The concept of recommended daily intakes (RDI) has been challenged, as it becomes clear that some nutrients assist in preventing several chronic diseases. Some vitamins may slow some of the physical deterioration that occurs with aging.

The Standard American Diet (SAD), or Western diet, does not always provide a consistent amount of the minimum quantities of vitamins or minerals that are needed to avoid "hidden" vitamin deficiency states. The modern, love affair with processed food commits every adult in America to think very seriously about regular vitamin intake. While vitamins are some of the body's best friends, they have to be given in optimum amounts. Excessive amounts of certain vitamins are best avoided, especially fat soluble vitamins A, D, E and K.

I recommend formulations of multivitamins that have the specific intent of providing generous amounts of safe health-giving vitamins. One should seek a comprehensive vitamin and nutrient formula, with a background content of REDOX balanced antioxidants, in a vegetable capsule presentation that will provide circumstances for good absorption of vitamins into the body. Many good vitamin supplements exist.

There are many cheap types of vitamin supplements which are presented in tablet form, or in preparations that have doubtful ability to be absorbed and utilized by the body. Superior vitamin supplements are presented in vegetable capsules to fulfill vitamin needs in a potent and versatile manner. I believe that several groups of people at risk must take daily vitamins. These individuals include: aerobic exercisers, smokers, prescription-drug users, people with diabetes mellitus, individuals with many chronic diseases and especially mature people, with special reference to the elderly. I have performed many studies on several prescription, or over-the-counter drugs that deplete nutrients from the body. Pharmaceuticals are an underestimated cause of nutritional depletion, which can be largely corrected by dietary supplementation with a well-formulated multivitamin product.

CHAPTER 2

SLEEP

SLEEP DEPRIVATION AND POOR HEALTH

ABOUT 65 million Americans do not sleep well. Most often, they have difficulty initiating sleep or staying asleep or early morning wakening. Sleeplessness is a grossly underestimated cause of mental and physical disability. Without the biorhythm of restful sleep, health cannot prevail. Recent scientific studies show that reductions in the quantity or quality of sleep contribute to premature aging, disability, obesity, impaired immune function, depression and death. Sleep problems cost the nation billions of dollars in loss of time from work and tragic events, such as road traffic accidents. I have highlighted the many problems of sleep deprivation in my book "Sleep Naturally" (www.wellnesspublishing.com).

Modern hypotheses suggest that lack of sleep may be responsible for hormonal imbalances and it may contribute to the modern epidemics of obesity, Syndrome X and maturity onset diabetes mellitus. While some sleep problems are caused by serious underlying disease, most cases of insomnia are related to simple issues, such as adverse lifestyle, anxiety, stress and poor diet.

The past decade has witnessed major advances in the diagnosis and management of sleep problems. "Medical Sleep Centers" have sprung up all over the country and every community hospital has at least one physician who has embraced a special interest in the treatment of sleep disorders. TV broadcasting is swamped by advertisements that encourage the premature use of drugs for sleep. In addition, recent media highlights the filing of lawsuits against drug manufacturers, as a consequence of some serious side effects caused by popular prescription sleep drugs.

LIMITATIONS OF DRUGS FOR SLEEP

There has been a widespread and unhealthy tendency for a large proportion of the population to rely on drugs to induce sleep. All pharmaceuticals used for sleep possess disadvantages or limitations, including cost and side effects. Tolerance to sleeping medication rapidly develops and addiction or "hangover" is a common problem. Short-acting, prescription drugs that are used for sleep problems are approved for use for a couple of weeks only, but many are used in a consistent and inappropriate manner, often for several years. Furthermore, over the counter (OTC) sleep drugs, such as antihistamines, can have serious side effects, especially in the elderly. These OTC drug side effects are under-reported.

There are promises made that newer types of sleeping tablets, such as Ambien® or Lunesta® are safer and perhaps more effective than older types of sleep drugs, such as Valium® or related drugs. At the time of writing, several law suits have been filed against the manufacturers of certain sleeping pills because people have experienced a "zombie-like" state, strange behavior and weight gain etc., alleged to be due to the use of these pharmaceuticals. Drugs that are purveyed for restless legs syndrome (RLS) have unpleasant side effects. Many physicians are rethinking their approach to the use of modern types of sleeping drugs, as their safety becomes increasingly questioned.

The common nature of disordered sleep and the drawbacks of conventional treatment approaches with drugs have caused many people to seek alternative, natural ways to healthy sleep. My book, "Sleep Naturally" (Wellness Publishing, Newark, NJ, 2003), presents a holistic lifestyle program to assist in the achievement of restful sleep. This program discusses many behavioral changes required to combat insomnia. I have described "The Sleep Naturally Plan," which proposes the concept of the use of natural, herbal, botanical and nutrient agents in dietary supplements for the nutritional support of the normal body function of sleep. Nutrients and botanicals present potential "first-line" approaches to help relieve sleeping problems, after positive lifestyle adjustments have been made.

SLEEP AND DIETARY SUPPLEMENTS

The application of synergistic formulations in dietary supplements led me to the development of complex formulations to support natural sleep. Such formulations have been used in millions of unit dosages with a high level of safety, tolerance and consumer satisfaction. It is increasingly apparent that natural substances, known to assist in the achievement of restful sleep, are best used in safe combinations. Sleep is composed of a complex cascade of body events, involving several body structures and functions.

I have proposed that a relatively small dose of a number of natural substances that promote sleep can work together, in concert. I believe that this approach produces a superior, safe, simple and effective outcome. This is the concept of synergy, where natural ingredients in supplements have "helper" effects on each other. A synergistic natural formula of nutritional agents may help avoid the tolerance that may invariably occur when a single natural substance or drug is used to promote sleep. There are several disadvantages when single supplements (e.g. melatonin) are used alone. Melatonin causes tolerance when used alone, often requiring increased dosage. High dosage melatonin triggers safety concerns.

I have proposed a proprietary product that combines herbal support for restful sleep with Valerian Root, Chamomile Flower, Passion Flower, Lemon Balm, Skullcap Whole and Ashwagandha Root. This synergistic formula also contains specific vitamins and minerals (Magnesium, Niacin, Vitamin B6 and Folic Acid), with the power of the sleep hormone melatonin and the natural effects of 5 Hydroxytryptophan (Table 1). This combination of natural substances should be avoided by pregnant women and children; and it should not be mixed with alcohol or used when driving or operating machinery. Dietary supplements that provide nutritional support for restful sleep with appropriate lifestyle changes are preferred first-line options in Integrative Medicine.

A Proprietary Blend of Valerian Root, Chamomile Flower, Passionflower, Lemon Balm, Skullcap Whole, Hops Whole and Ashwagandha Root
5 Hydroxytryptophan (5HTP)
Magnesium
Melatonin
Niacin
Vitamin B6 (Pyridoxine HCL)
Folic Acid

Table 1: Ingredients of a highly effective, safe formula for nutritional support of the normal body function of sleep (reproduced from www.holtmdlabs.com).

THE SLEEP NATURALLY PLAN™
(WWW.WELLNESSPUBLISHING.COM)

Restful sleep involves a multipronged or holistic approach in many people. Table 2 summarizes the principal components of the Sleep Naturally Plan that stress lifestyle changes.

- If sleep problems are long-standing, medical consultation is required.
- Abnormal sleep patterns or events, such as sleepwalking, narcolepsy and sleep apnea, are conditions that should not be self-managed.
- Individuals must adopt a regular sleep schedule. There are some new behavioral techniques that involve certain degrees of deprivation of time spent in bed. This approach can be valuable for insomniacs. Other behavioral therapies may help.
- Everyone must not take sleep for granted and they must engage in regular bedtime routines. Setting the mood for sleep is all-important.
- Restful sleep occurs only in the correct environment. Comfort, noise elimination and any safe "gadget" that works is worth a try.
- The importance of posture during sleep has been grossly underestimated in conventional medicine. The clever use of pillows to support various parts of the trunk or lower limbs can be quite valuable. New types of beds can be adjusted to help the adoption of optimal postures during sleep, but these are expensive interventions.
- Idle people cannot sleep. Regular exercise at the right time of day and attempts to reduce stress will benefit sleep patterns. Healthy sex promotes restful sleep.
- Many drugs interfere with sleep and many substances taken in an average American diet can cause wakefulness, especially caffeine.
- Alcohol, caffeine, smoking, illicit drug use, diet pills, natural weight control supplements and water pills are enemies of restful sleep. Caffeine comes in some foods, e.g., chocolate.
- If extra help is required with sleeping, one may consider nutritional support to assist and promote sleep.

Table 2: "The Sleep Naturally Plan," which suggests optimal pathways to improve simple sleep problems. (Excerpted with permission from Holt S, "Sleep Naturally," Wellness Publishing Inc., N.J., 2003).

PHARMACEUTICALS UTILIZED BY PRESCRIPTION OR OTC USE ARE BACK-UP PLANS ONLY. THESE DRUGS HAVE MANY DISADVANTAGES AND LIMITATIONS.

KEYNOTE SUMMARY ON SLEEP

There is a modern epidemic of sleeplessness that causes much mental and physical disability. Reductions in the amount or quality of sleep have been associated with many disorders, including: premature aging, disability and death from accidents, being overweight and poor control of diabetes – to name a few problems.

There has been a widespread unhealthy tendency for a large proportion of the population to rely on drugs to induce sleep. All pharmaceuticals used for sleep possess disadvantages or limitations, including cost and side effects. Tolerance to sleeping medication rapidly develops, requiring increased dosage and "hangover" is a problem. In 2005, there were 26.6 million prescriptions given by doctors for Ambien® (Sanofi-Aventis). The drug Lunesta® (Sepracor) is used by millions of people, sometimes without exercising first line options of lifestyle change, behavioral interventions or simple nutritional support.

All sleep drugs are best used for only a couple of weeks. However, as many as one third of all people taking sleeping pills consume them on a continuing basis, sometimes for years. There have been increasing reports of the occurrences of "zombie-like" states, strange behavior, eating disorders and weight gain with popular drugs used for sleep. The use of OTC (over the counter) sleep drugs is associated with an unknown amount of side-effects, especially in the elderly e.g. bladder problems, accidents and even disorders of heart rhythm. Antihistamines are popular OTC drugs taken for sleep promotion. These drugs are used for sleep because of their "side effects" of sedation. Using a drug for its side effects seems illogical.

There are many simple, gentle and natural options to achieve restful sleep. I have summarized many of these approaches in my book entitled "The Sleep Naturally Plan," Wellness Publishing Inc., Little Falls, NJ, 2003. Synergistic supplement technology has led to the formulation of synergistic nutritional products to modify complex cascades of events that occur during sleep. It is apparent that natural substances known to assist in the achievement of restful sleep are best used in safe combinations. Thus, a relatively small dose of a number of natural substances that promote sleep can work together, in concert. This produces a superior, simple and effective outcome. This is the concept of synergy where ingredients have "helper" effects on each other. This approach may help avoid the tolerance that may invariably occur when a single natural substance or drug is used to promote sleep. Whenever possible, people should "**sleep naturally**."

CONCLUSION

The average duration of sleep among several Western populations has been reduced by an hour or two over the past thirty years. This is a legacy of our "advanced lifestyle." Sleep deprivation turns on stress which ignites chronic disease. In particular, problems around the menopause or menstrual cycles and the nation's expanding waistline are aggravated by sleeplessness. Restoring sleep may itself result in better weight control in many people. Anyone who seeks wellness must restore the normal biorhythm of sleep.

RESTORATION OF RESTFUL SLEEP IS IMPORTANT IN THE MANAGEMENT OF MANY DISORDERS, E.G. MENOPAUSE, WEIGHT CONTROL ETC.

CHAPTER 3

MENOPAUSE AND PMS: THE MENOPLAN

MENOPAUSE, PERIMENOPAUSE, POSTMENOPAUSE AND PMS

THERE are two areas of major health concerns that face adult women through their lifetime. These concerns include problems that occur in relationship to menstrual cycles (Dysmenorrhea, Premenstrual Syndrome, or PMS) and life events in the perimenopause or the menopause. I have discussed natural ways to a healthy menopause and natural ways to combat PMS in my book entitled "Menopause and PMS Naturally" (2008, in press).

For more than 40 years, hormone-replacement therapy (HRT) has been used, most often by combining animal estrogens, derived from horses' urine, with or without synthetic progesterone. This HRT has been used to manage unpleasant symptoms of the menopausal transition. Unfortunately, the disadvantages and limitations of this conventional form of HRT have become apparent in recent medical research. It is now known that HRT can be potentially dangerous. While so-called "bioidentical hormones" are alleged to be safer than conventional HRT, clear evidence to support this position is still emerging.

I believe that current contraindications for bioidentical HRT are the same for conventional HRT… even though my opinion may be "unpopular" in alternative medicine circles. If a hormone preparation is used for menopause or PMS, I recommend a trial of topical progesterone creams, but I prefer always to recommend positive lifestyle change, nutrients, herbs, and botanicals as first line options to deal with unpleasant symptoms of PMS, the perimenopause and the menopause. It seems safer to avoid hormones, if you can!

RISKS OF HORMONE REPLACEMENT THERAPY (HRT)

While the menopause can herald unpleasant symptoms, such as hot flashes and lack of psychological well-being, the real significance for the postmenopausal years is the onslaught of age-related disease. Such diseases include breast cancer, cardiovascular disease, thin bones (osteoporosis) and age-related declines in brain function. There are many nutritional factors that can support body structures and functions. Such factors are involved intimately in disorders or diseases that emerge after the menopause.

There is no doubt that major hormonal changes occur around the menopause, but the idea that menopause is merely a deficiency of the female hormone estrogen is both a misleading and naïve concept. Unfortunately, this concept has been accepted, perhaps inappropriately, by many women and some physicians. The recent scientific information on the safety and effectiveness of certain kinds of conventional HRT is "spine-chilling." It appears that certain types or combinations of conventional HRT may actually cause or promote breast cancer and other diseases.

Conventional HRT does not seem to fulfill earlier promises of the protection of mature females against heart disease, or mental decline with age. In fact, some studies show that quality of life is not enhanced by taking conventional HRT. Both the timing of the start of HRT and the type of HRT (conventional or "bio-identical) may affect overall outcome. Because of doubts, many mature women are seeking natural and viable alternatives to hormone replacement therapy, at least to attempt to control unpleasant symptoms around the menopause.

In my book, entitled, "Menopause and PMS Naturally: The Menoplan," (www.wellnesspublishing.com), I indicate that there are natural pathways to healthy menstrual function or menopause (cessation of menstruation). I have often stressed the importance of positive lifestyle for a healthy menopause, together with the use of natural substances for improving a mature woman's experience during this transition of life and during the perimenopause, (age range 40-60 years, approximately). In fact, modern medical research implies that "well-adjusted" mature women, with a positive lifestyle, do not tend to experience unpleasant symptoms in the perimenopause. I hesitate, because some menopausal women have to question advice from an "andropausal man."

MENOPLAN, MENOPAUSE, PMS AND DIETARY SUPPLEMENTS

In a myriad of medical literature, scholarly physicians have examined the evidence behind the use of many dietary supplements for a healthy menopause or altered menstrual function. The science of nutritional support for menopause and PMS is evolving with a number of scientific studies that show evidence for the benefits of natural agents in the nutritional management of menopause or PMS. Conventional physicians have been slow to embrace the "natural approach."

Evidence-based dietary supplements can be designed to provide nutritional support for the perimenopause, menopause and PMS. Such supplements contain natural substances that have been associated with demonstrated benefits for menopausal women in the scientific literature. Menopause or PMS supplements should have a synergistic formula. Menopause is an example of complex cascades of body events that are often "lacking in harmony." Combination formulae of natural substances for menopausal wellbeing are more versatile and generally more complete than single or limited ingredient supplements for menstrual changes or disorders.

The ingredients of an evidence-based dietary supplement for PMS or menopause may include black cohosh as a standardized extract (2%), together with soy isoflavones. I have written about the benefits of soy inclusion in the diet in the perimenopause and PMS in my two books, "The Soy Revolution" (Dell Publishing, Random House, N.Y., 2000) and "Soya for Health" (Mary Ann Liebert Publishers Inc., N.Y. 1994).

Contained within superior menopause or PMS supplements are extracts of green tea, e.g. L-theanine, which assists in causing relaxation responses. Useful combination formulae include evening primrose oil (providing nutritional support for reproductive organ function and breast health), Dong quai (traditional female specific herbs) and Chasteberry (Vitex agnus-castus), for which there is a long precedent and history of use for female health. In addition, complete supplements for these female purposes contain the benefits of Ginkgo biloba, which supports central nervous system functions and blood flow. A sample formula for Menopause and PMS is shown in Table 3.

- Black Cohosh (Cimicifuga racemosa), standardized for triterpene glycosides
- Soy Isoflavones
- Red Clover
- L-Theanine
- Evening Primrose Oil
- Dong Quai (Angelica sinensis)
- Chasteberry (Vitex agnus-castus)

- Gingko Biloba (extract)

Table 3: Contents of Menopause or PMS formulae. Synergistic formulations provide nutritional support for menstrual function, menopause and perimenopause (reproduced from www.holtmdlabs.com). Many proposed formulae for menopause or PMS are incomplete in their ingredients.

METABOLIC SYNDROME X AND WOMEN'S HEALTH

Syndrome X is the combination or being overweight, having abnormal blood cholesterol (triglycerides) and/or high blood pressure, all linked by underlying insulin resistance. This entity of Syndrome X is associated with heart disease and stroke, but it can contribute to many other disorders including: irregular menstruation and polycystic ovary syndrome (PCOS). I have focused often on the major public health initiative presented by Syndrome X (the metabolic syndrome) and its far reaching adverse effects on women's health in my books "Menopause and PMS Naturally" and "Combat Syndrome X, Y and Z…" (www. wellnesspublishing.com).

In my book, "Combat Syndrome X, Y and Z ..." (www. wellnesspublishing. com), I emphasize the concept that Syndrome X has widespread health implications beyond its obvious role in the causation of cardiovascular disease. I have indicated that menopause may "load the gun" in terms of health problems for some women and I fear that the metabolic Syndrome X may "pull the trigger" in many mature females, or vice versa. Perhaps conventional HRT is sometimes the bullet in the gun..? (see Chapter 16)

A KEYNOTE SUMMARY: MENOPAUSE AND PMS

The science of nutritional support for menopause and PMS, using dietary supplements, is emerging with much strength. There are an increasing number of evidence-based studies showing variable benefits of a number of natural agents for the nutritional management of menopause.

Considering the management of the menopausal transition, most scientific support lies with the use of soy isoflavones and black cohosh, which form major ingredients and constituents of leading supplements used in menopausal transitions or PMS. There is good scientific agreement that red clover (which contains isoflavones similar to those found in soy) may help with relief from hot flashes and other symptoms in the menopause.

Promising information exists on the benefits of certain vitamins and the use of evening primrose oil and/or Dong quai for menopause and PMS. Though much of the support for the use of these latter substances is anecdotal, in comparison to the studies reported with soy, red clover and black cohosh, I believe that these are valuable constituents in dietary supplement support for PMS and menopause. They are "synergistic" additions.

CONCLUSION

Ideal supplements for menopause or PMS have versatile formulae. Constituents of formulae for Menopause and PMS (www.holtmdlabs.com) have antioxidant functions which can assist in nutritional support for anti-aging. Overall, synergistic menopause or PMS supplements, with recommendations for lifestyle change, present a useful first-line option for individuals experiencing uncomplicated transitions in the menopause and certain problems related to menstrual cycles. Much further research is required. All hormone therapies must be supervised by a knowledgeable healthcare practitioner. Nutritional and lifestyle approaches are first line options for Menopause and PMS; hormones are secondary strategies.

CHAPTER 4

ANTIOXIDANTS

BERRIES, FRUITS, VEGETABLES AND GREENS

MODERN medicine continues to research the health power of fruits, greens, vegetables, and berries. For almost 100 years, medical practitioners have been talking about the health benefits of fruit and vegetable intake in the diet, but inertia persists on this health initiative. Despite strong advice to improve Western diets, few people have adopted an adequate fruit, berry or vegetable intake.

Fruits and vegetables are distinguished by their content of many different natural substances that give them vibrant color. These substances are called phytonutrients (phyto=plant). Perhaps the most important health-giving components of fruits and vegetables are antioxidants and dietary fiber. The word "antioxidant" has confused many people. This subject of oxygen reactions and tissue damage should be understood by everyone. It is known that oxygen itself is absolutely necessary for life, but oxygen can be both a friend and a foe for health...vide infra.

Oxygen can be present in the body in a very "reactive" form (free radicals) and in this form it may damage tissues by causing oxidative tissue stress or damage. Fruits, berries and "veggies" provide powerful opposition to oxidative stress by supplying antioxidants that "mop up" reactive forms of oxygen, which are otherwise called "free radicals."

UNDERSTANDING OXIDATIVE TISSUE DAMAGE:
THE RUSTY NAIL CONCEPT (LARKHILL)

We can understand the process of oxidative stress by thinking about a "rusty nail." When a nail is left exposed to the atmosphere it ages and rusts. This occurs as a consequence of the combination of oxygen with the iron found in the nail. When we look at a rusty nail, we think about something that is weakened and aged. In simplistic terms, we can apply these thoughts to the human body where excessive oxidation is a key issue in body aging or tissue damage or disease causation.

Oxidation or oxidative stress can be at the root cause of many common diseases. Oxidative stress can attack and damage the heart, the brain, the bones and other vital organs of the body. In fact, not only is oxidative stress a key cause of aging, it is linked to the occurrence of many common diseases such as cancer, arthritis, peptic ulcer, osteoporosis, brain degeneration (e.g. Alzheimer's disease) and many other diseases.

Within fruits and vegetables are many antioxidants that can help counter the oxidative stress to which the body is exposed on a daily basis. The body itself produces reactive types of oxygen (free radicals) during normal events such as exercise. Even though the body has its own, built-in antioxidant mechanisms for dealing with reactive oxygen, good dietary antioxidant intake is a pivotal factor in health maintenance. Antioxidant activity in the body is a key factor in anti-aging (see Chapters 5 and 31).

Berries, fruits and greens confer many ancillary health benefits. For example, bilberry promotes healthy eyesight, cranberry is healthy for the urinary tract and many phytochemicals within fruits exert important anticancer effects. Some of these claims are not permitted by law, when describing dietary supplements, even though the evidence to support these statements is quite strong. Getting an adequate fruit and vegetable intake is no simple matter. If one was to purchase several punnets of berries, one would be spending many dollars. Few people can attain an optimal intake of several servings of fresh fruit, berries, or vegetables daily, for lifestyle or economic reasons.

SUPPLEMENTING FRUIT, VEGETABLE AND
BERRY INTAKE IN THE DIET

In order to overcome the inconvenience of gathering sufficient fruits and vegetables to put in a daily diet, I formulated products including Berry Supreme® or Berries and Greens Naturally Plus Supernutrition™ and Clinical Daily Prevention™. These products have different, but complete nutrient formulae.

These and other powdered supplements contain a valuable array of different types of berries and other key plant ingredients that have great precedent for the promotion of health and well-being.

In summary, Berry Supreme® or Berries and Greens Naturally Plus Supernutrition™ and Clinical Daily Prevention™ contain multiple antioxidants and vital nutrients including carotenoids found in spinach, sweet potatoes and spirulina, ellagic acid found in red raspberries and pomegranates, catechins found in green tea and bioflavonoids. In addition, Berry Supreme®, Berries and Greens Naturally Plus Supernutrition™ and Clinical Daily Prevention™ contain a group of healthy substances called phenolic compounds that are found in many different berries, fruits and vegetables (Tables 4A and 4B).

Table 4A: Contents of Berry Supreme® (Holt MD Labs Formulation).

- Strawberry powder
- Blueberry powder
- Raspberry powder
- Apricot powder
- Banana powder
- Pineapple powder
- Sweet potato powder
- Spinach powder
- Spirulina

- Beet powder
- Green tea
- Apple
- Elderberry powder
- Cherry
- Bilberry
- Pomegranate powder
- Blackberry
- Cranberry powder

Table 4B: Contents of Berries, Greens, Fruit and Vegetable Powders (Holt MD Labs).

Multivitamin and Multimineral Insurance:
Vitamin A, Vitamin C, Vitamin D, Vitamin E, Thiamin, Riboflavin, Niacinamide, Vitamin B6, Folic Acid, Vitamin B12, Biotin, Calcium, Zinc, Selenium, Copper, Manganese, Chromium (Vitamins at 100% RDI)

Holt MD Adaptogens and Body Cleansing Proprietary Blend™:
Soy Lecithin Powder, Carrot Powder, Fo Ti Root Powder, Pau D'arco Powder, Cinnamon Powder, Eleuthero Root Powder, Licorice Root Powder, Beet Powder, Cats Claw Powder, Ginger Root Powder, Astragalus Root Powder, Damiana Leaves Powder, Cumin Seed Powder, Royal Jelly Powder, Suma Root Powder, Jerusalem Artichoke, Cactus Powder, Yucca Juice Powder, Horsetail Powder, Milk Thistle Extract, Ginkgo Biloba Leaf Powder, Echinacea Angustifolia Herb Powder
Holt MD Greens Proprietary Blend™:
Alfalfa Powder, Barley Grass Powder, Spinach Powder, Parsley Powder, Spirulina Powder, Watercress Powder, Aloe Vera Leaf Powder, Chlorella Powder, Broccoli Powder, Green Tea Powder
Holt MD Functional Fiber Proprietary Blend™:
Oat Beta Glucan, Apple Fiber Powder, Oat Bran Flour, Apple Pectin Powder, Flax Seed Powder, FOS, Rice Bran, Guar gum
Holt MD Fruit Proprietary Blend™
Wheat Germ Powder, Citrus Bioflavanoids, Tomato Powder, Pumpkin Seed Powder, Acerola Extract Powder, Goji Powder, Mangosteen Powder, Grape Seed Extract, Acai Powder, Resveratrol Extract
Holt MD Berry Supreme™ Proprietary Blend™:
Strawberry Powder, Blueberry Powder, Raspberry Powder, Apricot Powder, Banana Powder, Pineapple Powder, Sweet Potato Powder, Spinach Powder, Beet Powder, Green Tea Extract, Apple Powder, Blackberry Powder, Sweet Cherry Powder, Cranberry Powder (Table 4A)
Holt MD Probiotics Proprietary Blend™:
Lactobacillus acidophilus, Lactobacillus bulgaricus, Lactobacillus rhamnosus, Bifidobacterium longum, Bifidobacterium breve
Holt MD Enzymes Proprietary Blend*:
Protease, Amylase, Lipase, Cellulase, Lactase, Bromelain, Papain
Holt MD Marine Nutraceuticals Proprietary Blend*:
Kelp, Marine Minerals, Dulse Powder, Sea Cucumber Powder, EPA/DHA Powder, Green Lipped Mussel

Other Ingredients:
Banana Powder, Strawberry Flavor, Raspberry Flavor, Stevia, Orange Powder, Spearmint, Cherry

SUMMING UP ON TARGETS FOR HEALTHY INTAKE OF FRUIT AND VEGETABLES

While many scientists and nutritional experts have been asking people to eat fruits and vegetables, the general public has not listened to this advice. Americans are "on the go" and they are not currently deriving the potential health benefits of many berries, fruits and selected vegetables.

Berries and Greens Naturally Plus Supernutrition™ (Table 4B) and similar products permit anyone to discover the power of berries with many fruit and vegetable extracts in a very versatile mix of many different berries, with extracts of fruit and selected health-giving vegetable extracts. Fruit, berry and vegetables are a necessary part of a diet for an active healthy lifestyle. Clinical Daily Prevention™ is an even more complex nutritional formula with mushroom extracts and immune stimulators (www.naturalclinician.com). The power of berries, selected fruits and vegetables benefits all age groups and it represents a major step forward in the promotion of health and well-being for many people. These formulations are popular in Integrative Medical practice as blanket-forms of nutritional insurance.

ANTIOXIDANT POWER®

While one can review the many benefits of antioxidant supplements, the best type of antioxidant supplement contains more than one antioxidant in a "balanced formulation." Antioxidants should be formulated in dietary supplements to act at different levels of antioxidant activities, in different areas of the body and its tissues. This concept is the use of antioxidants of different REDOX value. The term REDOX is best understood as the measure of the ability of something to become oxidized. I must reiterate that the major key to an efficient antioxidant effect is to have a supplement that contains antioxidants with the ability to access all different areas of body tissues.

Antioxidant compounds within a desirable antioxidant supplement must cover the water-containing segments of tissue and the fat-containing parts of tissues (fats and water in tissues). This technology is the basis of the concept of Antioxidant Power® which recommends antioxidant supplements that can function in both water and fat compartments of different tissues.

It should be noted that taking large doses of one antioxidant alone, e.g. vitamin E or vitamin C alone may not be healthy. For example, using vitamin C alone in high doses, given by injections, may actually cause an unwanted tissue stress causing oxidation (oxidative stress). This is why it is quite important to take more than one type of antioxidant at once, with a well chosen "REDOX balance." Well formulated antioxidants are highly desirable and they contain antioxidants that have been shown in corroborative scientific studies to exert potentially beneficial nutritional antioxidant actions. One key antioxidant is ellagic acid which has been extensively researched, especially in the areas of breast and cardiovascular health (Table 5). Ellagic acid is an example of how advanced literature exists on certain single antioxidant ingredients (Table 5) (cf. curcumin or turmeric extracts).

EFFECTS OF ELLAGIC ACID IN SCIENTIFIC STUDIES	REFERENCES
ANTI-CANCER EFFECTS: INHIBITION OF CARCINOGENICITY AND MUTAGENICITY	Ratnoff, O.D., Crum, J.D. (1964) J. Lab. Clin. Med. 63, 359; Bhargava, U.C., Westfall BA (1968) J. Pharm. Sci. 57, 1728
POWERFUL ANTIOXIDANT EFFECTS	Constantin A et al. Nutr. Cancer 23 (2): 121-30, 1995
REDUCTION OF BLOOD PRESSURE	Fiedler, V., Hildebrand, G.H. (1954) Arzneimittel Forsh 4, 426
INHIBITION OF THROMBOXANE B2 SYNTHESIS	Kimura, Y., Okuda, H., Okuda, T., Arichi, S. (1986) Planta Med. 52, 337
ACTIVATION OF HAGEMAN FACTOR	Ratnoff, O.D., Crum, J.D. (1964) J. Lab. Clin. Med. 63, 359; Bhargava, U.C., Westfall BA (1968) J. Pharm. Sci. 57, 1728
INHIBITION OF GLUTATHIONE TRANSFERASE	Dixit, H., Gold, B. (1986) Proc. Nat'l. Acad. Sci. USA 83, 8039; Das, M., Bickers, D.R., Mukhtar, H. (1984) Bio-Chem. Biophys. Res. Commun. 120, 427
SEDATIVE ACTION	Bhargava, U.C., Westfall BA, Sieta D.J., (1968) J. Pharm. Sci 57, 1728

INHIBITION OF ACID SECRETION BY THE STOMACH: BLOCKS GASTRIC PROTON PUMPS	Murakami, S., Kijima, H., Isobe, Y., Muramatsu, M., Aihara, H., Otomo, S., (1991), Planta Med. 57, 305-308

Table 5. Some of the versatile and potent effects of ellagic acid, found mainly in raspberries and pomegranates. Please note that this list of references is third party literature only and it cannot be used to make any claims for ellagic acid in specific disease prevention or treatment (at law).

Green tea polyphenols are often present in antioxidant supplements. Polyphenols possess a wealth of supporting information for their role in the promotion of wellness. In addition, grape seed extract, turmeric, lycopene and the powerful, indirect antioxidant elements selenium and zinc are important antioxidant supplements.

Direct and indirect antioxidant actions can benefit cardiovascular function, prostate health, immune function and they have potential anti-aging effects. I stress that many diseases and premature aging are linked to oxidative stress. For example, individuals with the metabolic Syndrome X or diabetes mellitus get disease complications as a consequence of continuing oxidative stress to the body. Table 6 lists the ingredients of a formulated antioxidant, with care to provide "blanket" coverage and REDOX balance.

- Ellagic acid (pomegranate and raspberry fruit)
- Lycopene from tomato
- Green Tea polyphenols
- Grape Seed extract 95% containing Oligomeric Proanthocyanidins
- Resveratrol
- Turmeric (curcumin) micronized
- Selenium (Amino Acid Chelate)
- Zinc (amino Acid chelate)

Table 6. The ingredients of well balanced antioxidant approaches (reproduced from www.holtmdlabs.com). Note other valuable antioxidant formulations exist, but the issue is range of access to body tissues and different REDOX potentials.

GREEN TEA MAX®

Green tea is emerging as one of the most important health-giving botanicals in the dietary supplement industry. Green tea is one of the oldest health remedies known to man; and its beneficial effects were documented thousands of years ago in traditional Chinese medicine. In fact, population studies indicate that green tea consumption in eastern Asia has been responsible for multiple health benefits, including anti-cancer effects, weight control and the promotion of cardiovascular health. These health claims for green tea are not allowed to be made to the same degree in the United States as they are in Japan.

In some Oriental nations, green tea is a staple in the diet. For example, Japanese and Chinese people may consume more than 10 cups of green tea per day as a refreshing drink. In contrast, in the U.S., the most popular hot beverage is coffee. Coffee contains polyphenols such as chlorogenic acid, which have been associated with beneficial effects on sugar metabolism and the prevention of type II diabetes mellitus.

Modern research on green tea is vast and impressive in terms of health benefits. In Japan, green tea is adopted and registered by the government as a disease preventive. In particular, it has a specific role in the potential prevention of cancer. These claims have not been made to the same degree in Western society, but the power of green tea is apparent in many recent scientific articles that describe benefits on body functions such as: immunity, cardiovascular function, brain function and even weight control.

For these reasons, I formulated a complex, green tea liquid concentrate for Holt MD Labs called Green Tea Max®. The formula of Green Tea Max® contains several other antioxidants that are given in a small amount, but in a balanced manner, for several potential health benefits. The liquid concentrate of green tea that is present in Green Tea Max® is organically grown and standardized for its content of powerful antioxidants or polyphenols. A principal ingredient of Green Tea Max® is a group of health giving compounds called catechins. The most potent Green Tea catechin has a complicated name, epi-gallocatechin gallate, otherwise known as EGCG.

THE UNIQUE FORMULA OF GREEN TEA MAX® (TEACHING EXAMPLE)

Green Tea Max® contains added antioxidants such as Turmeric, Red Clover, Grape Seed extract, Pinebark extract, Curcumin, Ellagic Acid, Magic Fruit extract (Lohan), Citrus bioflavonoids, Resveratrol, selected Oligomeric Proanthocyanidins, Stevia extract and Licorice. Each of these botanical and herbal additives has its own potential beneficial health profile including the nutritional support of cardiovascular, brain and general cellular function in the body.

Green tea has a poor reputation with the Western palate, largely because of its bitter flavor. Green Tea concentrations are presented in a convenient bottle with a dropper, where a few drops of green tea liquid concentrate can be added to hot or cold water to produce an energizing, refreshing, pleasant-tasting beverage. Aerobic fitness enthusiasts have enjoyed the benefits of Green Tea Max® by adding it to a water bottle. This provides a healthy perk for exercise and it may assist in reducing free radical damage to muscle tissue that causes muscle stiffness and discomfort following exercise.

KEYNOTE SUMMARY: ANTIOXIDANTS

The body generates free radicals on a daily basis and free radicals are found all over our environment. Free radicals are concentrated in cigarette smoke, exhaust fumes from engines and common household items e.g. chemical cleansers. The human body produces its own series of antioxidants. However, the body's antioxidant capacity is often overcome, resulting from our polluted environment. Many scientists believe that the health giving benefits of fruit and vegetable intake are mainly attributable to their antioxidant fiber content.

The first guiding principle of formulation of supplements with antioxidant functions is to make sure that the antioxidants go to all body tissues; and that they do not just concentrate their activity in water loving (hydrophilic) or fat loving (lipophilic) tissue zones. This concept is simple and it relates to antioxidants gaining access to as many body tissues as possible to prevent oxidative damage. The second guiding principle is to use antioxidants that work at different potentials of minute energy. This is the concept of REDOX balance.

I am convinced that much scientific data support the benefits of the daily taking of antioxidants, providing that antioxidants are taken in the correct manner. While I acknowledge the widespread need to increase fruit and vegetable intake to prevent disease, only a small proportion of the population achieves an ideal intake of fruit and vegetables. This reality of dietary inadequacies in modern society supports the use of dietary supplements in general, but I do not recommend a dietary supplement as a substitute for a poor diet.

The bottom line is that many human health needs are served by antioxidant activity. For example, damaged or wrinkled skin, muscle pain following exercise, tissue aging and the progression of almost every common, chronic medical disorder involves oxidative stress (e.g. diabetes, arthritis, etc). Fruit, berries, vegetables and greens powder mixes are replacing simple multivitamin use in the practice of Integrative Medicine.

CHAPTER 5

ANTIAGING: PREVENTING PREMATURE DISABILITY AND DEATH

ANTI-AGING METHODS

NATURAL approaches to anti-aging must take into account the modern theories of aging. The use of anti-aging methodologies is not a simple issue that is amenable to the use of a single drug or supplement (Chapter 31). There has been a tendency to look for "the fountain of youth," but the causes of tissue aging are many. Therefore, the approach to anti-aging must be multi-faceted. Dietary supplements and natural topical agents have become extremely popular anti-aging tactics in the U.S. These natural products play a viable role in the promotion of longevity, in combination with positive lifestyle changes (see Chapter 31).

"Anti-aging tactics" must be evidence-based and not merely fall into the category of "anti-aging antics." In brief, widely accepted theories of aging include oxidative stress, cross-linking of body proteins, altered immunity, changes in genetic codes, stress theories and repair-budget theories. Of all theories of aging, most attention has focused on the free-radical theory of aging, where the use of natural antioxidants offers great potential (see Chapter 4).

The selection of diets that have high antioxidant content or ORAC value is an important nutritional maneuver for anti-aging of all body systems. The term high ORAC means a high <u>O</u>xygen <u>R</u>adical <u>A</u>bsorbance <u>C</u>apacity; and it is a global measure of "Antioxidant Value" of foods or dietary supplements.

In contrast to nutritional and lifestyle approaches for anti-aging, focused interventions for body rejuvenation, such as the use of human growth hormone (HGH) or HGH releasers, and topical antioxidants are important complementary anti-aging methods. However, hormonal manipulations must be supervised by knowledgeable health care practitioners (Chapter 31). External manifestations of aging tend to mirror changes associated with tissue aging inside the body. Vitality and beauty comes from within the body, not from without. This concept has driven the use of oral antioxidant use, especially for skin health.

Adverse lifestyle accelerates aging. However, the investment in "behavior change today for health tomorrow" requires recognition (Chapter 31).

CONDITION SPECIFIC SUPPLEMENTS FOR ANTI-AGING

The quest for longevity must be seen as the eradication of common diseases that cause premature disability and death. Combat against these common diseases is the first stage of any anti-aging strategy. I believe that we can redefine the significance of certain chronic disorders in terms of their ability to cause premature aging. Table 7 lists examples of supplements that may provide nutritional support for changes in body structure and functions associated with aging.

Condition	Nutritional Considerations
Menopause	Evidence-based constituents (see Chapter 3)
Sleep Problems	Synergistic herbs and nutrients (see Chapter 2)
Obesity / Overweight	FucoseLean™ Hoodia Supreme®, Hoodia Supreme Plus®, Clinical Weight Management™
Oxidative Stress	REDOX balanced "blanket" antioxidants (see Chapter 4)
Syndrome X	Syndrome X Nutritional Factors®, (see Chapter 6)
Osteoporosis	Antiporosis®

Table 7. Common disorders associated with aging and useful categories of dietary supplements for nutritional support. These nutritional recommendations are not "magic bullets." They must be combined with positive lifestyle for anti-aging. Aging may not be fully reversed, but it can be slowed by positive health interventions. Products are mentioned for teaching comparisons. Readers are always encouraged to make product comparisons, based upon knowledge.

SYNDROME X AND DIABETES: DISORDERS OF PREMATURE AGING

The modern epidemics of Syndrome X (see Chapter 16) and maturity onset, Type II, diabetes mellitus are among the most important public health initiatives. These disorders form a common basis for premature aging (Table 8). It is time to move beyond focused anti-aging interventions and combat chronic diseases with the first-line options of positive lifestyle change. These first line options include important areas such as nutrition and the correct use of dietary supplements, or drugs where appropriate. Please note all mentioned products are examples. Other excellent supplement products exist. The importance of a combat against Syndrome X and its consequences are of pivotal importance in natural medicine. These issues are discussed in Appendix C (Metabolic Syndrome, Syndrome X or Syndrome X,Y and Z…).

COMPONENTS & ASSOCIATIONS OF THE METABOLIC SYNDROME X	FUNCTIONAL PROPERTIES OF SYNDROME X NUTRITIONAL FACTORS®
Insulin Resistance	Beta glucan fractions of oat fiber may lower blood glucose levels after sugar intake. Chromium may assist insulin function.
Abnormal Blood Lipids (cholesterol)	Oat beta glucan may reduce blood cholesterol levels (LDL and triglycerides) and may variably increase good cholesterol (HDL). Antioxidants and Chromium may exert favorable effects on blood cholesterol.
Obesity	Oat beta glucan may make people feel full when taken prior to meals and assist in dietary calorie control. The starch blocker found in white kidney bean extract may inhibit sugar absorption. Hoodia gordonii has non-stimulant appetite suppressing properties which can be applied alone or amplified with the metabolic advantages of green coffee bean extracts or green tea. FucoseLean™ or Clinical Fucoxanthin Complex™, seaweed fucoxanthin with metabolic enhancers.
Hypertension	Variable but small reductions in blood pressure result from weight control and lifestyle change. High blood pressure cannot be reliably controlled by dietary supplement use alone.

Oxidative Stress (advanced glycation end products)	The progression of Syndrome X and diabetes mellitus is linked to oxidative stress to body tissues. Antioxidants are beneficial for health, e.g. bioflavonoids, ellagic acid, anthocyanidins and alpha lipoic acid.
Homocysteine	Elevations of blood homocysteine levels are associated with cardiovascular disease, cognitive decline and osteoporosis. Vitamins B6, B12 and folic acid may reduce blood homocysteine levels. Methyl donors (see Chapter 31).
Inflammation	Several natural substances can variably suppress inflammation, particularly blood levels of C-reactive protein (CRP) e.g. curcumin, vitamin C, eicosapentanoic acid (EPA) in fish oil.

Table 8. Dietary supplement components that provide nutritional support for the many alterations of body structures and functions which occur in the metabolic Syndrome X, prediabetes and, in some case, established type-2 diabetes mellitus. No single drug or supplement can deal with the constellation of problems that occur in the metabolic Syndrome X. In this disorder, excessive body weight or obesity are often present. This complex approach is used as an illustration of the lack of "magic bullets" when supplements are used (supplied by Holt MD Labs) (see Appendix C).

To respond to the nutritional aspects of the major public health concern of the Metabolic Syndrome X and pre-diabetes, I have formulated two proprietary products for the adjunctive nutritional support of Syndrome X and early types of maturity onset diabetes, or pre-diabetes. Syndrome X Nutritional Factors® are available in mixed powder format or capsules and ingredients are shown in Table 9 A and B. The effects of these dietary supplements are highlighted in the preceding Table 8 and these products start to introduce the major complexities of synergistic formulations. Products are teaching examples.

A INGREDIENTS (Powder)
Patented glucocolloid, beta glucan fraction of oat soluble fiber
Chromium
A proprietary blend of alpha lipoic acid and guar gum
White Kidney bean extract
Vitamin B6

Folic acid
Vitamin B12
Vanadium
Sweetened with Erythritol (from glucose fermentation)
Mixed berry blend of strawberry, raspberry and blueberry with substantial antioxidant value (ORAC value 200 micromoles/g, anthocyanidin 0.25 mg, flavonoids 2.5% and ellagic acid 0.08%)
Beetroot blend (ORAC value 0.75 g, 100 micromoles /g, anthocyanidine 0.25 mg and mixed flavonoids 1%)
Natural flavor mix of pineapple, grape, strawberry, raspberry, orange and lime with citric acid

B INGREDIENTS (Capsules)
Fish Oil Omega-3 Fatty Acids, Eicosapentanoic Acid (EPA) and Docosahexanoic Acid (DHA)
Grape Seed Extract 95% Oligomeric Proanthocyanidins
Chromium (Polynicotinate)
Vanadium (amino acid chelate)
A proprietary blend of maitake mushroom, citrus bioflavonoids, alpha lipoic acid, white kidney bean extract, ellagic acid, cinnamon and CoEnzyme Q10 with 100% RDI of Vitamin B6 (pyridoxine HCl), Vitamin B12, folic acid, biotin, and zinc.

TABLE 9 A and B: Capsules and powder can be taken together. The powder product may have a greater effect on smoothing out blood glucose levels following meals because of its content of beta glucans, soluble fiber (Holt MD Labs).

ANTIOXIDANTS FOR ANTI-AGING (REVISION SECTION)

Many scientists have embraced the science behind the free-radical theory of aging by using REDOX-balanced, powerful antioxidants (Chapter 4). Examples of powerful antioxidant supplements are given in Chapters 4 and 31. Antioxidant supplements should combine antioxidants that access lipid and water compartments of tissues with antioxidant potential over a comprehensive REDOX range. Antioxidants are very important health-supporting substances and they can be found in liquid forms as organic green tea concentrates, to which other antioxidants may be added. Antioxidants are also available in powders and capsules (Chapters 4 and 31).

OSTEOPOROSIS: NEVER TOO EARLY, NEVER TOO LATE (SEE CHAPTER 6)

Osteoporosis is a devastating disease for the mature population (www.antiporosis.com). Bone fractures and impairments of skeletal functions occur in elderly people with osteoporosis. Bone fractures (especially fractured hips) are milestones for loss of quality of life, precipitation of institutionalization and sometimes premature death. One must prefer complete bone-boosting nutritional supplements which have complex evidence-based formulae. This is part of my proposal in "The Antiporosis Plan" (Holt S. The Antiporosis Plan, Wellness Publishing Inc., NJ, 2002) (see Chapter 6, Osteoporosis). Calcium alone is not enough to deal with osteoporosis prevention or management.

MINERALS AND LONGEVITY CORAL CALCIUM (CHAPTER 14)

Good mineral intake has been associated with longevity. This observation has been associated with the long and healthy life experienced by the inhabitants of the island of Okinawa, in Southern Japan (see Chapter 14). The longevity of Okinawans may occur for many reasons, other than the mineral enrichment of their environment from coral deposits (Table 10). Coral Calcium from Okinawa has a history of being the best-selling dietary supplement in the entire history of the US dietary supplement industry. Unfortunately, much misinformation was given about this valuable dietary supplement and many coral calcium supplements do not contain coral calcium from Okinawa.

Natures Benefit Inc. produces the best-selling brand of coral calcium without endorsing illegal treatment claims. These claims unfortunately damaged this valuable category of coral calcium supplements. Coral calcium is not just a calcium supplement. It is a versatile and valuable holistic mixture of minerals. This supplement remains very popular (see Chapter 14: Coral Calcium). While the role of coral calcium in anti-aging methods remains debatable, mineral supplementation in anti-aging protocols may have widespread benefits. There are several theories of aging which help the reader to understand that anti-aging must involve a multifaceted approach (Table 10) (see Chapter 31).

Aging programs	A program may exist in the genes for a specific number of cell functions.

Cross-link theories	Chemical links occur in collagen and other tissues. The basis of this process is aberrant mineral deposition and cross-linking of sugar and protein (glycation).
Free radical theories	Free radicals (reactive oxygen species) cause oxidative damage. Antioxidants of many types occur in the body or in nature.
Immunologic theories	Autoimmunity increases with age. The thymus shrinks. Many factors are involved.
Mutation and error theories	Mistakes in DNA replication or RNA function result in aging or age-related disease, e.g., cancer.
Repair budget theories	Environmental and lifestyle issues alter the investment of an organism in tissue repair. Tissue repair is dependant on nutrition.
Stress theories	Stress is cumulative and lifestyle-related. Nutritional deficiencies enhance stress.

Table 10: Seven theories of aging. Many complex factors operate (see Chapter 31).

KEYNOTE SUMMARY: ANTI-AGING

The widespread and effective use of natural anti-aging methods depend on public education, where the issues that cause tissue aging become clearly understood (Table 10). First-line approaches to anti-aging are rooted in natural medicine which includes change from adverse to positive lifestyle. Table 11 identifies several factors that may promote health and longevity (Chapter 31).

FACTOR	COMMENT
Balanced nutrient intake	Foods high in nutrients and essential trace elements, but low in calories, promote longevity.
Dietary restriction	Excessive animal protein intake is a physiological stress and is associated with excessive saturated fat intake and its sequelae - especially cardiovascular disease.

Economics	Poor people tend to die young.
Education	Intelligence is "environmental" with a genetic component. Intelligence correlates with survival.
Environmental influences	Urban living involves exposure to greater daily stress and pollution.
Exercise	A common factor for health promotion.
Genetics	Genetic influences on longevity remain unclear but operate to some variable degree.
High-fiber diets	Variable association with longevity. In non-deprived cultures, high-fiber diets can be shown to promote health.
Low calorie intake	Relationship in experimental animals very strong, emerging evidence in humans.
Marital status or loving relationships	Being married or in a close supporting relation-ship promotes health and statistics show a beneficial association between longevity and marriage.
Sociability	Getting along and reducing stress promotes health and well-being.
Trace elements in food	Populations living in areas where minerals are rich in the soil.

Table 11: Factors identified in medical research that contribute to longevity. The strength of each factor varies in different populations.

CONCLUSION

Aging cannot be considered a disease. Of all theories of aging, the role of oxidative stress in causing tissue damage, disease and premature aging seems to be very important. Antioxidant supplements must be regarded as a potential anti-aging tactic of merit (Chapter 31).

Age related diseases, such as osteoporosis, can be impacted by natural means, including bone-boosting substances. Nutritional approaches for diseases that cause accelerated aging such as Syndrome X and maturity onset diabetes may be highly effective. The educated diabetic has a better clinical outcome.

Syndrome X has emerged as perhaps the most important public health initiative facing Western nations, and a general consensus exists that the first-line option to deal with this constellation of problems should involve nutritional change, behavior modification and the judicious use of dietary supplements (Integrative Medicine) (Appendix C). Specific antiaging interventions are discussed in more detail in Chapter 31.

CHAPTER 6

OSTEOPOROSIS OR THIN BONES: THE ANTIPOROSIS® PLAN

THE CONCEPT OF THE ANTIPOROSIS® PLAN

OSTEOPOROSIS, or thin bones, is a tragic but preventable disorder. It robs quality of life from millions of mature Americans; and it has deadly consequences in the elite, elderly population. The first-line of attack against osteoporosis is the promotion of positive lifestyle changes combined with good nutrition and bone-boosting nutrients. (Prevention!)

Far too much trust has been placed in the value of calcium alone for both the prevention and potential reversal of thin bones. There are many nutrients, herbs, and botanicals that have bone building power and they complement the action of calcium and drugs that can be used to treat osteoporosis. A combination of these bone building natural substances is part of The Antiporosis Plan, which I have described in my book entitled "The Antiporosis Plan" (Wellness Publishing Inc., Little Falls, NJ, 2002).

I have stated that it is never too late or too early to attempt to combat osteoporosis. Rather than wait for the disease to become established in mature individuals, nutritional and lifestyle prevention of this disorder are key medical initiatives. Women should think about osteoporosis prevention in their thirties, at the latest!

Thin bones have reductions in their density which can be measured by simple, non-invasive, comfortable testing (bone density testing). Screening for bone density in mature females is a highly valuable way of detecting the silent disease of osteoporosis. Always remember that osteoporosis may progress and have tragic consequences in the elderly. Thin bones are more common in women than men; and they become a common problem after the menopause, when there is accelerated loss of bone in many women.

BUILDING BONES REQUIRES BUILDING BLOCK NUTRIENTS

In simple terms, building bone is like building a brick wall. Building a wall is not possible without bricks or building blocks. The idea of giving drugs that may help to build bone, without supplying the building blocks (bone nutrients), defies logic. Nutritional support for bone structure and function is often overlooked in routine medical practice. Prescriptions for bone building drugs (e.g. Bisphonates, Fosamax®, Merck Inc, etc.), are sometimes given with incomplete advice about lifestyle change and the value of dietary changes or nutrient supplementation with dietary supplements that provide the building blocks of bone.

LOVE YOUR BONES©

Many people tend to think about their bones when they are diseased, but skeletal structure of the body is a dynamic and it is a very active component of body chemistry. The skeleton contributes greatly to general well-being. These days many people are learning to "love their bones." Focusing on bone health and osteoporosis prevention is a key public health initiative for many nations, where dramatic increases in the elderly population are associated with increases in the occurrence and complications of osteoporosis. Several Asian countries are recognizing the importance of osteoporosis which is a legacy of westernized lifestyle, e.g. Indonesia, Japan, China, etc.

OSTEOPOROSIS OCCURS IN MEN AND WOMEN

I stress that osteoporosis is not just a "woman's thing." While the tragic consequences of thin bones, such as fractures and bone pain, are more common in women, the negative consequences of osteoporosis are more severe in elderly men. Modern research indicates the importance of assessing the risks for the development of osteoporosis. Some of these risk factors include poor diet, female sex, having blonde hair and blue eyes, being of Northern European descent, certain prescription drugs and indulging in substance abuse (smoking and alcohol consumption).

MORE THAN CALCIUM ALONE!

While life long deficiency of dietary intake of calcium has been associated with the development of thin bones, this is not the whole story. A greater nutritional understanding of osteoporosis prevention is required by the general population. There is an urgent need for the U.S. Government to educate the public on osteoporosis prevention. There are certain countries in the world where calcium intake is extremely high, e.g. Scandinavian countries, but these countries have among the highest occurrence of osteoporosis and hip fracture rates. In contrast, citizens of some third world countries, e.g. Thailand, have relatively low calcium intake, but osteoporosis seems much less common.

Many women are only starting to think about osteoporosis prevention during the perimenopause (age, over 40 years). This is a big mistake. Females should consider osteoporosis prevention after they have achieved peak bone mass in their early thirties, or even earlier! Studies show examples of alarming deficiencies of dietary calcium intake, and other nutrients that assist in maintaining bone structure, among all age groups. One major predisposition to osteoporosis is recurrent dieting, especially in young women. Again, it must be noted that there are many bone-boosting, nutritional substances, other than calcium, that have been shown to improve the density of bones. Aerobic exercise enthusiasts must build bone strength with muscle strength. Body builders often ignore skeletal structure. Supporting bone health involves more than taking calcium alone!

BONE BOOSTING DIETARY SUPPLEMENTS

Bone building dietary supplements can complement other specific interventions for osteoporosis, such as physical therapy or drug treatments. Users of these supplements are encouraged to speak to their doctors about their use of bone-boosting nutrition. Nutritional, bone building supplements are only one part of the Antiporosis Plan which calls for public education, appropriate exercise, good diet, elimination of substance abuse and regular bone density testing in mature people. The prevention of injuries must be stressed (especially in the elderly).

Dietary supplements that provide nutritional support for healthy bones should contain a versatile and potent nutritional formula (Table 12) including 100% of the recommended daily intake (RDI) of calcium. Dietary supplements for bone health should also contain a comprehensive array of bone-specific nutrients, including vitamins D3, B6, B12, folic acid, zinc, copper, manganese, boron and powerful antioxidants. Elevated blood levels of homocysteine contribute to osteoporosis. Some key ingredients in bone-boosting dietary supplements include plant substances that have been researched in the promotion of healthy bones, including soy isoflavones and active amounts of ipriflavone. I have favored more complete dietary supplement formulae as part of the Antiporosis Plan, (Table 12). My recommendations are <u>NOT</u> just for calcium supplements alone!

Calcium
Magnesium (oxide and citrate)
Vitamin C (ascorbic acid)
Vitamin D3 (cholecalciferol)
Zinc (amino acid chelate)
Copper (amino acid chelate)
Vitamin B6
Folic Acid
Vitamin B12
Vitamin K
Manganese (amino acid chelate)
Turmeric Root
Ipriflavone
Horsetail (Equisetum arvense L, herb)
Soy isoflavones
Boron (amino acid chelate)

Table 12. Combined ingredients in dietary supplements which provide nutritional support for healthy bones (Holt MD Technologies).

KEYNOTE SUMMARY: OSTEOPOROSIS

Osteoporosis or thin bones affects many more than 20 million Americans. About 80% of all individuals with osteoporosis are women and great risks exist for white females who are of Northern European descent. Almost every woman is at risk for osteoporosis, especially if they have engaged in poor dietary practices, lack of exercise, substance abuse or if they have reached the perimenopause.

"It is never too early or too late to combat osteoporosis," and this is the basis of what I have referred to as "The Antiporosis Plan." Fighting osteoporosis means never getting thin bones. I believe that osteoporosis is a preventable disease in the vast majority of cases. Men and women should engage in good nutritional practices, well-planned physical activity and supplementation of their diet with natural bone-boosting nutrients.

The Antiporosis Plan was created to educate the nation on natural pathways for the prevention and management of thin bones. Many bone building drugs have side-effects and they are expensive. These bone building drugs are unlikely to be fully effective unless dietary, bone-building nutrients are combined with these drugs.

There is a widespread misconception that calcium supplements alone are enough to support bone structure and function. Many scientific studies show that calcium supplements alone are inadequate to prevent or manage thin bones, and they do not provide complete support for bone structure and function.

CONCLUSION

In conclusion, the Antiporosis Plan can be summarized:

- Public education.
- Well-planned physical activity: anti-gravity exercises.
- A bone-boosting diet.
- Supplementation with natural bone-boosting nutraceuticals.
- Positive lifestyle change and remedies of natural origin are often compatible with standard drug treatments for bone and joint disorders.
- More use of bone-density testing.
- Prevention of injuries.
- Risk assessment and involvement of healthcare professionals.
- Use of prevention initiatives in early adulthood.
- Optimizing nutrition in pregnancy and childhood.
- Focus on the lack of safety of drug treatments is required. Commonly used drugs for osteoporosis treatment have serious side effects, e.g., renal damage, severe upper gastrointestinal ulceration etc.

CHAPTER 7

IMMUNE FUNCTION

THE BIODEFENSES OF THE BODY: IMMUNE FUNCTION

THE complex immune system is responsible for the biodefenses of the body. Cells of the immune system play a direct role in immunity; and some immune cells produce many substances such as antibodies and chemical messengers that play a role in the "complex cascade of immune events." These events involve intelligent communications within the immune system and throughout all tissues of the body. The complexities of the cascade of immune events help people to understand how difficult it may be to exert an effect on the immune system with a single drug or a single natural substance. Of all events in the body, immunity is best supported or modified by a combination of substances that act on the multiple components of immune structures and functions (synergistic supplement approaches).

Alterations in the balance of immune function are responsible for the cause or progression of many common diseases, including cancer, chronic inflammatory disorders, arthritis and specific autoimmune disease. People talk about boosting immune function, but most often they really mean balancing or modulating immune function. Independent laboratory studies of some dietary supplements show that complex combinations of herbs, botanicals and nutrients have an evidence base to support immune function (Holt MD Technologies).

OVERVIEW OF IMMUNE FUNCTION

Various types of white cells circulate in the blood or are found together in lymphatic tissues. Lymph nodes, the bone marrow, the spleen, and the thymus gland contain clumps of special white cells that are pivotal structures of the immune system. A complex series of chemical messengers is shared among cells in the immune system. Antibody production by specific types of white cells aids in clearing the tissue fluids of harmful intruders, e.g., antigens or microorganisms (viruses, bacteria and yeasts). The biodefenses within the immune system are not simple in their structure or function. Elaborate mechanisms of biodefense are present at entry sites into the body, including the nasal passages, throat and entire gastrointestinal tract.

Understanding the complexity of the body structure and functions involved in immunity is a difficult task for even the most knowledgeable health care giver. I reiterate that the complexity of the cascade of events that occurs during immune functions makes it highly unlikely that any single agent will have an efficient overall effect on balancing or promoting immune function. In other words, single drugs or nutrients or botanicals are not likely to be effective at correcting or promoting immune disturbances when used alone. This means that immune function may be best supported by positive lifestyle and the synergistic actions of combined substances, especially selected nutrients, herbals and botanicals.

THE POWER OF SYNERGY IN SUPPORTING IMMUNE FUNCTION

Single dietary supplements to "boost" immunity are limited in their effects (e.g., AHCC alone etc). "Boosting" certain aspects of the complex series of events in some immune-related diseases may sometimes do more harm than good. The additive benefits and versatile nature of many different natural agents in a dietary supplement that can work on different aspects of immune events may help modulate or balance many different immune functions (Table 13).

- Andrographis paniculata
- Acanthopanax senticosa
- Green tea
- Turmeric
- Grape seed extract
- Zinc
- Vitamin C
- Ashwagandha
- Oregon grape
- Shitake mushroom

- Echinacea purpurea
- Goldenseal
- Golden thread
- Aloe Vera
- Garlic
- Astragalus
- Korean ginseng
- Coriolus versicolor
- Active Hexose Correlate Compound (AHCC)
- Beta glucan

Table 13. Nutrients, herbs and botanicals with good scientific agreement of nutritional benefits for immune function. The basis of a patent-pending formula (Holt MD Labs).

SELF-RELIANCE FOR SELF-MANAGEMENT OF IMMUNE FUNCTION

Many people are seeking natural substances that will support immune function in the body and help with nutritional control of unwanted inflammatory responses. Some natural substances with immune-stimulating properties may have anti-viral properties. Modern research on remedies of natural origin has pointed to a number of remedies of natural origin that have complex actions on immune function. These actions occur at many different sites in the overall cascade of immune events.

COMPARISONS AMONG SUPPLEMENTS FOR IMMUNE FUNCTION

Single-agent approaches with one herb or nutrient possess disadvantages and limitations. For example, sterolins (Moducare®) or mushroom extracts (MGN3®,BRM4®) or active hexose correlated compounds (AHCC or ImmPower®), or Maitake Products®, are immune stimulators, but they have relatively focused and limited effects on only certain aspects of immune function. I have proposed that there is a way of producing an improved, synergistic, dietary supplement that can be used in combination to stimulate immune function, in a more global manner.

Any natural agent that exerts an antioxidant function can be potentially valuable in promoting healthy immune function. Oxidative stress (free-radical damage) to components of the immune system is a common reason for disordered immunity. In particular, the following antioxidants are of value for immune well-being: Vitamin C, zinc, green tea, turmeric, grape seed extract and other antioxidants that are found in a variety of herbs and botanicals (Table 13).

Botanical agents with specific immune-enhancing power include: several species of mushrooms; Coriolus versicolor, Shitake mushroom, natural components such as AHCC, plant or yeast sources of beta glucan, Echinacea, and the potent and versatile herb Andrographis paniculata (AP). Recent research implies that AP may be a very powerful stimulator of immune function by its specific actions on chemical signals in certain cells; and AP has reported antiviral properties, but this supplement is not approved for disease treatment, at law.

SYNDROME X, PREDIABETES AND DIABETES DEPRESS IMMUNE FUNCTIONS

Recent research links excessive intake of simple sugars in the diet with depressed immunity. Who would have thought that America's love affair with sweet foods would open the door for chronic disease, in a manner that has been unsurpassed in medical history? Syndrome X is the most important public health initiative facing Western society, and the practice of general medicine or the dietary supplement industry has still not woken up to the importance of Syndrome X, as a risk of death and disability risk from many causes (See Chapter 16: Syndrome X).

People with diabetes or Syndrome X often experience the consequences of diminished immune function. Early signs of diabetes in many people include recurrent infections, e.g. bacterial, yeast or Candida albicans. A reduction of the refined sugar intake in the diet may be a simple intervention to help restore balance to the immune system. Furthermore, many people with metabolic Syndrome X, prediabetes or diabetes mellitus may benefit from natural combinations of immune supporting substances, as well as specific nutrients to support insulin functions, smooth out blood glucose and help to promote healthy blood cholesterol (Syndrome X Nutritional Factors®). These are not disease treatment claims, but they are important general nutritional management principles for many people.

DIETARY SUPPLEMENT RESEARCH: IMMUNE FUNCTION

In the late 1990's and early parts of this century, many hundreds of millions of dollars worth of immune-stimulating, dietary supplements were sold. Among the most popular of these supplements was a product called MGN-3, now called BRM-4 (Lane Labs, NJ, Progressive Labs, TX and Daiwa Pharmaceuticals, Japan). Because of the popularity and reported benefits of MGN-3 (BRM4), comparative studies were made between a complex immune dietary supplement formula

(Holt MD Labs, Table 13) and MGN-3 (BRM4). The Holt MD Technologies product (Biodefense®) and MGN-3 have potential to alter immunity, by virtue of their biologically active contents. However, the mechanism of action of these two dietary supplements can be expected to be quite different, with the more comprehensive formula (Biodefense®) affecting more aspects of immune cascades.

The complex array of components in the Holt MD Technologies formula (Biodefense®) can be expected to act in a multi-faceted way on immune function (Table 13). This led to independent experiments that were designed to investigate the properties of this synergistic formula (Biodefense®) on the nutritional support of immune function.

In summary, independent laboratory studies performed by Gitte Jensen PhD and her colleagues at Natural Immune Systems Inc. (Ontario, Canada and OR, US), showed that the complex formula (Holt MD) is a potent stimulator of Natural Killer (NK) cells; and it is highly active in amounts where MGN-3 (BRM4) has no effects. While MGN-3 was shown to activate 60% of NK cells in lab experiments, the complex formula (Biodefense®) was shown to activate over 90% of NK cells, at maximum doses that could be tolerated by human lymphocytes (immune white cells).

In other words, the complex, Holt MD Technologies formula (Biodefense®) seemed to be much more potent in stimulating natural NK cells compared with MGN-3 (BRM4). The dietary supplement AHCC (e.g. ImmPower) has become popular as an immune stimulator, but its effects are quite similar to MGN-3 and they may not be as versatile as the synergistic, complex formula (Biodefense®), but no direct laboratory comparisons have been made. The compound AHCC is one of many components of the Holt MD formula (Biodefense®).

The actions of the complex formula (Biodefense®) have been studied in a small number of healthy volunteers by Natural Immune Systems Inc. and these studies show "homing" of NK cells, with apparent beneficial effects. All manufacturers of dietary supplements that promote healthy immune function have become conservative in their approach to health claims because MGN-3 (Lane Labs) (now called BRM4, Daiwa) was removed from the dietary supplement market as a result of the manufacturers (Lane Labs) making illegal treatment claims for the management of viral disease and cancer. I stress that there is no intention to make disease prevention or management claims for any immune supplement formulae. This dialogue is about immune function only.

CAUTIONS AGAINST TREATMENT CLAIMS

The general public has been scared about the outbreak of several different types of viral infections. There was a threat against the public that bioterrorists may use viruses; and the modern epidemics of AIDS, Hepatitis B or C and bird flu (H5N1 virus) are causing much public concern. Medical scientists are trying very hard to develop methods to prevent viral infections with drugs and vaccines, but in the case of AIDS and bird flu there have been some disappointments, especially with vaccination studies. Furthermore, it is known that the progression of many diseases may be related to disturbed immune function e.g. cancer. That said, readers must understand that dietary supplements have <u>not</u> been shown to prevent serious disease in a conclusive manner.

The circumstances of general threats to human immunity make the promotion of general levels of immunity in the population an appealing possibility, but this area of medicine remains under explored. **Therefore, it must be clearly understood that no dietary supplement can claim to have a beneficial effect in disease prevention or treatment, especially in the field of immunity**. I feel very strongly that illegal treatment or disease prevention claims about dietary supplements must be avoided, unless well constructed clinical trials show benefits and regulatory agencies endorse, evaluate and approve claims of benefits.

KEYNOTE SUMMARY

Any natural agent that exerts an antioxidant function can be potentially valuable in promoting healthy immune function; because oxidative stress or free-radical damage to components of the immune system is a common reason for disordered immunity. In particular, the following antioxidants are of value for immune support: Vitamin C, zinc, green tea, turmeric, grape seed extract and antioxidants found in a variety of herbs and botanicals (Table 13).

Botanical agents with specific immune-enhancing properties include several species of mushrooms, plant sources of beta glucan, Echinacea and the potent and versatile herb Andrographis paniculata (AP). Recent research implies that AP may be a very powerful stimulator of immune function by its specific actions on chemical signals in certain cells.

I believe that nutritional support for immune function must be multifaceted and formulations of dietary supplements that contain several different natural ingredients may be an optimal way to provide nutritional support for immune function. Companies that sell dietary supplements as nutritional support for immune function should produce their own research on their own products. This has not occurred often, and science is often "borrowed." All disease prevention and treatment claims must be avoided in the sale of immune-enhancing or modulating supplements.

CONCLUSION

I believe that nutritional support for immune function must involve a multipronged approach. Formulations of dietary supplements that contain several different natural ingredients are part of nutritional support for the complex cascade of events in immune function, but much further research is required.

DIETARY SUPPLEMENTS HAVE BEEN STUDIED IN INDEPENDENT LABORATORY EXPERIMENTS WHERE THEY HAVE BEEN SHOWN TO STIMULATE NATURAL KILLER CELL (NK) FUNCTION. MORE RESEARCH IS REQUIRED. COMPLEX FORMULAE ARE PREFERRED TO MODULATE COMPLEX CASCADES OF IMMUNE FUNCTION.

CHAPTER 8

JOINT CARE

DANGERS OF ARTHRITIS MEDICATION: THE NSAID

MANY millions of Americans with bone and joint problems are "gobbling" aspirin and non-steroidal anti-inflammatory drugs (NSAID). This is occurring in a manner that presents a major public health concern. This concern is a direct consequence of the common side effects of these drugs. Common side effects of NSAID include stomach upset that can herald the onset of peptic ulcer and the precipitation of life threatening bleeding from the upper or lower digestive tract. In addition, liver and kidney problems are relatively common with NSAID use. Certain types of NSAID are associated with a risk of stroke or heart attack. Unfortunately, the side effects of NSAID are sometimes fatal, especially in the elderly, who represent the main target population who take these drugs, and to whom these drugs are often selectively marketed.

For these reasons, many people have sought alternative management strategies for bone and joint health, including the use of dietary supplements. While dietary supplements for bone and joint health are not drugs or considered substitutes for drugs (at law), many doctors and their patients are using dietary supplements to manage simple arthritis, especially osteoarthritis. This approach can occur only with statements that stress the use of "nutritional support for bone and joint structure and/or function."

SUPPLEMENTS FOR JOINT HEALTH

Synergistic "joint" products use many natural agents in varying amounts to produce "additive benefits" for the nutritional support of joint function and mobility (synergistic formulation). Certain natural substances, such as glucosamine, have demonstrated nutritional benefits for joint structure and function, including the promotion of flexibility and the improvement of joint mobility during activity. Synergistic formulations have no rivals in terms of uniqueness and completeness of formulation, with overall nutritional versatility of various ingredients (Table 14).

- Glucosamine sulphate 2KCL
- Extract of Phellodendron Amurense
- Resveratrol
- Boron (Chelate/Fructoboron®)

In a proprietary natural composition of

- Barberry bark, Golden thread root, Fever few whole, Ginger root, Green tea extract 50%, Tulsi leaves, Hops flower, Oregano leaves, Rosemary leaves, Chinese Skullcap, whole Turmeric root, Nettle leaves, Boswellia serrata resin 60% extract, Devil's claw root, White willow bark, Sea cucumber, whole hydrolyzed type II collagen, Methysulfonylmethane, Cetyl Myristoleate, Chondroitin Sulfate and green lipped mussel (Perna canaliculus).

Table 14. The ingredients of a synergistic joint supplement, used for nutritional support for joint function. This product is a classic example of synergistic formulation and is used as a teaching example. This approach starts to uncover complex cascades of events that cause joint problems (Holt MD Labs). This formula contains herbs that may inhibit cyclo-oxygenase type 2 enzymes (COX-2 inhibitors).

SYNERGY IN JOINT CARE

The joint formulation (Table 14) has six potential, but different modes of potential action as a dietary supplement. This approach provides nutritional support for bone and joint health (Table 15). The formula contains full-dose, high-quality, low-sodium glucosamine. Glucosamine is a mainstay of joint nutrition that has been shown to have a clear benefit for the repair of cartilage in joints. Not only does glucosamine help repair cartilage in damaged joints, it promotes cartilage renewal and regeneration; and it may provide added advantages of improving lubrication within joints, by exerting beneficial effects on joint fluid. The formula also contains chondroitin which is another joint specific supplement that has variable, but demonstrable benefits in terms of improvement in joint mobility.

- Cartilage repair, renewal, regeneration and lubrication with glucosamine, cartilage and chondroitin.
- Inhibition of leukotrienes with Boswellia - a body function.
- Antioxidant actions.
- Herbal system for potential inhibition of Cox-2 enzymes - a body function.
- Independent benefits of boron
- Immune support with collagen.

Table 15: The six potential beneficial actions of natural ingredients for joint health. These ingredients are present in formulae created by Holt MD Technologies and they are used as a teaching example.

The above formulation strategy takes a lead over other beneficial joint supplements by employing the use of botanicals that have been used in traditional medical systems, as practiced in India and Asia. It utilizes the herb Boswellia serrata, which has been shown in laboratory experiments to antagonize or inhibit the production of substances (leukotrienes) that may promote inflammation in joints. This normal body function of the production of inflammatory substances (leukotrienes) is a key manner in which extracts of Boswellia provide nutritional support for joint structure and function. The proposed formula also contains the advantage of several antioxidants which can help minimize the oxidative stress that is put upon joints, as a consequence of "wear and tear" and other negative factors that cause oxidative tissue damage.

COX-2 INHIBITION WITH HERBS: A POTENTIAL ACTION OF SUPPLEMENTS

The most unique components of the proposed joint formula include a proprietary formula of herbal substances which are described variably in laboratory experiments to potentially inhibit COX-2 enzymes. COX-2 enzymes are produced as part of normal body function in the presence of inflammation; and they contribute to pain and disability that is experienced with inflammation, joint disorders, injuries, and arthritis.

There are a number of herbs which may inhibit COX-2 enzymes in the body. It is notable that the inhibition of COX-2 enzymes is the basic mode of action of popular and commonly used anti-arthritic medications that belong to the class of non-steroidal anti-inflammatory drugs (NSAID)(e.g., Vioxx® and Celebrex®). It is not possible to compare directly the herbal systems that may inhibit COX-2 enzymes with the drugs that inhibit these enzyme systems.

One important inhibitor of COX-2 enzyme systems that is found in the synergistic joint formula is the herb Phéllodendron amurense. Herbs or botanicals that have variable documentation of their ability to inhibit COX-2 enzyme systems include: Barberry bark, Goldenthread root, Feverfew Herb, Ginger Root, Green Tea extract, Polyphenols, Tulsi leaves, Hops flower, Oregano leaves, Rosemary leaves, Chinese Skullcap Herb, Turmeric root, Nettle leaves and Devil's claw root. A proprietary, synergistic formulation of these herbs is used in dietary supplements (Holt MD Technologies).

MORE POTENTIAL ACTIONS OF SYNERGISTIC, JOINT FORMULAE

The micronutrient "boron" that is present in the proposed formula has independent beneficial effects on joint health. Collagen contents in a joint supplement may provide indirect immune support for joint function. White willow bark is a tried and trusted herb used for nutritional support of joint function. Added to the completeness of the potential formula are sea cucumber, MSM, celadrine and New Zealand green lipped mussel (Perna canaliculus).

NUTRITIONAL SUPPORT FOR JOINTS
ENTERS MAINSTREAM MEDICINE

The benefits of dietary supplements for the promotion of bone and joint health have become a mainstay in medical practice of both alternative and conventional physicians. Many millions of people have used different nutritional ingredients, most often as glucosamine, for the nutritional support of their joint problems. Nutritional support for joint health may take several weeks to be maximally effective (up to 12 weeks). This means that individuals must be encouraged to continue taking dietary supplements for joint health for several weeks, before they conclude that they are not effective.

TOPICAL RUBS CAN ASSIST A SWITCH TO
NUTRITIONAL SUPPORT FOR JOINT FUNCTION

I believe that natural supplements and topical pain relief rubs can permit the reduction of the use of aspirin and NSAID, at least a reduction in drug dosage requirements. Since many of the side effects of NSAID may occur at high dosages of these drugs, a reduction in the amount of NSAID that are taken is a real advantage. A reasonable, natural approach to bone and joint problems is to use a topical agent that may help with pain and flexibility, while the action of simultaneously administered nutritional supplements are taking effect over a more prolonged period of time (up to 12 weeks).

This approach may spare the use of NSAID somewhat. An example of a bone and joint rub that is that beneficial in this context, is the topical product called Silver Emu™. The topical product Silver Emu™ is distinguished by its content of surface cooling agents with analgesic properties (menthol), and the presence of emu oil. Emu oil is a useful carrier substance with skin soothing properties. Several other natural ingredients that may help bone and joint problems include the use of natural substances that block substance P which gives "signals of pain" in the nervous system (e.g. capsaicin or salicylates). Blue dyes in topical bone and joint rubs are best avoided; they are toxic.

EMU NATURALLY: SILVER EMU™

Early explorers of the Australian continent were fascinated when they discovered the ancient flightless bird called the emu. Folklore told of stories of native aborigines who had used emu oil as a valuable treatment for wound healing, skin disorders, injuries and arthritis. The emu has been imported into the United States and it has become an important part of U.S farming. The emu is a source of delicious, low-cholesterol meat that is served in sophisticated restaurants.

Recent scientific studies have uncovered several health benefits of emu oil. This oil has a very special series of constituents which are fatty substances that present a natural way of penetrating the skin (carrier agent). Emu oil is particularly soothing under a number of circumstances, and it has become a valuable ingredient in natural cosmetics such as moisturizers, skin antioxidants, and anti-wrinkle creams or lotions.

EMU OIL: A CARRIER OF SOOTHING SUBSTANCES: SILVER EMU™

The health benefits of emu oil are most apparent when the oil is applied to the skin. Emu oil is available in some pain relief creams that can be used for the temporary relief of aches and pains in muscles and joints. These discomforts may be associated with arthritis, strain, simple backache, bruises, sprains and other disorders that result from physical activity.

Silver Emu™ is sold as a topical rub that is odorless, non-greasy and easy to apply. The formula is presented in a convenient form that provides a powerful, versatile soothing formula of emu oil, aloe, with valuable natural additives such as methylsulfonylmethane (MSM) and glucosamine.

Emu oil pain relief cream contains menthol. Menthol and camphor are immediate cooling pain relievers and methyl salicylate is an agent to help remove pain. Topical pain rubs contain variably other ingredients such as allantoin, aloe, calendula, chamomile, vitamin D, horse chestnut, comfrey root, glucosamine, and vitamin E. It must be understood that it is the cooling agents or inhibitors of pain signals that are considered the active ingredients in topical bone and joint rubs (at law). Other substances in these products are listed as inactive ingredients, even though some people believe they may be active.

SILVER EMU™: AN IMPROVED RUB

Silver Emu™ is a special type of emu oil product. There arc other commercially successful types of emu oil lotions or creams such as Blue Emu® and Blue Stuff® etc. These "blue" products contain many artificial ingredients and dyes with questionable safety. Remember emu oil is a carrier and it will help artificial dyes, such as those found in Blue Emu®, to penetrate the skin and enter the body. Many health food stores have refused to carry Blue Emu® or other emu oil rubs for these reasons. Silver Emu™ does not contain artificial dyes.

SPECIAL CONCERNS ABOUT TOXINS OR SYNTHETIC CHEMICALS IN TOPICAL PRODUCTS

There are increasing concerns among retailers and consumers about many potentially toxic substances that are found in topical products, such as cosmetics or pain rubs. Much concern has been expressed about the presence of artificial dyes in many lotions or creams. Of notable concern in FD&C Blue #1, a dye which has been associated with deaths in some circumstances. The skin is freely permeable to many synthetic chemicals and some extracted D&C dyes have been withdrawn or limited in their use following FDA rulings.

One major concern is the presence of parabens in topical products and trade associations have started to ban the display of allegedly "natural topical products" that contain large amounts or types of potentially toxic synthetic chemicals. Some bone and joint rubs contain not only blue dyes, but they contain both methylparabens and propylparabens. These parabens are fat soluble compounds which have shown an ability to penetrate the body and appear in body secretions. Other synthetic ingredients, such as diazolidinyl urea, found in some blue dye containing pain rubs have been associated with episodes of irritation to the skin and mucus membranes. The US FDA has been slow to regulate the use of some of these synthetic chemicals, which have been banned in several countries, including Japan.

There is a problem with the use of all natural ingredients in topical products. Synthetic chemicals produce ideal aesthetic characteristics by an appealing touch or feel. However, the price paid for these pleasant cutaneous experiences may be increasing "occult" toxicity in many people.

KEYNOTE SUMMARY: JOINT SUPPLEMENTS

Many of the 50 million or so Americans with arthritis or bone and joint health problems are at risk from the side-effects of pain killers, aspirin and non-steroidal anti-inflammatory drugs (NSAID). That said, dietary supplements are not drugs or proven substitutes for drugs.

Leading-edge, nutraceutical bone and joint formulations use many natural agents in varying amounts to produce "additive benefits" for the nutritional support of joint function and mobility. The use of many natural agents at one time produces an "additive benefit" that is referred to as "synergy." In other words, these agents add to each other's range of nutritional benefits for joint structure and function, including flexibility and the improvement of joint mobility during activity.

Synergistic formulations have no known rivals in the dietary supplement industry, in terms of uniqueness and completeness of formulation, with an overall projected versatility of their various ingredients.

CHAPTER 9

DIGESTION

DIGESTIVE HEALTH IS A KEY TO GENERAL HEALTH

Without healthy function of the digestive tract, general health cannot prevail. Every bathroom cupboard in America contains one or more digestive aids, including laxatives, antacids and other concoctions for "tummy problems." I have described many natural pathways to digestive health in detail in two of my books entitled, "Natural Pathways to Digestive Health" (M. Evans Publishing Inc., N.Y., 2000) and "Digestion Naturally" (Wellness Publishing Inc., Little Falls, N.J., 2008, in press, www.wellnesspublishing.com).

Digestive upset is notoriously recurrent in many people, because it is often triggered by adverse lifestyle. While symptoms of digestive disturbance can spell serious disease such as cancer or inflammation, most common digestive symptoms are due to altered function of the digestive tract. These disorders are called "functional digestive diseases;" and they are often associated with "stress" or disturbance of "mind-body functions."

I reiterate that the most common causes of digestive upset represent an imbalance of the digestive function ("dysharmony") and they are not due to serious tissue inflammation or cancer. Restoring the balance and providing nutritional support for digestive structure and function are possible with lifestyle changes and selected synergistic dietary supplements. Formulations are used as teaching examples of ranges of dietary supplement ingredients for digestive health.

Classic examples of functional digestive upset include the irritable bowel syndrome (IBS) and upper abdominal pain in the absence of peptic ulcer, a disorder that is often called "functional dyspepsia." Natural Medicine is ideal for "functional" digestive upset and restoration of the harmony of digestive structure and functions.

THE HARMONY OF THE GUT

The controls of digestive function are highly complex. Drugs and surgery for digestive disease do not work generally to restore the harmony of the gut, but these approaches are necessary for diseases that alter the structure of the bowel, e.g., cancer, certain serious types of inflammation and occasionally complicated peptic ulceration or serious gastroesophageal reflux disease (GERD).

I have proposed that functional upsets of the digestive tract are prime targets for the use of remedies of natural origin. For example, education and relaxation techniques including hypnotherapy, together with natural substances, provide simple, gentle and safe first-line options for functional dyspepsia and irritable bowel syndrome (IBS). Peer-review medical literature supports this approach. Natural options may be applied before an individual reaches for an over-the-counter drug or a drug prescription for digestive upset, providing that serious or significant organic diseases of the gastrointestinal tract have been excluded. Symptoms of simple or benign gastrointestinal disease may be similar to symptoms of serious digestive disease and self management must involve caution or medical advice.

TRADITIONAL USE OF NATURAL REMEDIES FOR DIGESTIVE UPSET

Several approaches exist in natural medicine to attempt to balance digestive function. Many individuals believe in the benefits of colon or body cleansing, the use of enzymes to promote digestion, and attempts to detoxify the body.

Friendly bacteria can grow in the lower bowel. These healthy bacteria are called "probiotics" (pro=for, biosis=life); and they can be taken in dietary supplements, with the result that they can implant themselves in the lower digestive tract and promote health in a variety of complex ways (probiotics) (Table 16).

- Assistance with digestion.
- Alleviation of digestive disorders, e.g. colitis, IBS, peptic ulcer (arguable).
- The synthesis of several vitamins in the colon (especially B complex).
- Enhanced mineral absorption, especially calcium.
- Protection against pathogenic bacterial infections, e.g. E. coli infection.

- Reduction of symptoms of lactose intolerance, permits limited reintroduction of dairy products.
- Reduction of yeast overgrowth (candidiasis), notable reduction in vaginal thrush.
- Improvement in immune function, "primes" the gut immune system.
- Anti-carcinogenic effects, some good evidence.
- Prevention of Helicobacter pylori infection and its association with peptic ulcer.
- Acne prevention.
- Cholesterol reduction (modest and unpredictable).
- Benefit for opportunistic gut infections in immunodeficiency states (e.g. AIDS)

Table 16 Major benefits of probiotic therapy, some physicians or scientists argue about these potential benefits.

Conventional medicine has argued that colon cleansing may not be a valuable intervention. However, the idea that the bowel can be a source of toxins is a concept that is being increasingly accepted, even though this concept has been challenged. Simple constipation is extremely common and many people report a favorable outcome from the appropriate intermittent use of laxatives or colonic irrigation (Chapter 11 Colon Cleansing). There is emerging evidence that colon cleansing helps to detoxify the body; and it may contribute to the elimination of environmental poisons, such as heavy metals.

SEEDING THE GUT: PREBIOSIS AND PROBIOSIS: HEALTHY BACTERIA

The value of using healthy bacteria (probiotics) in dietary supplements for gastrointestinal and general health is well recognized in medical practice. This process of reseeding the lower intestines with friendly bacteria is called "probiotic therapy." Probiotic usage is considered to be evidence-based in medical practice.

Scientific literature has described many circumstances in which probiotic therapy may be beneficial including: the nutritional management of simple digestive upset, disturbance of the gut in AIDS, inflammatory bowel disease and other digestive disorders… to name a few. However, treatment claims for dietary supplements are to be avoided, even if there is clear evidence of treatment potential. This is what I have described as the enigma of modern medicine where natural medicine is looking for a pathway of integration of the "natural" with the "conventional" (or the application of medical pluralism). The readers may now understand how terms like "Integrative Medicine" have emerged in the modern practice of medicine in the United States and worldwide.

One can assist the growth of friendly bacteria in the colon by using specific "foods" (often complex carbohydrates) that are metabolized by friendly bacteria, such as *Lactobacilli* and *Bifidobacteria*. These foods that promote the growth of friendly bacteria are called prebiotics, and they include dietary fiber and fructo-oligosaccharides (FOS). Fiber and FOS are found commonly in cereals, fruit, vegetables and they are concentrated in specific foods such as bananas and onions. Fiber and probiotics are best taken together, producing a powerful health synergy (see Fiber, Chapter 12).

Friendly gut bacteria promote the normal structure and function of the lining of the intestines, and they prime the immune system in both the gut and the body overall. Friendly bacteria (probiotics) have far reaching health benefits (Table 16).

DETOXIFICATION AND ENZYMES

Many herbs have been proposed for body detoxification. The liver is a principal organ of detoxification. Liver detoxification involves breaking down compounds and preparing them for elimination in the urine or digestive tract. The liver metabolizes many drugs and botanical compounds. Milk thistle (silymarin) has been shown in several studies to assist in the process of detoxification of chemicals by the liver and to exert a liver-protective effect, by partially guarding the liver against damage from toxins. Milk thistle works to increase glutathione levels in the liver.

Supplementation of the diet with food (digestive) enzymes has become a popular part of natural medicine. There are many different enzymes that can be taken in supplements. Certain enzymes may assist in the digestion of food. These enzymes include: protease, amylase, lipase, cellulase, lactase, and pepsin. Digestive enzymes digest food and they are distinct from systemic enzymes that exert other effects such as anti-inflammatory or healing actions, e.g. bromelain and papain (see Enzymes, Chapter 13). There are new concepts emerging about the use of enzymes. In brief, enzymes either exert their effects in the digestive tract (digestive enzymes) or exert their effects in the body itself (systemic enzymes).

ENZYMES: THE FOOD ENZYME CONCEPT

Enzymes are absolutely necessary for the normal absorption of nutrients from the diet. It has been suggested that "you are what you eat," but it is more accurate to say, "you are what you absorb into your body." The idea of supplementing a diet with enzymes, in order to improve digestion and health, has become popular in the practice of Integrative Medicine. In states of enzyme deficiency, such as failure of the pancreas to secrete enzymes (e.g. chronic pancreatitis), the value of enzyme supplements is unquestionable. There are proponents of enzyme supplements who believe that everyone may benefit from enzyme supplements, but conventional medicine may disagree.

USING FOOD ENZYME SUPPLEMENTS

The notion of eating "live foods" which contain active enzymes is of growing interest in Naturopathic and Alternative medicine. This concept has led to the widespread sale of "green foods" and mixed fruit, berry and vegetable supplements, such as berry powder or extracts (e.g. Berry Supreme®, Berries and Greens Plus Supernutrition™, Clinical Daily Prevention™, Chapter 4). These dietary supplement powders contain an array of vegetable and plant sources of enzymes which are considered very healthy and very versatile in their application. Furthermore, dietary supplements such as berry powders have many valuable phytochemicals that provide nutritional support for the structure and function of many organs of the body, including the brain, the eyes, the gastrointestinal tract; and they may have anti-cancer benefits. These fruit and vegetable powders are sold in powder to make beverages by addition to juice or pure water and they can be added to many foods. These berry and vegetable or greens supplements are good sources of vital nutrients, and their antioxidant contents have significant health potential (Chapter 4).

CHOOSING ENZYMES (REVISION)

Some enzymes work to facilitate important chemical reactions in the body (systemic enzymes), whereas digestive enzymes are absolutely necessary to break down food for its efficient digestion from the gastrointestinal tract. Thus, I reiterate that there has been an arbitrary classification of enzymes into two different types. The first type of enzymes is those that act within the body to govern the chemistry of life. These are called systemic enzymes or "metabolic enzymes" and they are increasingly popular as dietary supplements, even though research on some of the "systemic" enzymes is quite limited (see Enzymes, Chapter 13).

SYSTEMIC OR METABOLIC ENZYMES

There are several thousand metabolic enzymes that cause vital chemical reactions in the body. Key examples of metabolic enzymes include: superoxide dismutase (SOD), catalase and glutathione-S-transferase – to name a few. These important metabolic enzymes play a major role in the body's own ability to detoxify itself. In this chapter, I concentrate on the second type of enzymes called digestive enzymes which are found in abundance in various regions of the tubular digestive tract.

DIGESTIVE ENZYMES

Pancreatic enzyme supplements are reported in observational studies to provide valuable nutritional support in a variety of diseases (e.g. cancer, diabetes, "malnutrition"). However, these alleged benefits have not gained acceptance in conventional medicine. Lipase has been proposed as beneficial for cardiovascular health, but it should be taken in a continuous manner, in order to attempt to overcome its inactivation by acid in the upper gut. Lipase functions in the digestive tract to break down fat that is found mainly in dairy products and meat. Adding lipase to fish oil supplements is naïve and without any clear advantage.

The enzyme lactase breaks down lactose that is found in several milk products, such as ice cream and milk puddings. Amylase is found mainly in saliva and it breaks down carbohydrates and starches which are commonly found in fruits and vegetables. The enzyme cellulase assists in breaking down fiber in the diet; and it is a common ingredient in high quality digestive enzyme supplements. An array of enzymes is added to well formulated dietary supplements. Such supplements should have the added benefits of prebiotics, probiotics and the detoxifying herb, Milk Thistle (silymarin). Combining these natural substances that balance the gut or help restore "digestive harmony" is a highly cost effective approach to supplement formulation.

Table 17 gives a more complete list of enzymes that act on various foods.

FOOD	ENZYME ACTING ON SPECIFIC FOOD
Fruits and Vegetables	Glucoamylase, Cerealase, Alpha galactosidase, Amylase, Malto- diastase, Cellulase
Sweets	Invertase (or sucrase), disaccharidases
Butter, Oil and Other Fats	Lipase
Cereals, Breads and Other Foods	Malto- diastase, Amylase, Glucoamylase, Cellulase

| Dairy Products | Lipase, Lactase, Protease |
| Chicken, Fish and Meat | Lipase, Protease |

Table 16: Foods and examples of the endogenous (inside the body), or supplemental enzymes that digest them. These are examples of "digestive enzymes."

DIGESTIVE HARMONY: COMBINING PROBIOSIS, PREBIOSIS, DETOX, AND ENZYMES

Many people have used probiotics (healthy bacteria), prebiotics (food for healthy bacteria), detoxifying herbs and enzymes in separate supplements. Taking these supplements individually is inconvenient and expensive, with poor compliance. Compliance with dietary supplements or medications is a huge issue in the effective use of health giving substances. To promote digestive balance, the repeated use of natural substances is important for the achievement of any benefit. In other words, probiotics, enzymes, and detox substances must be taken with regularity. In fact, the regularity of their use may be more important than the amount delivered in daily or single dosages. The "strength" of probiotics measured in counts of organisms may be a marketing "ploy" in some supplements.

Poor compliance with dietary supplements is likely to occur if many capsules have to be taken in complicated daily routines, or if the presentation of the supplement is not readily acceptable to the user. Other factors operate to prevent people from "sticking with" the regular use of supplements. These factors include excessive cost, unpleasant taste or sensations that may occur with some supplements, e.g. bad breath with liquid fish oil.

Dietary supplements should be formulated with a view toward improving compliance in taking supplements for specific health benefits. It is advantageous to provide a cost effective alternative to the use of many different digestive supplements at the same time. If one were to attempt to purchase every ingredient present in the synergistic formulae that I propose on an individual basis, the cost would exceed U.S. 100 dollars or more.

I have proposed a dietary supplement formula that combines the four mainstays of balancing digestive function by providing probiosis, prebiosis, detoxification and enzymes, together. This "one-stop digestive shop" is a cost-effective way of helping to provide natural balance for digestion (Table 18). Again, the value of synergy in supplement formulations becomes apparent. This approach is the future of dietary supplement technology and specific product examples of complex formulae is the key to the teaching experiences in this book.

- Milk Thistle extract (80%) (detoxifier)
- L-Glutamine (heals the lining of the gut)
- Omega 3 Fatty Acids (stabilized, high quality, pure fish oil)
- Turmeric root (lipophilic antioxidant)
- Fructoligosaccharides (prebiotic)
- Proprietary Enzyme and Probiotic Blend: Protease, Amylase, Lipase, Cellulase, Lactase, Bromelain, Papain, Pepsin and Lactobacillus Acidophilus (4billion/g) (digestive enzymes plus probiotics)
- Quercetin (key antioxidant)
- In a proprietary base containing: Mastic Gum (gum mastica), Green Tea extract (50% polyphenols), Oregano leaves, Oregon grape root, Barberry bark, Cloves, Slippery Elm bark, Fava bean powder, Garlic, Grape seed extract, (95% oligo-proanthocyanidins), Licorice root, Thyme (leaf), Tansy (bark), Rhubarb (root), Jalapeno(fruit), Terminala spinosa (fruit), Cinnamon(bark), and Peppermint leaves (multi-functional blend).

Table 17: Ingredients in a synergistic, digestive supplement formulation that provides nutritional support for digestive functions. Please note the extensive inclusion of different ingredients that are used to support the harmony of digestive function. This combination is unique (Holt MD Technologies Inc).

HELICOBACTER PYLORI CAUSES DYSPEPSIA, PEPTIC ULCER AND STOMACH CANCER

Peptic ulcer is often caused by an infection with a bacterium (bug) called *Helicobacter pylori*. Several herbal and botanical agents or extracts have shown promise in fighting *H. pylori*, e.g. gum mastica (mastic gum, an ancient Greek remedy), peppermint and oregano oils. However, the effective eradication of *H. pylori* can only be considered to occur with drugs, including those that reduce acid secretion (proton pump inhibitor drugs) and antibiotics. Unfortunately, *H. pylori* has shown resistance to several antibiotics and the drugs used in conventional treatments for the eradication of this infection cause common, unpleasant side effects.

Modern nutraceutical approaches to *H. pylori* infection, proposed by my research group, stress the role of antioxidants in reversing the oxidative damage caused to the lining of the digestive tract by H. pylori infection. I believe that specific combinations of antioxidants can alter the clinical course of functional dyspepsia and acid-related disease of the upper digestive tract in a beneficial manner, but conventional medicine may not agree. Again, one must avoid treatment claims with dietary supplements. These disclaimer statements are important for compliance with all laws, rules, regulations and ethical guidelines that govern the use of dietary supplements. People taking acid lowering medications may benefit from the addition of ingredients found in complex natural formulae (Table 17).

ANTIBIOTIC USE AND DIGESTIVE BALANCE

The frequent use of antibiotics results in significant changes in the bacterial populations of various regions of the gastrointestinal tract. Antibiotics can kill or inhibit the growth of many different bacterial species; and they may kill both friendly and unfriendly bacteria. The elimination of friendly bacteria from the intestines, including the colon, leads to disruption of the ecology of the gut and gives damaging bacteria an opportunity to grow and cause problems. Friendly bacteria elaborate a number of chemicals that can actually kill or interfere with the growth of damaging microorganisms, including yeast (Candida albicans) and bacteria that cause disease or are "unhealthy."

The overuse of antibiotics can result in the overgrowth of yeast, which can be very difficult to eradicate. There is a serious disorder of the bowel that can result from antibiotic administration and this disorder is called antibiotic colitis or pseudomembranous colitis. This disorder can cause severe inflammation of the bowel with bleeding and diarrhea that can even be life-threatening. It is caused by a "nasty" bug called Clostridium difficile. Of course, simple diarrhea is probably the most common side effect of general use of antibiotics and it responds favorably to restoring digestive harmony, especially with probiotics.

One can now understand just how important the friendly bacterial populations of the bowel are in health maintenance. A strong recommendation exists among many medical practitioners that a course of antibiotic treatment should be followed or perhaps accompanied by the administration of friendly bacteria as probiotics. The formula shown in Table 17 is a more complete approach in these circumstances. Anyone who has developed bowel upset following the use of antibiotics must consider natural ways of restoring harmony to the function of the gut, especially the colon.

KEYNOTE SUMMARY: DIGESTIVE HARMONY

While everyone must be concerned about cancer or inflammation of the digestive tract, the commonest causes of upper or lower digestive problems involve alterations in the functions of the digestive tract. Upper abdominal pain and sour stomach is most often called "dyspepsia." There are about 25 million people with "functional dyspepsia" where upper abdominal pain and digestive upset occurs in the absence of peptic ulceration or other serious tissue disease.

The most common disorder of the gastrointestinal tract is the irritable bowel syndrome (IBS). The IBS is another example of a functional disorder of the gut which affects the lower gastrointestinal tract. Scientific studies show that irritability or disordered function of the upper and lower digestive tract may occur together. In simple terms, disorders of function of the bowel represent a lack of harmony of the complex functions of the digestive tract and they often affect the entire tubular digestive system, to a variable degree. Restoring digestive balance in IBS is important, but fiber, probiotics and peppermint oil (enteric-coated) seem to have special roles in the management of IBS.

Every bathroom cupboard in the nation contains one or more digestive aids, including anti-acids and over-the-counter (OTC) pills that reduce the secretion of acid by the stomach. These popular digestive medications are used often in a premature or inappropriate manner without attention to positive changes in lifestyle and nutritional support with dietary supplements. Many supplements can help to restore balance to gastrointestinal function (Table 17).

Symptoms such as difficulty in swallowing, significant change in bowel habit or bleeding from the gastrointestinal tract should cause an individual to seek medical advice and avoid self-medication. That said, a number of dietary supplements can be combined together to support many different functions of digestion and to support the structures of the gut (see Chapters 10, 11 and 12). Formulations are mentioned to provide a teaching experience about many excellent supplement ingredients that are ignored, despite evidence of their benefit.

There are six major ways of supporting digestive function and if anyone were to seek separate supplements for the support of each function, then individuals may be taking at least six different dietary supplements. Natural ways to digestive health with supplements include:

- **PROBIOTICS**: Taking healthy bacteria that can grow in the lower bowels and produce a variety of the local and general health benefits.
- **DIGESTIVE ENZYMES**: Taking a variety of different enzymes that can help to digest food and help to improve general nutritional status. These enzymes can be combined with systemic enzymes which have several health benefits (see Chapter 13).
- **PREBIOSIS**: Feeding the healthy bacteria (probiotics) which cause a healthy environment in the colon.
- **DETOXIFICATION**: Taking herbs or botanicals that can support the

role of the digestive tract, especially the liver, in eliminating toxins from food and the body.

- **STRUCTURE SUPPORT**: A variety of natural substances can help support the lining of the digestive tract which is a very active interface of the body (e.g. glutamine).
- **OPTIMIZING THE DIGESTA:** Many clinicians have underestimated the value of antioxidants, contained within several botanicals, for the promotion of digestive and general body health.
- **MAINTAINING REGULARITY:** Assistance in evacuating the colon, a form of body cleansing, can be achieved with several herbs.

Revolutionary dietary supplements that provide holistic support for digestive function are available increasingly. Combinations of probiotics, prebiotics, enzymes, detoxifying substances and natural agents that support digestive function are to be preferred because of cost effectiveness and improved compliance.

CHAPTER 10

HEARTBURN

STOMACH ACID

WE are all aware that stomach acid can cause heartburn, upper abdominal pain or discomfort, and feelings of a sour stomach. Drugs used to control upper digestive complaints and hyperacidity are among the most commonly used of all medications (H2 receptor antagonists and proton pump inhibitors). The option of providing metal or mineral containing antacids that can immediately neutralize stomach acidity, together with a drug that can have a delayed and later effect on reducing acid secretion, has become quite popular (e.g. Pepcid Complete®). This approach has typically involved the combination of a mineral antacid with the acid suppressing ability of drugs, such as H2-receptor antagonists (e.g. Zantac®, Tagamet® or Pepcid® etc). This action is described as a "bimodal" effect on acid secretion.

I reiterate that an initial neutralization of stomach acid with a more prolonged delayed effect on acid secretion by the stomach has been referred to as a biphasic or two-phase mode (bimodal) of action of drug treatments for heartburn and symptoms of dyspepsia. This dual action may provide initial relief of upper digestive upset as a consequence of immediate acid neutralization, with more prolonged relief as a consequence of inhibiting acid secretion by the stomach. These drug effects are a novel approach to immediate and more prolonged control of upper digestive upset, but I have hypothesized that similar effects on stomach acid secretion may be achieved with natural substances.

I stress that natural substances have not been subject to the same degree of research that has been applied to verify the effectiveness of drugs. Again, it is important to note that I want to restrict my discussions to the approved use of dietary supplements. My discussion can only involve "solid comments" about changes in body structure and function, without any disease prevention or treatment claims. In the present circumstances, one must accept that the production of acid by the human stomach is a normal body function, involving stomach tissues that have a structure to elaborate and secrete acid (the stomach lining).

Modern dietary supplement technology has evolved to present natural substances that may both act like an antacid which immediately neutralizes stomach acidity and may also act to inhibit acid secretion with a more delayed and prolonged effect. I am purposely cautious how I present information on dietary supplement use, because I do not want to confuse supplements with drugs or make direct comparisons of supplements with drugs. Again, one must reflect that dietary supplements cannot be used to prevent, treat, diagnose or cure any disease – at law (a legacy of lawyers). My work is subject to patent applications.

ARE THERE ADVANTAGES IN THE NATURAL CONTROL OF STOMACH ACID?

There are disadvantages and limitations with the use of standard, mineral antacids that are presented in "chalky" tablets or liquids, containing calcium, magnesium or aluminum in oxide or hydroxide form (e.g. Tums®, Maalox®, Aludrox®, Mylanta®, etc) For example, calcium-containing antacids may cause constipation and magnesium may cause diarrhea. Several drugs that are used to block acid secretion are powerful in their effects. The complete abolition of stomach acid with powerful drugs (proton pump inhibitors) may not result in a healthy circumstance, especially over the long term. Abolition of stomach acid may "deplete" certain nutrients.

I have produced a natural dietary supplement which provides nutritional support to alter or change the normal body functions of acid secretion by the stomach. This supplement contains components with immediate acid neutralizing functions, including the completely natural component of Fava bean, with relatively small amounts of calcium, magnesium and sodium bicarbonate, to rapidly neutralize acid. Fava bean flour has been shown in the laboratory to neutralize stomach acidity, in a "similar" manner to standard antacids that are available for over-the-counter use. In fact, fava bean flour has USP standards for acid neutralization (Table 19).

ın Tea

neric

ıstic Gum

- Ellagic Acid (from raspberries and pomegranate)
- Apple Pectin
- Lecithin
- Gastric Mucin
- Fava Bean
- Vitamin E
- Beta Carotene
- Zinc
- Sodium Bicarbonate (2% RDI of Sodium)
- Vitamin C (100% RDI)
- Calcium (carbonate)
- Magnesium (chelate)

Table 19: Ingredients in a product formulation that is subject to a pending patent (Holt MD) for combinations of natural agents for the nutritional support of structures and functions of the upper digestive tract.

INHIBITING THE PUMPING OF ACID IN THE STOMACH

Certain antioxidants have been shown to alter acid secretion in the stomach of animals by blocking the proton pumps in stomach. It is these "pumps" (proton pumps) that are found in the lining cells of the stomach that push acid into the stomach. This acid-blocking effect is well described with the use of proton pump inhibitor drugs such as Prilosec®, Prevacid®, and Nexium®. Recently, these stomach-acid pump inhibitor effects have been associated with the use of natural substances (e.g. ellagic acid and other specific types of antioxidant containing botanicals) (see Table 5, Chapter 4).

I stress that the description of the inhibition of acid secretion, by certain antioxidants, may appear to be similar to the mechanism of actions of some drugs (e.g., Prilosec®), but readers must understand that dietary supplements are not to be used to prevent or treat disease. That said, third party literature has been published that does suggest that there are natural proton pump inhibitors, found in plants, that have a mechanism of action in the stomach that is similar to the actions of commonly used proton pump inhibitor drugs. Natural proton pump inhibitors appear to have a desirable, "weaker effect" on reducing stomach acid than proton pump inhibitor drugs that completely abolish stomach acid.

LIFESTYLE AND HEARTBURN RELIEF: THE HEARTBURN NATURALLY PLAN©

The readers of this book should appreciate that the author is not proposing dietary supplements as any form of "magic bullet" to deal with health problems. That is why this book raises the importance of positive lifestyle change as an absolute need for a dietary supplement to exert measurable health benefits. Likewise, it is wrong to promote the use of any dietary supplement or <u>any drug</u> for the complete treatment of heartburn or dyspepsia. All medications and dietary supplements possess variable degrees of disadvantages and limitations.

It is known that changes from negative to positive lifestyle, such as smoking cessation and correction of alcohol abuse, play a major role in managing heartburn and other upper digestive complaints. However, I believe that natural interventions are often the best first- line approaches to functional upper digestive problems and simple heartburn or dyspepsia. I state with confidence that positive lifestyle changes in disease prevention or management are much more valuable in many circumstances than any food, dietary supplement or drug.

HINTS FOR HEARTBURN AND DYSPEPSIA RELIEF

Heartburn can respond favorably to dietary changes. Orange or tomato juices, as well as some acidic foods, are direct irritants to the lower esophagus. Multiple small meals are advisable, with the avoidance of eating heavy meals late at night. Sleeping propped up and wearing loose fitting garments are valuable ways of avoiding heartburn. The use of acid-fighting substances or substances that provide nutritional support for digestive health may be beneficial. However, it must be noted that serious gastrointestinal disease can be present with very simple symptoms and individuals are not advised to self-medicate in cases of doubt. Checking with a health care practitioner is a must sometimes (especially in the elderly or if symptoms are prolonged or difficulty in swallowing is present).

I emphasize that my work on natural medicines has not received the same kind of controlled clinical scientific study as drug treatments for altering digestive function. However, good scientific agreement exists that natural substances may provide help in the nutritional support of upper digestive function.

KEYNOTE SUMMARY: HEARTBURN AND DYSPEPSIA

Many Millions of Americans are troubled by burning upper abdominal discomfort or a burning sensation behind the breast bone. This symptom is called heartburn. Heartburn is most often caused by the backwash of stomach acid into the lower gullet or esophagus (acid reflux). The underlying causes of heartburn and sour stomach or upper abdominal pain or discomfort remain poorly defined in many individuals; and they are due often to functional upsets or a lack of harmony in digestive functions. Individuals who deny the importance of excessive acid in upper digestive symptoms are misguided.

Complex scientific studies show that there is often abnormal function of the upper digestive tract in people with upper digestive complaints. In the case of heartburn, there is often a weakening of the small muscles that close the lower esophagus, at the entrance to the stomach (lower esophageal sphincter). This predisposes people to the backwash of acid from the stomach into the lower gullet (esophagus). This is what is commonly called "acid reflux", "GERD" or gastroesophageal reflux disease or disorder. This disorder can be associated with an internal hernia (hiatal hernia of the stomach through the diaphragm).

In simple terms, stomach acid is linked to heartburn, dyspepsia and functional disorders of the upper digestive tract. Some people with these symptoms have serious diseases in their upper digestive tract including peptic ulcer, inflammation of the lining of the esophagus or cancer. Therefore, any symptoms that are persistent should cause an individual to seek medical advice, especially if they are elderly.

The most common causes of upper digestive symptoms include poor dietary habits and poor lifestyle, both of which should be corrected. Millions of Americans take prescription or over-the-counter (OTC) drugs to treat upper digestive symptoms. Many of these drugs include H-2 receptor antagonists (e.g. Tagamet®, Pepcid®, Zantac®, Axid® and others) or proton pump inhibitor drugs (e.g. Prilosec®, Nexium® etc.) These drugs are available often without a prescription (OTC) and they all work by reducing the secretion of acid by the stomach, to a variable degree. These drugs carry some disadvantages.

Drugs like Prilosec® have become particularly popular because they reduce symptoms and work generally by completely abolishing stomach acid. Many scientists have expressed concern about the long term use of potent drugs that diminish the presence of acid in the stomach in a potent manner. These drugs that reduce acid secretion in a powerful manner are highly effective in reducing symptoms of heartburn, but they have not been shown to be consistently effective in managing "functional disorders" of the digestive tract. Functional types of digestive upset are by far the commonest types of simple digestive disorders and symptoms. While the drive to use acid-suppressing drugs is symptom relief, the relief of symptoms alone may permit the individual to engage in the adverse lifestyle that caused the functional digestive upset in the first place. People who "pop" acid suppressing drugs prior to alcohol drinking or dietary indiscretions, in order to avoid symptoms of dyspepsia, are hurting themselves. Furthermore, proton pump inhibitor drugs do not work immediately on initial dosing. Their effects may take several hours.

Recent research has shown that certain antioxidants can alter acid secretion by blocking stomach pumps (a proton pump inhibitor effect). In contrast to proton pump inhibitor drugs, such as Prilosec®, these antioxidants are likely to have a much milder effect on acid secretion and do not completely abolish stomach acid. These circumstances result in a potentially healthier circumstance, where gastric acid can continue periodically to exert its important functions in the digestive process.

Much inflammation in the linings of the upper digestive tract is caused by oxidative stress. Common infections with the bacterium Helicobacter pylori, cause free radical damage (oxidative damage or stress to tissue). This oxidative damage may result in inflammation of the lining of the digestive tract, peptic ulcer and precancerous changes in the lining of certain parts of the upper digestive tract. Useful digestive supplements contain powerful antioxidants including ellagic acid, green tea extract and turmeric. Ellagic acid has been shown in laboratory experiments to suppress acid secretion by the stomach, by a mechanism of action similar to that of proton pumping inhibitor drugs, but, to date, there have been no controlled human studies using ellagic acid for this purpose.

The problem with acid-suppressing drugs or supplements is their lack of immediate action in suppressing simple symptoms of simple heartburn or sour stomach. This is why many people favor mineral antacids (e.g. Rolaids® or Maalox® or Mylanta® etc) for rapid symptom relief. These mineral antacids can cause bowel upset in high dosage, but there are natural antacids that can immediately neutralize stomach acid. Novel supplements contain flour from fava beans which has USP standards described for acid neutralization, similar to those standards described for commercial mineral antacids. Supplements benefit from a content of calcium and magnesium in a 2:1 ratio which is not only a way of neutralizing acid, but also a way of partially supplementing two important minerals in the diet.

Complete digestive nutraceutical formulations offer ingredients that may soothe the lining of the upper digestive tract. These ingredients include lecithin, mastic gum, apple pectin and gastric mucin. These soothing agents help improve the barrier to the penetration of acid into the lining of the upper digestive tract. Mastic gum has been researched in Helicobacter pylori infection. Other ingredients provide the added benefit of classic antioxidant vitamins A, C and E, with the indirect healing and antioxidant potential of zinc or carnosine. Again, the importance of synergy is apparent by learning about product compositions.

The products that I propose are pleasant chewable tablets which can be taken as required, up to twice daily. The formulation of these supplements is designed to have natural effects on the normal body function of acid secretion by the stomach. This formulation may have an immediate effect on acid neutralization followed by a more delayed and gentle effect on the secretion of acid by the stomach, but further research in humans is desirable. A particular advantage of the proposed synergistic formulation is its antioxidant power as nutritional support for the structure and function of the lining of the upper digestive tract.

> **FOR MORE INFORMATION ON STOMACH UPSET AND HEARTBURN INDIVIDUALS CAN READ TWO OF DR. HOLT'S BOOKS ENTITLED "NATURAL WAYS TO DIGESTIVE HEALTH" AND "DIGESTION NATURALLY," AVAILABLE AT WWW. WELLNESSPUBLISHING.COM.**

CHAPTER 11

COLON CLEANSING

BACKGROUND

EVERY day of everyone's life, thoughts are triggered about bowel function or bowel activity. The colon is "hard wired to the brain" and there is a highly complex pathway of intercommunication between the bowel and the mind. This is part of the "**gutmind**" or "**mindgut**." When one thinks about the colon, one most often thinks about its contents. The contents of the colon are somewhat transient. These contents come and go, but the overall time (duration) that these contents reside in the colon may be an important factor in general health and wellbeing. "Friendly" bacterial inhabitants of the colon are responsible for general health and well-being. For many years, the colon and its contents were viewed as a source of potential toxins to which the body was exposed, especially in the presence of constipation. These days, conventional medicine often rejects these ideas.

There is no doubt that these thoughts of "colon toxins" led to the common belief that everyone should open their bowel, at least on a daily basis. However, it is recognized that a healthy bowel habit involves, generally, the opening of one's bowel less than three times daily, but more than once in three days. That said, many people suffer from uncomfortable changes in their bowel habit, most often in the form of temporary constipation due to lifestyle or environmental changes. Constipation makes many people feel lousy.

Conventional medicine has been rather unwilling to acknowledge any benefit of intermittent colon cleansing. While there is surprisingly little research on the benefits of colon cleansing, there are thousands of people who claim they derive an improved sense of well-being by restoring the regularity of their bowel habit. Achieving a regular bowel habit involves a healthy lifestyle, including: regular exercise, adequate fluid intake and good nutrition (especially adequate dietary fiber intake).

An important aspect of regular bowel habit depends on the amount of unabsorbed fiber that is taken in the diet. There have been many studies that show the benefits of insoluble types of dietary fiber (and combined soluble fiber intake) on the promotion of healthy bowel function. Examples of healthy dietary fibers include mixtures of fiber (see Chapter 12). Dieters should consider ways of supplementing fiber in their diet because fiber provides a great "feel-full weight-loss trick". Dietary fiber is not absorbed, but it is subject to fermentation by the healthy bacterial inhabitants of the colon (prebiotic effects). Furthermore, dietary fiber may provide added benefits, due to its ability to cleanse the colon and assist in detoxification of the body. Fiber can mop up "toxic forms" of bile acids and other toxicants that are present in colonic contents.

STOOL WEIGHT AND SIZE

Elegant studies of the weight of stools show that the size and weight of an individual's stool is most often related to the amount of fiber taken in the diet. There is a widespread deficiency of dietary fiber in Western diets and not only can fiber improve bowel function, it has other far-reaching benefits such as helping to control weight, lowering cholesterol and preventing certain types of cancer. Scientific literature confirms a strong basis to make health claims about the inclusion of extra fiber in the average diet.

One famous study compared the weight of stools in certain African natives with the weight of stools in elderly females in Great Britain. African natives have stool weights that may sometimes exceed 1 kilogram in a 24 hour period, whereas many elderly ladies in Western society may only average the production of a couple hundred grams of stool daily. This major difference in stool weight is readily explainable by differences in dietary fiber intake between these groups of individuals.

So powerful are the health benefits of dietary fiber that every person should consider meeting the recommended intake of dietary fiber for adults which is at least 25 grams of dietary fiber on a daily basis. Few people reach this expectation. Even fewer people understand that many of the health benefits of fiber involve the way that the bacterial contents of the colon interact with fiber during the "tail end" of the digestive process. This interaction of fiber in the colon with bacteria is why I recommend that fiber supplements be taken with probiotic supplements. This forms the basis of my recommendations for BioFiber® or Probiotics Plus Fiber™.

DANGERS OF STRONG LAXATIVES

While regularity of bowel habit must involve positive lifestyle principles, a large proportion of the population requires temporary help in overcoming constipation. There are many over-the-counter (OTC) laxatives available, but some laxatives can be quite dangerous in some people. Laxatives that cause excessive purgation can actually damage the function of the bowel. There is a disease entity that is well described among people who use powerful, stimulant laxatives on a regular basis. This is called "cathartic colon." The word "catharsis" means forced exit of stool from the bowel.

Strong laxatives are unpleasant to take because they can cause griping abdominal pain and they may stimulate imbalances of body fluids or chemistry and cause excessive discharge of sticky mucus in the colon. Continuing to "purge the bowel" causes a "lazy bowel" that will only respond to the continuing use of strong laxatives. Over a period of time, strong laxatives can damage the nerve supply to the colon and the bowel cannot engage in normal movements that cause easy evacuation of stool. There is a common type of constipation that seems to be related to lack of coordination of muscles around the back passage (anus and rectum). This lack of coordination can be overcome to some degree by increasing insoluble dietary fiber intake. Fiber helps to treat hemorrhoids and it lowers "pressure" inside the colon.

Many people have experienced an unpleasant initial reaction to increasing fiber in their diet. Delivering large amounts of fiber to the "untrained" colon often results in increased frequency of bowel habit and gas. This situation is fortunately short-lived. The biggest problem encountered in the healthy recommendations for increasing fiber intake is lack of compliance, because of these early adjustments that are made by the colon and digestive tract to the presentation of a "fiber load." Some experimentation is always required when extra fiber is consumed in the diet; and I advise people not to "give up" prematurely on fiber supplements. I advise individuals to keep adjusting the amount of fiber that they take in supplement form until their colon becomes agreeable and accepting of its new healthy contents.

COLON CLEANSING

As a gastroenterologist with a major interest in alternative medicine, I believe in the need for simple, natural and gentle ways to engage in the healthy habit of colon cleansing. There are complicated but effective ways of intermittent colon cleansing with colon hydrotherapy. Colon hydrotherapists can improve the outcome of their treatments by the correct use of well formulated dietary supplements for digestive health. However, I stress that the supplements that they use should have a clear evidence-base for an effect on digestive functions. Again, this raises the important question "Who formulated the supplements that you may wish to use?"

The products that I propose have an effective formula for supporting regular bowel function, in a simple, gentle and natural way. The complex nutrient and botanical formula in Table 20 is more versatile than many other colon cleansing formulas.

Artichoke Leaf	Ashwagandha Root
Beet Leaf	Burdock Root
Chlorella	Corn Silk
Dandelion Root	Arabinogalactans
Milk Thistle 80%	Mullein Leaf
Red Clover Flowers	Turmeric Root
Aloe Vera 200: 1 Concentrate	Rhubarb Root
Slippery Elm Bark	Marshmallow Root
Fennel Seed	Ginger Root
Triphala	Magnesium (Hydroxide)
L-Glutamine	Fish Oil 50% Powder

Table 20: Ingredients of an effective colon cleansing formula. This complex formulation is designed to support the principle function of the colon in the act of evacuation of stool. The formula draws upon several traditional medical systems that have focused their attention on the colon as a source of health and wellbeing. The formula uses an Ayurvedic herbal system for body cleansing (Triphala) and it utilizes recommendations from master herbalists on a variety of different botanicals that can support or modify colon structure and function. Some ingredients do provide gentle purgative actions (Fennel Seed, Rhubarb Root), but some ingredients are designed to support the lining of the colon or work by mild astringent properties (Aloe Vera,

Slippery Elm Bark). Supporting nutrients for the colon lining include Fish Oil and L-Glutamine. In simple terms, soothing agents for the lining of the colon include Mullein leaf and Ginger root. One principle mechanism of action of this formula is to hold water in the bowel to make the stool softer and easier to pass (courtesy of Holt MD Technologies). Medical practitioners continue to argue about the benefits of colon cleansing. Once relegated to the world of quackery, the act of colon cleansing as a part of detoxification of the body is emerging as increasingly valuable in the promotion of well-being. Simple, gentle ways of colon cleansing are preferred and this is the basis of the concepts of colon cleansing that I support.

KEYNOTE SUMMARY: COLON CLEANSING

Conventional medical practitioners cling to concepts that were proposed in the early part of the 20th century, where the colon was characterized as a mere receptacle for undigested food. In some respects, this made the colon appear to be a "dumping ground." Researchers in the 1920's made a living by trying to show how boring and unimportant colon contents were in general health. Opinions have changed. Over the past 50 years, the ecology and structure of the colon have been redefined and "the medical wheel has turned." Colon cleansing may be a much more important health initiative than hitherto supposed.

Colon cleansing was once called "the royal pathway to health" because of its popularity among kings, queens and the aristocracy of the Victorian era. Members of the French aristocracy were the strongest proponents of stool evacuation for health. For a while, this activity was considered to be an "embarrassing joke." These days individuals are more willing to talk about normal body functions in an open and constructive manner.

It is interesting to note that the optimal way to keeping the colon healthy may be to use the simple, gentle and natural options that have been used in ancient medical practices, such as traditional herbalism and Ayurveda. Certainly, opening the bowel in a regular way is a great pleasure of life and it forms the basis of constructive conversation, in the correct context.

CHAPTER 12

FIBER

BACKGROUND

MEDICAL science continues to unravel the versatile health benefits of dietary fiber. Many supplement users have been confused by the different types of dietary fiber that occur in foods and dietary supplements. It is puzzling to many people why something as apparently simple and inert as dietary fiber, can exert so many different health benefits. In my books entitled "The Natural Way to a Healthy Heart" and "Natural Ways to Digestive Health" (M. Evans Publishers Inc., N.Y., 1999 and 2000, respectively), I review many health benefits of soluble and insoluble fiber and explain their mechanisms of action. Fiber promotes both gastrointestinal and general health. The importance of dietary fiber for health has been grossly underestimated by all disciplines of medicine; and even by the dietary supplement and food industries (see the book, "Combat Syndrome X, Y and Z…," www.wellnesspublishing. com).

CHARACTERISTICS OF DIETARY FIBER

What is dietary fiber? Dietary fiber is best understood as material that is responsible for the structural integrity of most plants and their constituent parts. In essence, dietary fiber is made from many different carbohydrate units, but fiber resists digestion by the human gastrointestinal tract. In other words, fiber in the diet is not digested, even though it has carbohydrate content. Insoluble forms of dietary fiber pass into the lower bowel where they exert many different beneficial actions in the colon. Dietary fiber acts as a prebiotic, by promoting the growth of healthy bacteria (probiotics). Fiber is fermented in the colon.

I see very little point in taking dietary fiber without a good source of healthy bacteria that can implant themselves in the colon (probiotics). It is the interaction between the friendly bacteria of the colon and the dietary fiber that accounts for the health benefits of probiosis and fiber supplementation (prebiosis). Again, this is important synergy for the harmony of life. Healthy bacteria can be found in certain foods such as "raw yoghurt." This is not the kind of sugar-loaded, fruit flavored yoghurt that fills the shelves of supermarkets. Probiotic dietary supplements are the best way of ensuring a supply of healthy bacteria for growth in the colon. A poor supply of healthy bacteria in the diet is one of the major inadequacies of the Standard American Diet (SAD).

SOLUBLE AND INSOLUBLE DIETARY FIBERS

There are two principal types of dietary fiber, namely "soluble" and "insoluble" fiber. Fiber has a number of complex effects on body metabolism. Soluble types of dietary fiber exert beneficial effects in altering body metabolism. Soluble fiber can often lower bad types of blood cholesterol and smooth out blood sugar responses, after a meal. In fact, soluble fiber lowers the glycemic index of other foods, when they are taken at the same time. On the other hand, insoluble fiber is often regarded as a stool-bulking agent; and it can exert a laxative effect by holding water in the lower bowel. Retaining water in stool contents makes stools bigger, softer and easier to pass. In contrast, soluble fiber plays more of a "balancing act" in the digestive tract and certain types of soluble fiber, such as pectin, may actually help regulate loose bowel actions, in some circumstances.

The chemistry of dietary fibers is extremely complex and not always apparently relevant to an understanding of how to apply different types of fiber for general health and wellbeing. Several of the actions of different types of fiber are related to their physical characteristics and the end products of fiber breakdown in the colon.

"SMOOTHING-OUT" GUT FUNCTION WITH FIBER

There are obvious advantages of dietary fiber intake in terms of smoothing out gastrointestinal function. Insoluble fiber holds water and results in the bulking of stools or relaxation of the bowel. These effects can counter bowel spasms that occur in the irritable bowel syndrome (IBS) or in individuals with diverticular disease (pockets in their bowel). There are more than 20 million people with

IBS and even more people with diverticular disease. Diverticular disease is often present, but asymptomatic, in older people.

All types of fiber can reside in the colon and promote the growth of healthy bacteria. Bacteria in the colon use dietary fiber as a source of food and energy which permits them to grow and multiply. Healthy bacteria have been termed probiotics and dietary fiber is one of several examples of food for probiotic organisms. This is why fiber is called prebiotic material.

The consequences of the promotion of the growth of healthy bacteria in the colon are many, and healthy bacteria can have far-reaching health benefits such as the manufacture of vitamins for use by the body and the dilution of toxins taken in the diet. Many toxins "end up" in the colon (Tables 21 A and B).

A. REASONS WHY CONSUMERS USE PROBIOTICS.

CONDITION	COMMENT
Yeast infection	Assists in reduction of Candida overgrowth, but action not immediate and recurrence common with cessation of probiotics.
Antibiotic therapy	Broad spectrum antibiotics "knock out" friendly and unfriendly bacteria. An advantage from reseeding the guts with probiotics.
Digestive disease	Uncertain benefits in some disorders, e.g., Helicobacter pylori infection, but a real advantage in Clostridium overgrowth is documented.
Acne	Possible benefit.
Hypercholestrolemia	Unpredictable effect.
Colon cleansing	The idea of cleansing and reseeding is interesting, but its attributed health benefits require research.
Immune dysfunction	An underestimated potential for probiotics. Promising research data.

B. PROPOSED BENEFITS OF PROBIOTIC THERAPY

- Assistance with digestion.
- Alleviation of digestive disorders, e.g., colitis, IBS, peptic ulcer, HIV.
- Enhanced mineral absorption, especially calcium.

- Enhancement of the synthesis of several vitamins (especially B complex).

- Protection against pathogenic bacterial infections, e.g., E. coli infection.

- Reduction of symptoms of lactose intolerance; permits limited reintroduction of dairy products.

- Reduction of yeast overgrowth (Candidiasis); notable reduction in vaginal thrush.

- Improvement in immune function; "primes" the gut immune system.

- Anticancer effects, some good evidence.

- Prevention of *Helicobacter pylori* infection and its association with peptic ulcer, dyspepsia and gastric cancer.

- Acne prevention (?)

- Cholesterol reduction, modest and unpredictable.

Table 21A and B: Table 21A lists reasons why people have used probiotic supplements. The author is not attempting to make treatment claims, but many of the reasons listed in 21A are applications of natural probiotics used by healthcare givers who practice natural medicine. Table 21B includes a list of proposed benefits of probiotic therapy. Some of these benefits have been reported in peer-review scientific literature. Probiotics have entered mainstream medicine.

SPECIFIC FORMS OF PROCESSED OAT BRAN: SUPERIOR, COMPLEX FIBER SOURCES

Oat bran is a superior type of dietary fiber with several active components. One special constituent is a fraction called a beta-glucan or oat bran hydrocolloid. Not only can this fraction of oat bran fiber promote a healthy blood glucose level, it can lower blood cholesterol by a factor of up to 20%. In addition, this form of dietary fiber has been reported to cause weight loss and modest reductions in blood pressure, by unknown mechanisms. Oat beta-glucans found in special forms of processed oat bran fiber are produced by a patented process that was developed by the United States Department of Agriculture. These superior types of dietary fiber are often not present in many fiber products, but they are used as an ingredient in Syndrome X Nutritional Factors®.

Dietary fiber, in general, has found a special adjunctive role in the management of weight control and it is particularly valuable in the nutritional management of the metabolic Syndrome X. There is no doubt that soluble fiber has a special role in management of diabetes mellitus, of both the type I and type II varieties; but soluble fiber, in the form of oat bran hydrocolloids (beta-glucans), can make real differences to levels of blood sugar that occur after meals.

Therefore, I caution that these dietary supplements can reduce medication needs in some diabetics. These effects may precipitate requirements for adjustments of insulin dosage and adjustments of oral hypoglycemic drugs (blood sugar lowering medications). Individuals with diabetes mellitus are strongly advised to have their blood sugar monitored to avoid episodes of low blood sugar and they should talk to their healthcare-giver about any need for the adjustment of diabetic medications. The self-management of diabetes should always be disclosed and supervised by a medical practitioner.

FIBER AND PROBIOTICS PROVIDE HEALTH SYNERGY

There are special types of oat bran fiber that are not only rich in the health giving soluble fiber (beta-glucan component), but they also contain the added benefit of insoluble oat fiber. This type of fiber is found in superior fiber supplements. Probiotics Plus Fiber™ can provide nutritional support to help promote a healthy blood glucose level, a healthy blood cholesterol level, healthy digestive function and healthy immune function. It is not commonly recognized that glucans are among the most common natural promoters of healthy immune function that are found in nature (present also in mushrooms and yeast).

Probiotics Plus Fiber™ can be used as a dietary adjunct for calorie control diet by virtue of its ability to produce the sensation of fullness in the stomach, when taken prior to meals. This is a "feel-full," weight-control trick. Probiotics have emerged as important in weight control tactics.

KEYNOTE SUMMARY: FIBER

There are thousands of scientific studies that show the general health benefits of dietary fiber and healthy bacteria in the colon. However, there have been few attempts to leverage the power of fiber and probiotics together (an important synergy). Combining probiotics with fibers produces a quintessential fiber supplement, presented in a convenient format, to be taken with at least 8 oz of pure water or a healthy beverage. I caution individuals that fiber swells in the digestive tract and people with swallowing disorders must check with their physicians. There have been rare cases where fiber may block the upper portions of the tubular digestive tract. Furthermore, fiber cannot exert its physical benefits in the digestive process without holding water and a daily intake of eight, 8oz. glasses of pure water per day is a healthy recommendation for many people.

CONCLUSION

In summary, the mixed fiber components of probiotics plus fiber provide food for the growth of healthy bacteria, as well as providing the major versatile and potent health benefits of soluble and insoluble fiber components. Probiotics plus the best types of fiber form a unique, new generation of dietary fiber supplements that has great potential in the promotion of health and well-being of many different body functions. There is little reason to take fiber or probiotics alone, they are synergistic in dietary supplement formulations.

CHAPTER 13

ENZYMES

WHAT ARE ENZYMES?: A REVIEW

ENZYMES are naturally occurring chemicals that accelerate or facilitate chemical reactions in the body. Enzymes are sometimes called catalysts, and they are a fundamental component of the chemistry of life. Readers have learned that there are two broad types of enzymes that need to be defined. The first types are termed "digestive" enzymes which are secreted by the gastro-intestinal tract and are responsible for the digestion of food. These types of enzymes are discussed in Chapter 9. The second types of enzymes are referred to as systemic or "metabolic enzymes" and they are the focus of the present discussion. The words metabolic or systemic enzymes imply that these enzymes support body chemistry and these enzymes are the most common types of enzymes that drive body functions and support body structures.

FUNCTIONS OF ENZYMES

Enzymes act in a manner that causes many different changes in body structures and functions. Examples of the vital role of enzymes include growth of tissues, repair of tissues, chemical alteration of drugs or chemicals in the body, regulation of hormone secretion and even the balanced transmission of nervous impulses in the brain. When cancer or inflammation occurs in the body, different types of enzymes exert many different effects on body tissues. Enzymes must be present for breaking nutrients down into forms of building blocks that support the structure of the body. The function of enzymes themselves is often dependent upon the presence of vitamins and minerals, or other nutritional co-factors.

ENZYME HARMONY

There are several thousand metabolic enzymes that work in harmony to run chemical reactions in all body tissues. A very important group of metabolic enzymes are antioxidant types of enzymes that remove free radicals or potentially damaging substances such as hydrogen peroxide. These free radicals are a common by-product of oxidative reactions, which damage tissues in many ways (see Antioxidants, Chapter 4). These enzyme antioxidants are manufactured by the human body and examples include superoxide dismutase (SOD), catalase and peroxidase. These three enzymes are very important in the body's ability to detoxify itself and defend itself against oxidative damage. Such damage causes much disease and disability.

A simple example of oxidative damage to the body is muscle pain that occurs after heavy exercise. Muscular activity generates free radicals and that is why antioxidants are used increasingly by aerobic fitness enthusiasts and "weekend warriors" in the gym. These circumstances has lead great popularity of using green tea liquid concentrates in water bottles that accompany anyone involved in fitness pursuits (Green Tea Max®). The use of balanced antioxidants is a favorite selection among professional trainers in the gym and their clients. Running to the gym is fun, but "hobbling home" is not!

METABOLIC ENZYMES

One concept of nutritional support with enzymes involves how enzymes may actually go into the body and perform important functions in the nutritional support of a variety of body structures and functions. Again, disease treatment claims have to be avoided, but there is no doubt that metabolic enzyme support is used increasingly by practitioners of Integrative Medicine to alter body structures and functions in disease states. This kind of "metabolic enzyme" support remains in its infancy in terms of conclusive research. Metabolic or systemic enzyme support has been reported in medical literature as useful in many diseases such as, inflammatory disease, autoimmune disorders, cardiovascular disease, infectious disease and even cancer management. (Again, disease treatment claims must be avoided for dietary supplements.)

Conventional medicine has tended to reject the value of metabolic enzyme supplementation, otherwise called "systemic enzyme" support. Again, the idea is to give enzymes in supplements that go into the body (systemic) and cause beneficial effects on certain tissue functions, but this concept is close to a treatment concept. These circumstances make "in-detail" discussions of metabolic enzymes somewhat problematic, in any commercial or conventional medical context.

A major problem in acceptance of metabolic enzymes by modern science is the question: Whether or not "metabolic" enzymes are adequately absorbed by the human gastrointestinal tract? Some, but not all, well-conducted studies show that many types of enzymes are absorbed, including: combination enzyme preparations containing bromelain, chymotrypsin, pancreatin, papain and trypsin, even though their absorption is incomplete. Dietary supplements have been produced containing very important enzymes that are found in the human body, such as SOD, catalase and peroxidase, but these enzymes may not be efficiently absorbed, or they are unstable in their regular chemical forms.

The story of systemic enzyme support is not so simple because many factors alter the activity of enzymes, especially when such enzymes are used in dietary supplements. Several important factors affect enzyme activity in supplements or enzyme activity in the body. These factors include: the amount of material present that an enzyme can act on (substrate), acidity or alkalinity of the body, body temperature and the presence of other nutritional factors that are required to make enzymes function effectively, such as essential vitamins and minerals (co-factors).

It seems quite obvious that many enzymes are destroyed by stomach acid when they are taken as dietary supplements (e.g. lipase). This circumstance can be overcome to some extent by increasing the amount of enzymes that are administered in oral supplements; and in some cases by applying special coatings to the capsules that contain enzymes in dietary supplements (enteric-coating). These types of supplement formulations can be used to improve the tolerability of enzyme supplements and their absorption. I have taken this approach to formulate enzyme supplements this approach may be superior in several ways to existing enzyme products.

ENZYMES DIFFER IN ACTIVITY AND EFFECTS

There is a wealth of literature on the use of metabolic enzymes, but enzymes from different sources that are manufactured by different methods have variable biological activity. Therefore, quality enzyme supplements are made with checks on the activity levels of the enzymes that are used in the supplements. Enzyme supplements should be tested for the activity of their enzyme content.

POTENTIAL USE OF NUTRITIONAL SUPPORT
WITH METABOLIC ENZYMES

The most common and effective use of several metabolic enzymes is in the management of inflammatory disease. It is believed that in these circumstances enzymes can trigger repair mechanisms and alter blood circulation to inflamed tissues. These effects can be considered to be alterations of normal body functions or structures. This mechanism of action has led to favorable reports of systemic enzyme supplements in conditions such as arthritis, viral infections, sports injuries and sinusitis … to name a few conditions. However, the science that supports these reports of beneficial activity has been questioned by some physicians.

Reports of the successful use of metabolic enzymes in the nutritional support of cardiovascular health are of major interest because heart disease remains the number one killer in America. It has been suggested that several metabolic enzymes can balance body functions such as blood clotting or exert effects such as natural blood thinning (nattokinase). However, any attempts to self-medicate to alter blood clotting must be performed with much informed judgment and the supervision of a medical practitioner. Readers must understand that the maintenance of the balance between blood clotting and blood thinning in the body is critical for the prevention of clogging of blood vessels, both veins and arteries. Significant attempts to self-manage cardiovascular function may be associated with hazards, in some people.

ENZYMES AND IMMUNITY

There are a host of immune disturbances where the body's own defense mechanisms may attack body tissues (autoimmunity). This type of self-attack by the body's own immune system is called autoimmune disease. In this circumstance, immune reactions occur in an uncontrolled manner that cause a variety of types of inflammation and damage to body tissues. It is believed that some enzymes can inhibit the complexes or chemical consequences of immune reactions, but this is not an easy area of nutritional, self-management. In these circumstances, one may appreciate the real concept of food or nutrients as "medicine," a dictum of Hippocrates, the father of modern medicine. In other words, some metabolic enzymes may inhibit several complicated cascades of immune events, especially when antibodies are deposited in tissues as immune complexes. These are complicated issues that are best discussed with knowledgeable healthcare givers.

There is a growing body of scientific evidence that provides good scientific agreement that enzymes can provide nutritional support for tissue and cellular health, in a variety of circumstances. It would be illegal to state that enzymes can prevent or cure any diseases, but metabolic enzymes are increasingly used in the nutritional support of many disorders. These disorders include those that are encountered with alterations in body structures and functions, e.g. in circumstances such as tissue repair, inflammation and cancer. Throughout this book, I am very conscious of complying with regulations and laws. Readers must understand that limitations exist on the information that can be discussed – at law. I reiterate that dietary supplements cannot be used to prevent or treat any disease, even though some medical practitioners may justifiably use supplements in this manner. The problem is that using supplements in this manner is not considered by some people to conform to usual and customary standards of medical practice.

ENZYMES COMBINATIONS

A review of literature on the health benefits of enzymes has led me to develop combination enzyme supplements. These dietary supplements contain a combination of enzyme preparations including bromelain, chymotrypsin, pancreatin, papain, trypsin, amylase, lipase and elastase, together with bioflavanoids, including rutin from biologically active sources. In comparison with other enzyme supplements that are quite popular (e.g. Wobenzym®) the formulae that I propose are more complete with added contents of small and safe dosages of nattokinase and serratiopeptidase. Wobenzym® is a registered trademark of Mucos Emulsions GmbH, Germany and it has been licensed to Marlyn Nutraceuticals Inc., Scottsdale, AZ, US.

I believe that enzyme combinations have many advantages over single enzymes because of a broader range of action, under different conditions, on many different tissues. This is the concept of synergy when applied to combined digestive and metabolic enzyme supplements. In brief, this approach may make systemic or metabolic enzymes more effective in their ability to alter body structures and functions in a favorable manner.

Systemic enzyme supplements have been used with apparent safety for many years, both in the practice of medicine and in freely available dietary supplements.

SAFETY ISSUES WITH METABOLIC ENZYMES

There are no significant side effects to be expected with oral enzyme supplements, used at recommended dosages, in individuals who are not known to be allergic to the components of the enzyme supplements. There is good scientific agreement that enzyme preparations obtained from suitable sources are quite safe when used in supplements.

Enzyme supplements are not to be used in pregnancy and their use in children must be supervised by a knowledgeable medical practitioner. Any signs of allergic reaction should result in immediate discontinuation of enzyme supplements and any individual with a bleeding tendency from any cause, including drugs or diseases, should avoid metabolic enzyme supplements, unless prescribed by a physician for a specific, valid reason. Enzymes should not be administered by enema, in topical applications or by injection without prescription and supervision by a medical practitioner.

KEYNOTE SUMMARY: ENZYMES

There are several combination enzyme products that claim health benefits and some of these products are accompanied by illegal treatment claims. Enzyme deficiencies have been variably associated with many disorders including: hardening of the arteries, increased blood clotting tendencies, high blood pressure, low blood sugar, obesity, fatigue, leaky guts, constipation, bad breath, allergies and skin problems… to name a few. Of course, this does not necessarily mean that enzyme supplementations can prevent or treat any of these diseases, in any consistent manner.

Manufacturers of bulk enzymes from various natural sources recommend enzymes as nutritional support for many conditions including indigestion, sugar intolerance in the diet, fatigue and general nutritional disorders, but evidence of the benefit of enzymes in several of these conditions may not be complete in scientific literature.

The most popular combination enzyme containing dietary supplement is Wobenzym® which may not be as complete in its composition, compared with my recommendations. Table 22 compares the components of my formula with Wobenzym® N. Cost advantages are present with my proposed formula and the biological range of activity of the enzyme contents of my formula is superior to Wobenzym®.

AMOUNT PER SERVING AMOUNT PER SERVING

WOBENZYM® N		HOLT MD TECHNOLOGIES	
Pancreatin	300mg	Pancreatin	330mg*
Papain	180mg	Papain	200mg*
Bromelain	135mg	Bromelain	150mg*
Trypsin	72mg	Trypsin	100mg*
Chymotrypsin	3mg	Chymotrypsin	3.5mg*
Rutosid	150mg	Rutin	160mg*
		Nattokinase	30mg
		Serratiopeptidase	9mg
		Amylase	
		Lipase	
		Lactose	
		Cellulose	
		Protease	
		Mixed Bioflavanoids	
		Plus a proprietary blend of 150mg	

Table 21: A comparison of the contents of the dietary supplements Wobenzym® N and the author's proposed formula. The content of the Holt formula is much more complete than the enzyme profile of Wobenzym® N. The new formula has selected extra digestive enzymes and metabolic enzymes. There are more enzymes in the Holt formulation compared with Wobenzym® N. *All ingredients in the author's proposals are at high concentrations. Some value added ingredients in the proposed formula are not present in Wobenzym®. The Holt formula is enteric coated to protect the enzymes from degradation by gastric acid.

CONCLUSION

The science of metabolic enzyme supplementation is emerging and one cannot divorce the effects of digestive enzymes entirely from metabolic or systemic enzymes. These concepts are used in revolutionary, combination, enzyme, dietary supplements.

CHAPTER 14

CORAL CALCIUM

CORAL CALCIUM PRODUCTS

CORAL calcium from Okinawa, Japan, is one of the best selling dietary supplements in the history of natural approaches to wellness. Confusion has prevailed on the subject of coral calcium and the reputation of this valuable dietary supplement has been tainted by exaggerated claims of health benefits. However, many thousands of people have experienced the health benefits of this supplement and continue to use it with confidence and satisfaction.

Coral calcium is much more than just a source of calcium. It is a holistic mineral supplement that is rich in calcium and magnesium, but it also contains more than 70 trace minerals that may be of value for general health. There are many different types of coral calcium products in the market that are promoted in both honest and misleading ways. The tried and trusted, best-selling brands are Natures Benefit Coral Calcium and some private label brands. There have been hundreds of millions of unit dosages of Natures Benefit Coral Calcium used, with much consumer satisfaction.

The only documented benefits of coral calcium supplements relate to coral sand that is derived from the pristine waters or land masses of Okinawa in the South of Japan. If a coral calcium product does not certify its place of origin in Okinawa, Japan, it does not carry any precedent for a health benefit. Much material sold as coral calcium in the US did not come from Okinawa, Japan.

Consumers must also be aware that limestone or other calcium containing material derived from land masses in the United States, the Dominican Republic and waters or land masses around Brazil may have been mislabeled as coral calcium from Okinawa. Some of this "fake" coral calcium has been and is still sold in dietary supplements in health food stores and chain stores. Natures Benefit Coral Calcium, is authentic and preferred by most consumers. (www. naturesbenefit.com)

THE RETAIL CATEGORY OF CORAL CALCIUM

Natures Benefit, Inc. was responsible for starting the major retail category of coral calcium supplements several years ago with its product Coral Calcium Plus. Natures Benefit, Inc. made a commitment to collaborate and engage in substantial research and development on coral calcium, and it signed research, development and supply agreements with the Japanese producers of quality, science-backed coral calcium. Natures Benefit has not supported exaggerated claims of benefits for coral calcium made by others, but there is widespread belief in the versatile health value of authentic Okinawan coral calcium (www. naturesbenefit.com).

SORTING SCIENCE ON CORAL CALCIUM

In my writings, I have attempted to separate fact from fiction concerning the origin, characteristics and the potential health benefits of coral calcium. It is fair to say that many testimonials have emerged on the striking health benefits of coral calcium, but testimonials do not provide sufficient evidence to back exaggerated treatment claims. Coral calcium remains lacking in clinical research, even though it has been recognized by many people as providing health benefits. I believe that coral calcium has been very poorly understood by many individuals and by members of the dietary supplement industry. The name coral calcium is somewhat misleading because coral calcium is more than just a calcium supplement. I reiterate that it possesses a holistic mineral profile with dozens of micronutrient elements that may promote cellular health (cell salts).

RESEARCH WITH OKINAWAN CORAL CALCIUM

Premium types of coral calcium are well-absorbed sources of calcium and other minerals, especially magnesium. However, statements that coral calcium is 100% absorbed are ludicrous. Studies in healthy volunteers show that coral calcium-treated water may induce relaxation of the body. Some studies have used electrical recordings of brain activity in healthy volunteers given coral calcium. These studies showed a change in brain waves associated with relaxation.

There have been emerging studies on the potential anti-cancer benefits of coral calcium in animals, but the evidence of this effect is not clear in humans. However, there are dozens of studies that show benefits of calcium, per se, in potential cancer prevention, especially the prevention of colon cancer or colon polyps. Furthermore, calcium enrichment of diets has been associated with weight control, lowering blood cholesterol and lowering blood pressure, in addition to calcium's obvious role in the promotion of healthy teeth and bones.

Exciting research has shown that certain ratios of calcium and magnesium in coral calcium supplements (land coral sand) may control hormone release. Studies show this effect in relationship to the release of the hormone insulin which controls blood sugar and several other body functions. These observations may explain why some people have produced testimonials on the improvement of their blood sugar levels while taking coral calcium, but these matters have not been defined in controlled clinical trials. Interesting information has emerged on the ability of the calcium content of coral calcium to help improve symptomatic heartburn; and well-conducted studies in Japan have shown coral calcium supplements may help improve bone health.

In one study performed in Japan, the administration of coral calcium together with an exercise program improved bone density. This has led to the suggestion that coral calcium may be a valuable form of calcium and mineral supplementation in the nutritional support of bone health, particularly in relationship to osteoporosis or thin bones.

HOW DOES CORAL CALCIUM EXERT A HEALTH BENEFIT?

There have been a number of suggestions concerning how coral calcium may exert a health benefit, but its wellness-promoting actions remain under-explored. The real issue in the potential benefits of coral calcium, as a dietary supplement, rests in its quality in supplying a holistic micro-mineral profile, as well as its contents of calcium and magnesium to a variable degree.

Coral calcium supplements must conform to the regulations that exist concerning heavy metal content. In this regard, Natures Benefit has committed itself to use only material collected and processed in Okinawa, which is not contaminated with unallowable levels of heavy metals. Okinawa is the world leader in coral calcium research and production and Natures Benefit Coral Calcium is the best selling brand (www.naturesbenefit.com).

CONCLUSION

Coral calcium, from Okinawa, Japan, is a valuable dietary supplement that was once "down staged" by unscrupulous marketing promotions. There is a major revival in interest in authentic coral calcium as a nutritional supplement. Coral calcium has a "new lease on life" to support multiple body structures and functions, given emerging research and continuing, customer satisfaction (www.naturesbenefit.com). Natures Benefit, Inc. is the rightful owner of certain trademarks and these trademarks have been subject to commercial piracy and some degree of misrepresentation. These matters are of teaching significance where dietary supplement counselors should check the origins of products that they recommend.

The premium best-selling brands of Okinawan coral calcium are Natures Benefit Coral Calcium which contains high quality authentic coral calcium and other coral calcium formulae that contain premium coral calcium with added micronutrients and vitamins. Plain forms of coral calcium supplements are preferred by people who are already taking vitamin supplements because they may not require the added vitamins and nutrients that are present in Coral Calcium Plus™. I strongly advise consumers to be aware of "fake" coral calcium supplements. Readers should note that there is no evidence to support that land-derived coral sand from Okinawa is any less effective than marine (below sea) collected coral sand, despite the rhetoric. I have been disturbed that some major retailers of their own brand of coral calcium may not have shown sufficient interest in checking the authenticity of the coral calcium that they sell.

CHAPTER 15

WEIGHT MANAGEMENT

OBESITY OR OVERWEIGHT STATUS: A MAJOR PUBLIC HEALTH INITIATIVE

MANY people are tired of being told that they are overweight and sedentary, but any complacency about weight gain or excess must not be encouraged. Modern medicine has shown us the serious increase in premature disability and death due to obesity or being overweight. Obesity has rapidly become the number one preventable cause of premature death and disability in Western society, most notably the US.

Recent statistics and trends on obesity are alarming, especially in children. The US has the most idle and obese children in the world. Individuals have tended to focus on the cosmetic aspects of obesity without considering its tragic and devastating effects on physical and psychosocial wellbeing. Recent studies show that a large proportion of infants and toddlers cannot fit into standard, safety, car seats, and if they do, many are unable to fasten their seat belts!

The real significance of obesity to Western nations and some Third World countries is the occurrence of many obesity-related diseases, together with mounting, obesity-related death rates (Table 23).

High Risk	Moderate Risk	Lower Risk
Diabetes mellitus	Heart Disease	Cancer of womb, breast, colon

Insulin Resistance	Peripheral vascular disease	Hormonal disorders: especially sex hormones
Hypertension	Stroke	Infertility
Abnormal Blood Lipids	Arthritis, osteoporosis, gout	Congenital defects in children of obese mothers
Gallstones	Polycystic Ovary Syndrome	Increased Accident Rates
Sleep Apnea	Low Back Pain	Depression
Decreased aerobic fitness potential	Fibromyalgia, medical risk in surgery	Social isolation

Table 23: Illnesses that have been clearly associated with being overweight or obese. Risks for these diseases tend to increase by degrees of obesity. Overlap of disease risk exists in the spectrum of being overweight ("degrees of fatness"), and prominent factors in the high risk column constitute the definition of Syndrome X.

DIETS ARE NOT "STAND-ALONE" INTERVENTIONS FOR WEIGHT CONTROL IN MANY PEOPLE

Obesity does not usually present itself as a single medical problem, requiring focused management. Low-carb diets are certainly effective for short-term weight loss in people who wish to lose a few pounds of body weight, but low-carb diets, such as the Atkins diet have often failed to achieve sustained weight control. My friend, Robert Atkins MD (deceased) was a Titan in the science of weight control; and it troubles me that his valuable diet has experienced a recent decline in interest, when used as a short-term, weight loss measure. Dr. Atkins modified his approach to carbohydrate restricted diets with the specific intention of trying to combat the metabolic Syndrome X (see Syndrome X, Chapter 16).

Silly marketing and mixed messages confused the public about Atkins diet. The promise of prolonged weight control with the "Atkins Lifestyle" diet was unfounded. I have discussed these issues in my book entitled "Enhancing Low-Carb Diets" (Wellness Publishing Inc, Little Falls, NJ, 2004). The big problem with carbohydrate restriction alone is that it does not overcome insulin resistance consistently in overweight people with Syndrome X. Insulin resistance, resulting in high insulin levels, is a principal trigger to fat storage by the body. Excessive circulating insulin in the presence of insulin resistance generates several components of the metabolic Syndrome X. These issues are discussed in more detail in Chapter 16, where it is obvious that overcoming insulin resistance is a principle task for many people who are overweight or obese (see Appendix C).

National registers that keep information on people who have lost weight, and managed to keep the weight off, imply that weight control occurred by many means other than diet alone. Successful dieters use modification of eating behavior, positive lifestyle change and exercise to sustain weight control. In other words, few people can achieve sustained weight loss by diet alone. Weight management must be holistic with diet, exercise, behavior modification and other lifestyle changes. The long term approach to weight control must involve the adoption of a diet that serves an overall health objective, not just a simple weight loss objective (see Appendix C).

OBESITY, METABOLIC SYNDROME X, PRE-DIABETES AND TYPE II DIABETES

Before one starts to assess the overall negative effects of obesity and its related disorders, one must understand the relationship between obesity and the modern epidemics of Metabolic Syndrome X and Type II diabetes mellitus. There are 70 million Americans who have a condition called the Metabolic Syndrome or Syndrome X. This syndrome is a common forerunner to type II diabetes mellitus (Appendix C).

The simplest definition of Syndrome X is the variable combination of obesity, high blood pressure and abnormal or high blood cholesterol, all linked by resistance to the hormone insulin (Chapter 16, Syndrome X).

CALORIE CONTROL IS IMPORTANT

Energy is taken into the body in the form of calories that are delivered by and contained within food. This energy is utilized by the body for day-to-day living and to support physical activity. It is true that if people eat too many calories, they will tend to become fat. These facts reveal that many "diet books" are just "nonsense literature." However, the equation of "energy in and energy out" (the law of thermodynamics) does not fit perfectly with weight control tactics in humans.

There are a small number of people who can consume large amounts of energy (calories in food) and not gain weight, even though their level of exercise is not particularly high. That said, calorie control is generally a very important aspect of weight control. Calories do count! Contrary to unsubstantiated back chat!

AN OVERALL HEALTHY WEIGHT CONTROL INITIATIVE

A combat against the modern pandemic of obesity must involve positive lifestyle change with increased levels of exercise and modification of eating behavior, including the selection of smaller, meal-portion sizes. Excess dietary intake of simple sugars, together with environmental toxins, lack of physical exercise and poor lifestyle tend to cause insulin resistance. There is no simple drug approach to combat insulin resistance and its principal associated diseases or disorders in a comprehensive manner (abnormal blood cholesterol, high blood pressure, etc. see Chapter 16). The side-effect profiles of drugs, used to manage the individual components of the metabolic Syndrome X make dietary supplement and "functional food" interventions attractive "first-line options" for management strategies, e.g. some insulin sensitizing drugs can damage the liver or cause weight gain.

OVERWEIGHT: MANY CAUSES REQUIRING
MULTIPLE INTERVENTIONS

The overweight status of Western nations is due to many causes (Table 24). When the reader reviews the recognized causes of obesity, they must conclude that a combat against weight gain has to be complex series of interventions with many different management aspects that must be applied over a prolonged period of time, perhaps a lifetime! Clearly, a holistic approach to combat weight gain is required to address the most serious public health initiatives (obesity and Syndrome X) that threaten the future health of Western nations (Appendix C).

Recognized Causes	Medical Causes
Social gluttons (USA)	Drugs
Family predispositions	Surgery
Genetic obesity	Brain Disease
Diet composition	Endocrine causes
Eating patterns	Abnormal metabolism
Emotional factors	INSULIN RESISTANCE, EXCESS

Table 24: The most common form of obesity is "simple obesity," which is a lifestyle disorder. Insulin resistance is a much more important and common cause of obesity than previously supposed; and insulin resistance is the pivotal factor that underlies

the metabolic Syndrome X (see Chapter 16). Individuals, who are overweight or obese, with the metabolic Syndrome X, must consider a combat against the multiple components of Syndrome X. This combat may help to reduce premature disability and death that occurs from obesity and its related disorders or diseases.

KEYNOTE SUMMARY: WEIGHT MANAGEMENT: HOLISTIC HINTS

Many citizens in industrialized nations, including urban areas of third world countries, have expanded or expanding waistlines. While many people see the global epidemic of obesity as a cosmetic issue, the circumstances of obesity are a serious "medical or public health emergency" which requires active correction. Americans are tired of being told that they are fat and idle; and the psychology of weight control involves self-defeating attitudes in many people. Everyone is looking for a quick fix for their weight problem, but no quick fix exists!

Despite these matters of fact, billions of dollars have been spent on diet books that promise an easy way out. Many people can lose weight in the short term, but sustained weight control is a difficult target for many people. I have written extensively on this subject in the book entitled "Enhancing Low Carbohydrate Diets." Weight gain in the majority of mature people is associated with insulin resistance or the metabolic Syndrome X. These circumstances commonly affect mature adults, but children are not spared.

It is the presence of obesity related disease and disordered body chemistry that are the real problems in the overweight individual. Weight control is a function of several important factors:

- Diet involving reduction of calorie intake and, for short term weight loss, restriction of simple carbohydrate intake is important. A weight control diet for the long term should be a balanced diet with rotating modest intake of protein from fish, lean meats and vegetables (soy), restriction of saturated fat and liberal use of healthy fats e.g. omega 3 fatty acids (Fish Oil, see Chapter 18).
- Complex carbohydrates and dietary fiber are healthy inclusions in any diet (oat bran hydrocolloids (beta glucan), fiber, see Chapter 12). Salt restriction is particularly important in many people with the metabolic Syndrome X, for blood pressure control. Anyone who reduces calorie intake using standard Western food must take a multivitamin supplement (see Multivitamins, Chapter 1 and Antioxidants, Chapter 4) because much food is processed and lacking in vital nutrients.

- Without behavioral change, there will be no sustained weight loss. Excessive eating over short periods of time, such as public holidays, causes cumulative weight gain. The idea of getting fat over the holiday and slimming down afterwards does not work. Food selection and portion sizes are often subject to distorted thought, especially in the US (Food-Portion-Distortion, FPD). Dieters should learn to leave food on their plate or order one portion for two people. Americans and others may have sometimes developed "eyes that are bigger than their bellies."

- Without exercise, the body cannot expend energy that it has derived from food; and this excess energy is stored as body fat. Many American adults and children do not move. There can be no weight control without exercise.

- Modern research shows the role of sleep deprivation in causing nocturnal eating disorders, promoting insulin resistance, altering appetite, hormone regulation and fuelling the nation's problem with an overweight status. Without restful sleep and an established daily biorhythm, weight control cannot occur. All individuals who are trying to control their weight must deal with their sleeplessness (The Sleep Naturally Plan, see Chapter 2).

- Dietary supplements used for weight control must be seen as adjuncts. There is no drug or nutritional supplement that can cause weight loss without lifestyle changes, such as control of calorie intake, behavior modification and aerobic exercise. Some drugs and some supplements that have been or are currently used for weight control are not safe. Many dietary supplements that are used for weight control attempt to suppress appetite without stimulation (Hoodia) or induce thermogenesis (Seaweeds, fucoxanthin, FucoseLean™). This approach is to be commended because calorie control in the diet is mandatory for weight control. Hormonal and metabolic adjustments with certain supplements are very exciting options for weight management.

- Weight Management supplements should go beyond attempts to control appetite by providing substances that may help to combat insulin resistance and alter sugar metabolism in a favorable manner. Individuals who have Syndrome X should consider using the many supplements that can impact the constellation of problems that comprise the Metabolic Syndrome X (see Syndrome X, Chapter 16).

WEIGHT MANAGEMENT (A LEARNING APPROACH)

The formulations of some valuable weight loss supplements are energizing, but they should not be used in combination with supplements that "stimulate" (Chapter 26). The presence of green tea and green coffee bean extract in weight control supplements may favorably affect sugar metabolism in the body and the presence of chromium assists insulin in its complex actions. There has been a great deal of medical literature that highlights the value of chromium supplements in weight control, management of cholesterol problems and the facilitation of the effects of insulin on the body. In contrast, the important research on green coffee bean extract has not been highlighted to any significant degree in popular healthcare literature.

Garcinia cambogia, guarana and gotu kola provide a perk and assistance with behavior modification for controlled calorie intake. The dosages of these agents should be modest because of their stimulating activity. Anyone with significant blood pressure problems is advised to avoid stimulant supplements, or check with their healthcare giver, prior to their use. I believe that ephedra (Ma huang) is not generally safe for use as a weight control supplement and I have never endorsed the use of ephedra for weight control.

MODERN CONCEPTS IN WEIGHT CONTROL

Healthcare practitioners are not providing a good service to clients who wish to control weight by promising unrealistic outcomes from diet or drug or supplement administration, used in isolation. Promising approaches with supplement use include the appetite suppressing effects of Hoodia gordonii, which works without strong stimulant effects. Thermogenic effects of fucoxanthin may be valuable as an adjunct to weight control. Some members of the dietary supplement industry used ephedra in an incorrect manner. The serious side effects of ephedra occurred mainly in people with cardiovascular or stroke risk factors because of the powerful stimulant actions of ephedra at high dosage. In fact, many people who received ephedra had metabolic syndrome X, where high blood pressure and cardiovascular risk factors often co-exist.

Calorie control is a very important principle in weight control and non-stimulant ways of controlling appetite are quite attractive. In fact, the continuous administration of special types of soluble fiber (Syndrome X Nutritional Factors® powder) can result in a simple, feel-full, weight loss approach. The beta glucan fraction of oat fiber holds water and expands in the stomach. If this special type of soluble fiber is taken 20 to 30 minutes prior to a meal, then two beneficial effects occur. First, the oat beta glucan induces a sensation of satiety with zero calorie delivery. Second, the oat hydrocolloid fiber reduces blood glucose levels following a meal and blunts insulin responses. This latter effect is useful in the presence of insulin resistance, which is often present in syndrome X and obesity in mature individuals.

The use of thermogenic supplements has become quite popular and in Chapter 31, I discuss the role of fucoxanthins (found in certain seaweeds) as "fat-burning" agents. There are several supplements that have been proposed as fat burners, but all of these approaches to weight control must be associated with the correct diet, exercise and behavior modification. Altering sex hormone profiles (e.g. diindolylmethane, DIM) and detoxification are innovative weight control tactics.

CONCLUSION

If one was to assemble all "modern diet gurus," one would witness a "free-for-all" in opinions. A general consensus would probably emerge that "diets alone," regardless of their type, must be "calorie-controlled," but all diets fail in the long term, without exercise programs and behavior modification (a holistic, weight control approach). Many "diet books" are just gobbledygook.

INDIVIDUALS WHO REQUIRE FURTHER ADVICE ON WEIGHT MANAGEMENT MAY REFER TO ONE OR MORE OF DR. HOLT'S BOOKS ON LOWCARB DIETS OR SYNDROME X (www. wellnesspublishing.com)

CHAPTER 16

SYNDROME X AND NUTRITIONAL FACTORS

INSULIN AND BLOOD GLUCOSE

Insulin is known to push glucose into tissues of the body. Glucose is used as fuel for life and abnormalities of glucose handling are associated often with loss of energy. Fatigue is probably the most common symptom of the metabolic Syndrome X, pre-diabetes, and diabetes mellitus. Insulin resistance occurs when the body does not take the command of insulin. When insulin resistance is present, the body reacts by making more insulin and so insulin levels become high in the blood. This situation is the hallmark of Syndrome X. As this situation progresses with insulin resistance, the body "gives up" producing insulin and Type II diabetes occurs. This is an oversimplified explanation of how Type II diabetes may occur in many people.

Insulin resistance is the underlying problem that generates the combination of problems found in the condition called the Metabolic Syndrome X (Figure 3). While all of us recognize the ability of insulin to help the body handle glucose, it is not quite as apparent to many individuals that insulin in excess can give signals to many organs of the body to make them function in a negative manner for health.

> THE METABOLIC SYNDROME X AFFECTS 70 MILLION AMERICANS AND IT IS THE SINGLE MOST IMPORTANT PUBLIC HEALTH PROBLEM IN THE USA. THIS SYNDROME IS OFTEN OVERLOOKED BY ALL TYPES OF HEALTHCARE GIVERS, AND IT IS STILL A HIDDEN EPIDEMIC! THIS DISORDER IS INCREASING IN CHILDREN AND IT IS ASSOCIATED WITH MANY DISEASES! (APPENDIX C)

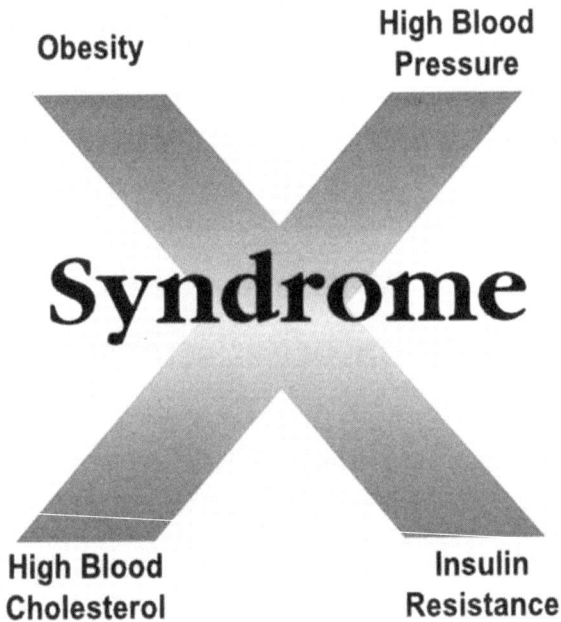

Obesity   High Blood Pressure

Syndrome

High Blood Cholesterol   Insulin Resistance

Figure 3: The multidimensional components of Syndrome X that account for cardio-vascular risks. Note: each of the four components of the metabolic Syndrome X and other associated disorders can be variably present. The manifestations of this disorder are many and complex. The constellation of problems that is part of the metabolic Syndrome X account for much premature death and disability. Syndrome X is a common forerunner to the development of type II diabetes mellitus. Please understand the concept of Syndrome X, Y and Z... (Figure 4) (see Appendix C).

INSULIN'S ACTIONS: BEYOND GLUCOSE HANDLING

Insulin gives strong signals to the fat storage cells of the body to store more fat. Hence, obesity or overweight status goes hand in hand with insulin excess and resistance in the metabolic Syndrome X. Insulin can "tell" the liver to make cholesterol and it can "tell" the kidneys and blood vessels of the body to act in a manner that raises blood pressure. One can now see, in somewhat simplistic terms, why obesity, high blood pressure and abnormal blood cholesterol (high triglycerides) occur together under the umbrella term "Syndrome X," or the metabolic syndrome (Figure 3).

This is not the whole story. Insulin has many other functions in the body which are not widely appreciated. Insulin can "tell" the ovaries to secrete male-type hormones, "tell" the body to make inflammatory messenger molecules and even "tell" genetic material to express cancer growth. Thus, insulin resistance and excess causes a diverse array of diseases (Figure 4). The extension of the concept of the metabolic Syndrome X beyond its role in creating cardiovascular risks (Figure 3) is shown in Figure 4. Thus, the metabolic Syndrome X causes many other diseases and this is what I have called "Syndrome X, Y and Z..." Let me explain further.

THE CONCEPT OF SYNDROME X, Y AND Z...

Syndrome X is associated variably with more than abnormal blood cholesterol, high blood pressure and an overweight status. Syndrome X, with its characteristic component of insulin resistance (Figure 3), can contribute to: cardiovascular disease, stroke, infertility, irregular menstruation, polycystic ovary syndrome (PCOS), fatty liver, declines in brain function (Alzheimer's disease), inflammation in the body and the development of certain types of cancer.

> **SYNDROME X PRESENTS A UNIFYING CONCEPT ON THE EMER-GENCE OF CHRONIC DISEASE. OUR "ADVANCED LIFESTYLE" OUTPACED THE SPEED OF OUR METABOLIC EVOLUTION?**

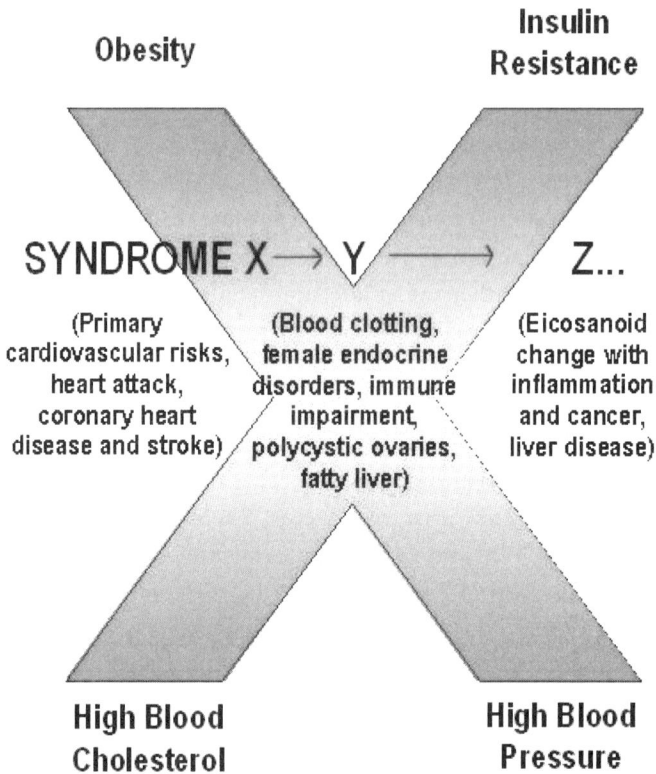

Obesity

Insulin Resistance

SYNDROME X → Y ⟶ Z...

(Primary cardiovascular risks, heart attack, coronary heart disease and stroke)

(Blood clotting, female endocrine disorders, immune impairment, polycystic ovaries, fatty liver)

(Eicosanoid change with inflammation and cancer, liver disease)

High Blood Cholesterol

High Blood Pressure

Figure 4: Combat Syndrome X, Y and Z ... the X in the diagram has the four cardinal components of obesity, glucose intolerance, abnormal blood cholesterol and high blood pressure, causing cardiovascular disease. The Y and Z are polycystic ovary syndrome, immune impairment, fatty liver, inflammation, "sticky blood" and cancer— all of which occur in association with the four cardinal components that are attached to the symbol X in this diagram. This diagram is an attempt to conceptualize the notion of Syndrome X, Y and Z ... These concepts go beyond the metabolic Syndrome X. This is a unifying concept of disease that is related to altered functions of the hormone insulin. One can see that our "advanced lifestyle" has caused us to evolve with conditions that may cause extinction of some members of our species. Perhaps I should have called Syndrome X, Y and Z... the "Do Do" disease or the "Human Dinosaur Disorder"!

WHAT CAUSES SYNDROME X?

Syndrome X is caused by many factors including: poor lifestyle, excess simple sugar in the diet, lack of exercise, environmental toxins and hereditary tendencies. For effective management of Syndrome X, pre-diabetes, and Type II diabetes mellitus, one must address the constellation of disorders that occur together. Recent research has focused on the alarming rate of occurrence of the metabolic Syndrome X. This disorder affects as many as one in four of the population (at least 70 million U.S. citizens) and it occurs at all ages. Overcoming health problems in many overweight people is only possible by addressing the many components of Syndrome X. The next time you think about weight control, ask yourself if you or someone else has the metabolic Syndrome X?

SYNDROME X: A FORERUNNER OF TYPE II DIABETES

Type II diabetes mellitus is the commonest type of diabetes (about 95% plus of all cases). The metabolic Syndrome X is a common forerunner to Type II diabetes and one can often see the variable combination of obesity, hypertension and abnormal blood lipids (cholesterol) in people with pre-diabetes and Type II diabetes. While maturity-onset Type II diabetes occurs most often in adults, a striking increase has been noted among young children and teenagers, in recent years. Either type I or type II diabetes can cause similar medical complications, such as cardiovascular disease, nerve damage (neuropathy), eye disease (retinopathy) and kidney disorders (nephropathy). In essence, obesity or Syndrome X progresses often through stages to Type II diabetes mellitus, in many people. Many people have type II diabetes and do not know it! (Table 26).

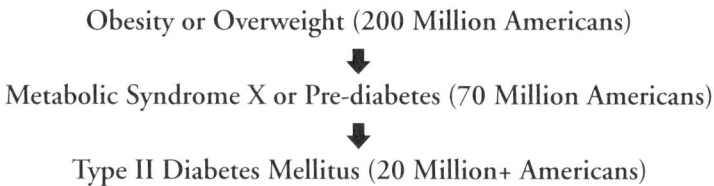

Obesity or Overweight (200 Million Americans)
⬇
Metabolic Syndrome X or Pre-diabetes (70 Million Americans)
⬇
Type II Diabetes Mellitus (20 Million+ Americans)

Table 26: A hypothetical progression from obesity to Syndrome X to diabetes that occurs commonly among Americans of many age groups. This is an oversimplified concept showing the progression of the nation's obesity to type II diabetes mellitus. Not all individuals with Metabolic Syndrome X will develop diabetes and some individuals may die from Syndrome X related diseases, before they develop type II diabetes! Being overweight goes along with a whole spectrum of diseases which are part of the concept of an expanded definition of Metabolic Syndrome X to Syndrome X, Y, and Z…. (see Figures 3 and 4) ("Do Do Disease" or the "Human Dinosaur Disorder").

FIBER AND DIABETES

Diabetes mellitus is the oldest dietary fiber-deficiency disease observed in humans. In 1979, my colleagues and I described the physiological effects of soluble fiber on the absorption of glucose and model compounds in humans (Holt S. et al., Lancet, 1, 636-9, 1979). In our study of acute dosing of soluble fiber, we observed the rate of sugar absorption was slowed and blood glucose tolerance curves tended to flatten. This research forms the basis of an understanding of what is popularly termed the "Glycemic Index." Thus, soluble fiber makes absorption of glucose smoother and efficient. Soluble fiber delays the metabolic incorporation of ingested glucose into the body (Figure 5). In other words, it "smoothes-out" blood glucose responses, following meals.

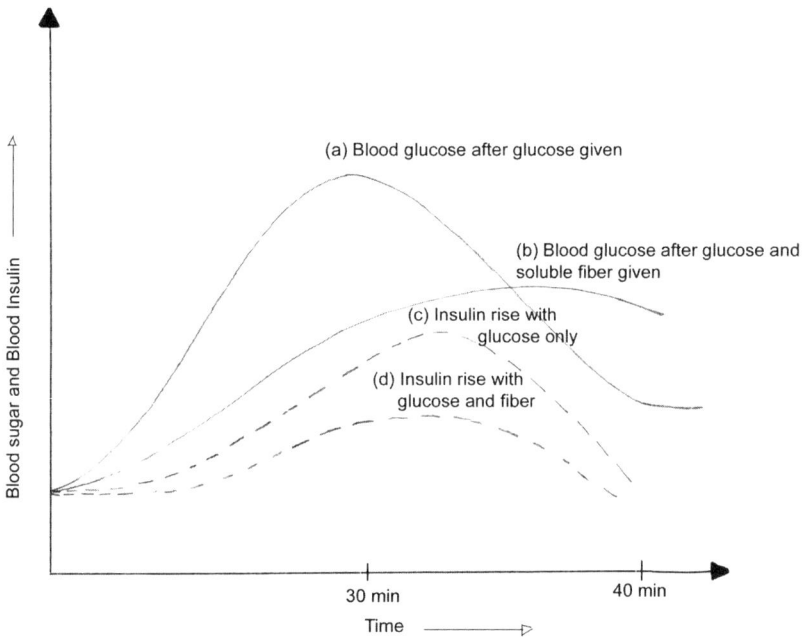

Figure 5: "Blunting" of blood glucose and insulin responses following a meal or the ingestion of glucose. Derived in part from data presented by Holt S. et al, Lancet, 1, 636-9, 1979 and reproduced in a "diagrammatic" form. When soluble fiber is taken with glucose the blood glucose curve over time is "flattened" to a major degree. This "blunts" the rise in blood glucose and, secondarily, the rise in insulin levels after fiber is taken. These observations explain the Glycemic Index of foods, to a major degree.

Recent studies have shown the ability of the extracts of soluble oat fiber (beta glucans) to significantly lower blood glucose levels following meals and reduce blood cholesterol levels in a favorable manner (lower LDL, lower triglycerides, with a tendency to raise HDL). Beta glucans are a special type of dietary fiber, made by a patented process, that function to control blood glucose levels and other abnormal body chemistry that occurs as a consequence of insulin resistance in the metabolic Syndrome X and some early cases of type II diabetes mellitus.

Diabetes mellitus is often associated with multiple risk factors for cardiovascular disabilities, such as obesity, hypertension and high blood cholesterol. Extracts of soluble oat fiber, or beta glucans, have an important role to play in controlling these risk factors. Enhanced intake of both soluble and insoluble dietary fiber is a grossly underestimated natural option that can improve health in both Type I and Type II diabetes (Syndrome X Nutritional Factors® and Fiber, see Chapter 12). Selected soy foods are valuable, despite the back-chat of the "soy critics."

ANTIOXIDANTS AND OMEGA-3S

Antioxidants of many types may benefit an individual with obesity, pre-diabetes, premature aging and diabetes. I coined the term **"obesitis."** It must be emphasized that many of the consequences or complications of diabetes are due to oxidative stress on the body, or the generation of free radicals, with resulting inflammation (**obesitis**). In diabetes and Syndrome X, cross-linking of sugar and protein causes advanced glycation end products (AGES) which, in turn, damage vital organs. In simple terms, sugar and proteins may combine in damaging ways. Of course, this whole situation is made worse by poor lifestyle and substance abuse, such as excessive alcohol consumption and tobacco use. Antioxidants may interfere with damaging, cross-linking of sugars and protein which form AGES (see Chapter 31).

In these circumstances, antioxidant compounds, e.g. vitamins C, E, beta-carotene, selenium and coenzyme Q-10 and many plant or animal antioxidant compounds (phytonutrients, phytoantioxidants), can exert beneficial effects. Of particular interest is the dietary supplement alpha-lipoic acid (thioctic acid). This potent and versatile antioxidant plays a specific role in glucose oxidation in many body tissues. Alpha-lipoic acid may improve the body's sensitivity to insulin and it has been used in the prevention of complications of diabetes and liver damage. In some countries in Western Europe, alpha-lipoic acid has been used as a prescription drug, but it is classified as a dietary supplement in the US, where it is available without a prescription. There is no need to give alpha-lipoic acid by injection. It is well absorbed.

EPA: AN EMPEROR OF FATTY ACIDS

Much interest has focused on the omega-3 fatty acid EPA (eicosapentanoic acid) because of its vital role in balancing favorable eicosanoid production in the body. Eicosanoids are chemical messages in the body that drive many different body functions and they are particularly relevant in the inflammatory process. EPA is found in high concentrations in well formulated fish oil supplements (see Fish Oil, Chapter 18). It is well documented that EPA can exert beneficial effects in common cardiovascular diseases. Scientific studies show the ability of fish oil to lower blood cholesterol, lower blood triglycerides, and it affords protection from sudden death as a consequence of common heart attacks. In addition, some studies imply that fish oil may help people with angina as a consequence of established coronary heart disease, including individuals who have undergone cardiac bypass surgery.

The fatty acid EPA is readily converted to DHA, which is found in large amounts in cell membranes, especially in the nervous system. EPA is an effective inhibitor of the development of "undesirable" forms of eicosanoids from arachidonic acid. Undesirable chemical messengers (some eicosanoids) may promote blood clotting and inflammation. In other words, EPA stops the body from producing bad chemical messengers that promote disease. For these and other reasons, EPA must be considered the "Emperor of fatty acids." Fish oil has been underestimated in its role in the management of diabetes mellitus and Syndrome X (see "Combat Syndrome X, Y and Z …," Holt S, www.wellnesspublishing.com and Fish Oil, see Chapter 18). There are many fish oil capsules available; some are cheap, some are weak and some are useless. The advantages of enteric-coating of fish oil capsules are quite obvious (see Fish Oil, Chapter 18).

OMEGA 3 FATTY ACIDS ARE INSULIN HELPERS

Evidence has accumulated that the active omega-3 fatty acid, EPA, can favorably affect the PPAR (receptor complex), which is involved in insulin action, carbohydrate metabolism and the body chemistry of blood lipids (cholesterol or triglycerides). Thus, EPA has emerged as a very important potential way of combating insulin resistance, by regulating certain components of the PPAR receptor. EPA (found in fish oil) appears to be a natural and powerful antidote to insulin resistance. Fish oil is emerging as a first-line option for nutritional support of the metabolic Syndrome X (with its cardinal components of glucose intolerance, hypertension, abnormal blood cholesterol and obesity). I am particularly impressed by the use of coenzyme Q-10 combined with relatively high doses of EPA in the management of diabetes-related cardiovascular disease. Diabetes and heart disease "go hand in hand."

YOU CANNOT UNDERESTIMATE
THE IMPORTANCE OF SYNDROME X

I remain passionate about the need to educate the public and the dietary supplement industry on the metabolic Syndrome X. This syndrome is able to be managed by good nutrition and positive lifestyle changes. In fact, I believe the management of Syndrome X represents a real future for a major impact of the use of food and dietary supplements on the health of Western society. The solution to Syndrome X is not readily found in a drug or conventional medical treatment. Table 2 shows a lifestyle and nutritional approach to Syndrome X (see APPENDIX C).

1. Lifestyle Change—with specific avoidance of substance abuse, including smoking cessation, reduced alcohol and simple sugar intake. (see Anti-Dependence, Chapter 28).

2. Behavior Modification—change of eating patterns and amounts; extinguish adverse lifestyle.

3. Exercise—matched to the level of aerobic fitness; medical or professional training advice recommended for "couch potatoes."

4. Diet—reduced in simple sugars, salt and saturated fat with controlled protein intake and more liberal healthy fats, e.g., fish oil (EPA). (Fish Oil, Chapter 18) Consider more fruit and vegetables (Berries and Greens Naturally Plus Supernutrition™, see Antioxidants, Chapter 4) and vegetable protein (soy) in the diet.

5. Syndrome X Nutritional Factors—oat beta glucan, antioxidants from berries, alpha-lipoic acid, chromium, biotin, vanadium, starch blockers, antihomocysteine vitamins and foods with low Glycemic Index properties.

Table 2: A lifestyle and nutritional program to combat the metabolic Syndrome X (courtesy of Holt MD Technologies).

MORE PUBLIC EDUCATION REQUIRED ON METABOLIC SYNDROME X

I am saddened that the importance of Syndrome X as a forerunner to the modern epidemic of type-II diabetes mellitus remains a mystery to many people. When individuals talk about reversing diabetes, they are often referring to turning back to the early phases of type II diabetes mellitus. There is a transition phase that occurs between a status of obesity, insulin resistance (the hallmark of Syndrome X) and deficiency of insulin (the hallmark of type II diabetes mellitus) (Table 26). In 2001, the Bush administration allotted several hundred million dollars to the office of the Secretary of Health and Human Services in order to educate the nation on diabetes prevention. Despite this investment, the terms metabolic syndrome, Syndrome X and pre-diabetes are still overlooked to a major degree in public health education.

KEYNOTE SUMMARY: SYNDROME X

Taking obesity for granted can be a deadly habit. Excess body fat located in and around the organs of the body (visceral obesity or "apple-shaped" obesity) presents an independent risk factor for cardiovascular disease and many other diseases. The "pot-belly" is a useless, dangerous "endocrine organ" composed of abdominal fat that creates hormonal havoc. This belly fat stores toxicants (organochemicals).

The metabolic Syndrome X is associated with more than abnormal blood cholesterol, high blood pressure, insulin resistance and obesity. The metabolic Syndrome X can contribute to infertility, irregular menstruation, polycystic ovary syndrome (PCOS), fatty liver, inflammation in the body, Alzheimer's disease and the development of certain types of cancer (Syndrome X, Y and Z…).

Syndrome X is caused by poor lifestyle, excess simple sugar in the diet, lack of exercise, environmental toxins and hereditary tendencies etc. In general health care, it is important to consider the whole constellation of obesity-related disorders. Careful attention must focus on the health-challenging components of obesity related diseases. These concerns must not be divorced from considerations of weight problems or obesity alone, remember "obesitis."

CHILDHOOD OBESITY

If ever there were tears in the eyes of the US nation, these tears must be shed for our tragic problem with overweight or obese children. Obese children often become unhappy and unhealthy, obese adults. It is estimated that one in three children born in the year 2000 will develop type II diabetes mellitus in their lifetime. Childhood obesity is one of the most difficult problems to treat in medical practice. In fact, the outcome of many research studies, aimed at the treatment of childhood obesity, show that the prevention of further weight gain is a very common outcome. In other words, reversing weight gain in children is sometimes a monumental task.

I can recommend few, if any, drugs or dietary supplements as safe management of childhood weight problems. I believe that children may benefit in many ways from fiber supplementation, especially supplementation with soluble fiber. Syndrome X Nutritional Factors® contain significant amounts of soluble fiber from oat bran that is presented in a powder that can be mixed into a healthy smoothie, "The X-Smoothie™" for children. In strict terms, the use of these nutritional factors for Syndrome X cannot be considered to be a true meal replacement, but taking soluble fiber tends to promote a feeling of fullness when it is taken 20 or 30 minutes prior to a meal. This is what I have referred to previously as the "feel-full, weight-loss trick". This approach has no signified adverse effects when applied with reasonable care..

Soluble fiber and antioxidants provide nutritional support to promote healthy blood cholesterol and healthy blood sugar levels. This effect is particularly valuable because there is an increasing number of children and teenagers with the metabolic Syndrome X. Observations in some groups of high school students show that as many as one in ten, or 10% of teenagers may have significant obesity, with variable components of the metabolic Syndrome X.

Syndrome X Nutritional Factors® also provide nutritional support for healthy immune function and it has a beneficial antioxidant profile derived from berry flavoring (significant ORAC) with phytonutrients (e.g. ellagic acid, anthocyanidins and flavonoids). ORAC is Oxygen Radical Absorption (Antioxidant) Capacity. All of these supplement or food products should be used with lifestyle changes that support healthy body structures and functions that are involved in effective weight management and the metabolic Syndrome X (where relevant).

CONCLUSION

I believe that the metabolic Syndrome X is the most important public health initiative facing Western society. This syndrome accounts for much obesity-related disability and death.

CHAPTER 17

BLOOD SUGAR

UNDERSTANDING DIABETES

I start this Chapter with a strong warning that I do not recommend that individuals with established diabetes take drugs or dietary supplements to alter blood sugar levels without the advice of a knowledgeable healthcare giver. However, the careful, self-management of the many facets of diabetes mellitus is extremely important. This approach requires intense patient education. Many studies show that education about the control of blood sugar in people with diabetes results in favorable clinical outcomes. In other words, an education in the effective management of diabetes is a key factor in keeping the individual with diabetes in a zone of wellness.

DIAGNOSING DIABETES

I emphasize that everyone with diabetes must become a student of the comprehensive management of this disorder. There are more than 50,000 searches in the U.S. on the internet on a monthly basis made for people who are seeking information about the diagnosis or warning signs of diabetes. A large, and still unknown, number of people in the US have type II diabetes that has not been diagnosed.

Reasonable estimates of the number of people with undiagnosed type II diabetes may be 7-10 million US citizens. Below is a simple questionnaire that is used in screening for diabetes. This questionnaire was constructed by the American Diabetes Association (ADA), for general public use.

Instructions: *Write down the number of points next to each statement that is true for you. If the statement is not true for you, place a zero in the space. Then add up your total score. See below for evaluation.*

1. I believe that I am more than 20% overweight.	Yes (score 5 points if true)	_____
2. I am under 65 years of age AND I get little or no exercise in a typical day.	Yes (score 5 points if true)	_____
3. I am between 45 and 64 years old.	Yes (score 5 points if true)	_____
4. I am 65 years or older.	Yes (score 5 points if true)	_____
5. I am a woman who has had a baby weighing more than nine pounds at birth.	Yes (score 5 points if true)	_____
6. I have a brother or sister with diabetes.	Yes (score 5 points if true)	_____
7. I have a parent with diabetes.	Yes (score 5 points if true)	_____

Evaluate Your Score: *This test is meant to educate and make you aware of the serious risks of diabetes. Only a medical doctor can determine if you do have diabetes.*

3-9 Points: *If you scored 3 to 9 points, you probably are at low risk of having diabetes now. But just don't forget about it – you may be at higher risk in the future. Maintaining a healthy weight and regular exercise can help reduce your risk.*

10 Points or More: *If you scored more points, you are at high risk for having diabetes. Only a doctor can determine if you have diabetes. See a doctor and find out for sure.*

TYPES OF DIABETES

Diabetes mellitus is a common disease in which the body cannot handle sugar efficiently; and excessive levels of blood glucose (sugar) often result. In simple terms, diabctes is generally due to an absence or lack of function of insulin. Two common types of diabetes are described. The first type (Type I diabetes mellitus) has been called "juvenile onset diabetes," where there is damage to the cells in the pancreas that secrete insulin. This type of diabetes occurs from a lack or absence of insulin and it tends to occur in young people.

The second type of diabetes (Type II diabetes) is commonly called "maturity onset diabetes" (MOD). Type II diabetes is much more common than Type I diabetes, accounting for more than 95% of all known cases of diabetes. This type of diabetes is sometimes associated, in its early phase, with a resistance to insulin (Syndrome X) and high levels of insulin (hyperinsulinism). Please review table 26 (Chapter 16) and help to understand how type II diabetes mellitus may evolve from pre-diabetes or Syndrome X.

Some insulin may be present in the body at the onset of Type II diabetes, but it is not able to do its job of driving glucose into cells. Type II diabetes is the type of diabetes that is most relevant to our understanding of the abnormalities of body chemistry (metabolic disturbances) that cause Syndrome X. Although maturity onset (Type II) diabetes occurs most often in mature people, a striking increase in this type of diabetes has occurred in children in recent years. This disorder has been called maturity onset diabetes of the young (MODY), a strange disease label!

While there are at least two distinct types of diabetes, each type can cause similar medical complications. These complications are due to elevated blood sugar which is common to both types of diabetes. Oxidative stress plays a role in the progression of diabetic complications ("**diabetitis**"). The complications of diabetes include cardiovascular disease, nerve damage (neuropathy), eye disease (retinopathy) and kidney disorders. While much of our discussion will address Type II diabetes (maturity onset diabetes), one cannot completely separate Type I and Type II diabetes; some overlap exists between them.

A SHORT OVERVIEW OF DIABETES

In the disease Diabetes Mellitus, the body does not produce enough insulin or the body does not respond to insulin (insulin resistance). Common symptoms in Type I or II diabetes include:

- Constant thirst and/or hunger
- Frequent urination
- Blurred vision
- Lack of energy
- Obesity (Type II)/ Weight loss in some people
- Inability to lose weight on a "low fat diet" (mainly Type II)
- "Low blood sugar" symptoms when meals and snacks are missed: headaches, blurry vision, nervousness (Type I and II)
- Fatigue (Type I and II)

Type II diabetes is closely associated with obesity, hypertension, abnormal or high blood cholesterol and triglycerides and early heart disease (also noted in the killer combination of Syndrome X). It is a disease of premature aging. Our "Westernized lifestyle" seems to be a major cause of insulin resistance and its progression Type II diabetes mellitus. (Table 26, Chapter 16). The **American Diabetes Association** (ADA) makes it very clear that the goals of treatment of Type II diabetes involve:

- Meal planning with nutritional intervention
- Exercise
- Weight loss or control
- Drugs as a "back-up plan"

Did the ADA forget dietary supplements?

SYNDROME X: A FORERUNNER TO TYPE II DIABETES MELLITUS: A REVIEW

Syndrome X is often confused with diabetes mellitus. While the factors that cause diabetes are similar to those that cause Syndrome X, the two conditions are distinct. Factors common to the cause of Syndrome X and diabetes include hereditary (genetic) tendencies, lack of exercise, obesity and excessive refined sugar in the diet (Holt. S. et al. Nutritional Factors for Syndrome X, and Holt S. Combat Syndrome X, Y and Z…, www.wellnesspublishing.com).

The real distinction between Syndrome X and Type II diabetes mellitus is that in Syndrome X, insulin resistance with insulin excess is the key problem. In early stages of Type II (maturity onset) diabetes, insulin resistance may exist and blood sugar "goes high" along with the high circulating, blood levels of insulin. In the later stages of progression of Type II diabetes, the pancreas may become "exhausted," and insulin levels may drop. Thus, in established type II diabetes the problem is insulin lack or absence.

While the differences between Syndrome X and Type II diabetes mellitus are more complex than I describe, it is clear that Syndrome X is often a forerunner to Type II maturity onset diabetes mellitus. In other words, insulin resistance and excess is often a preceding event in the development of maturity onset diabetes mellitus (Type II diabetes mellitus). My statements are oversimplifications.

INSULIN RESISTANCE	INSULIN LACK
Elevated blood sugar	Very elevated blood sugar
Pre-diabetes or Metabolic Syndrome X	Established Type II diabetes

SYNDROME X AND DIABETES RUN IN FAMILIES

It is estimated that at least 6% of the entire U.S. population has diabetes mellitus, but as much as 25% or more of the population may have the metabolic Syndrome X (obesity, abnormal blood cholesterol or hypertension, all linked by insulin resistance or pre-diabetes). Much of the discussion in this book focuses on Syndrome X and Type II (maturity onset) diabetes, but the risk of Type I diabetes (juvenile onset diabetes) is clearly linked to genetics. While genetics figure strongly in the cause of diabetes mellitus and Syndrome X, environmental influences also play a major role.

Understanding the genetics of Type II diabetes (the commonest type of diabetes, accounting for 95% of all cases) is quite difficult and information is incomplete. In most individuals with maturity onset diabetes, more than one type of gene (components of the body's genetic code) is apparently at fault. Moreover, in different families with Type II diabetes (maturity onset diabetes) different combinations of genes may be involved. Certain types of genetic material seem to limit the body's ability to produce enough insulin to overcome insulin resistance. When this happens the control of blood glucose goes "haywire" and diabetes emerges. Inflammation is also involved in the genesis of insulin resistance.

HERBS AND BOTANICALS REGULATE BLOOD SUGAR

Several herbs have been used in traditional medical practices to manage or even "treat" diabetes mellitus, but botanicals cannot be used to treat established diabetes, as part of usual and customary medical care. I stress that herbs or botanicals, that have been used in non-conventional medical disciplines, have not received the same degree of research and development or scrutiny, compared with prescription drugs that are used to treat diabetes mellitus (oral hypoglycemic drugs).

Some botanical extracts have significant effects on lowering blood sugar and their mechanism of action is not always entirely clear in medical, folklore, herbal or scientific literature. There is a possibility of serious interactions between herbs that lower blood glucose and drugs (anti-diabetic medications, oral hypoglycemic drugs or insulin). It is important to use potent herbal or botanical remedies, in the presence of diabetes, only with the supervision of a healthcare giver that is skilled in the management of diabetes mellitus.

CINNAMON BARK

There has been much recent research on components of the spice cinnamon that seems to act like the hormone insulin. In fact, components of cinnamon, called methyl-hydroxychalones, mimic the actions of insulin in promoting glucose utilization in the body. Cinnamon has a very long history of safe use in baking. It is used as a spice for buns and apple pies etc. It is very fascinating that cinnamon would be the selected spice for placement on sweet deserts containing simple sugars. This may be a marvelous trick of nature where the taste preference for mixing cinnamon with sugar laden food helps the body to handle the sugar laden food.

While studying the effects of chromium on glucose control, researchers started to look at extracts of the spice cinnamon. Extracts of cinnamon with low levels of chromium were found to have a strong insulin-like response in the stimulation of the burning of glucose (glucose oxidation). This has led to the proposal that cinnamon may have components within it that are "insulin mimetics."

Recent scientific articles present clear evidence that an extract of cinnamon referred to as "hydroxychalone" is an effective mimic of insulin. Cinnamon may be very useful in the nutritional management of insulin resistance and Type II diabetes and further studies are justified. Studies have been performed to define the ability of cinnamon extracts to assist the tissue responses to the hormone insulin.

BITTER MELON (MOMORDICA CHARANTIA)

Known by many names (Balsam pear, Karela, Bitter Gourd), Bitter Melon has been described as an "insulin mimic" which seems to lower blood sugar only when blood sugar is elevated, at least in experimental animals. Several human clinical trials, performed on the Indian subcontinent, imply that bitter melon can decrease the absorption of sugar and enhance glycogen stores in the liver, with an added benefit of modest lowering of blood cholesterol.

Bitter melon can be taken as a specially prepared drink or in supplement tablets or capsules that often contain dried bitter melon combined with other herbs that may regulate blood glucose. Few physicians in Western communities have great experience with the use of this botanical; and the optimal doses of bitter melon required for a desired response on blood sugar are not clear. The advice of an Ayurvedic physician, naturopath or master herbalist is recommended with the use of "anti-diabetic" herbs or botanicals. Bitter Melon can be quite potent at reducing blood sugar; and it may enhance the effect of drugs used to treat diabetes or insulin. Therefore, there is a possibility of drug interactions exists with bitter melon and other botanicals or drugs that lower blood sugar.

FENUGREEK (TRIGONELLA FOENUM-GRAECUM)

Fenugreek powder has been described as effective at balancing blood glucose and supporting a healthy, blood cholesterol. It appears to be a safe botanical and it is a popular food ingredient in Southern Europe and Asia. Fenugreek has a long history of safe use in the food chain.

GYMNEMA SYLVESTRE

This bitter tasting herb has been used widely in Ayurvedic medicine to treat diabetes. Clinical experiences using Gymnema have reported benefits in supporting a healthy blood sugar in people with Type II diabetes, in comparison with placebo. There are few comparisons of the use of the herb Gymnema with anti-diabetic drug therapy, but Ayurvedic physicians extol its superiority to drug treatments. More research is required to define the described effects of Gymnema on balancing glucose, lowering cholesterol and reduction of AGES (advanced glycated protein end products formation) in Type II diabetes. The acronym AGES refers to cross linking of sugar and protein that causes tissue damage in people with diabetes.

MULBERRY FRUIT

Mulberry fruit belongs to the genus of Moraceae (Morus species). It grows in many locations in Eastern and Western countries and it has a colorful folklore history as a traditional medicine. Mulberry fruit has been classified in traditional Chinese medicine as a blood tonic that nourishes "the yin." Mulberry contains several nutritional components including minerals and water soluble vitamins.

Mulberry fruits are rich in antioxidants called anthocyanins. Mulberry has been used in combination with other herbs to manage thirst, dry mouth and deficiency of body fluids, especially in individuals with diabetes mellitus. It is believed to act by helping the body to normalize its fluid content, but, of course, individuals with diabetes are recommended to maintain their fluid intake. Thirst is best counteracted by the consumption of pure water. Mulberry has no clear documented ability to control blood sugar by itself.

CHROMIUM

In several areas of this book, I have reviewed the good scientific agreement that exists on the use of chromium to assist in blood sugar regulation.

OAT BRAN BETA GLUCANS

I have discussed the major nutritional value of special types of soluble fiber, such as oat beta glucan in the nutritional support of obesity, metabolic Syndrome X, pre-diabetes and type II diabetes mellitus.

ALPHA LIPOIC ACID

The potent and versatile antioxidant, alpha lipoic acid, has been discussed in detail, elsewhere in this book. Alpha lipoic acid has a role in preventing oxidative stress and helping insulin to function.

BIOTIN

Biotin is known to play a special role in blood sugar regulation, as one of the relatives of the B group of vitamins. Extra supplementation of this vitamin is recommended as an ingredient in the nutritional support of a healthy blood glucose level.

GARLIC (ALLIUM SATIVUM)

Garlic has been studied extensively for its benefits in cardiovascular disease but results of some studies show inconsistent benefits. This problem may be related to the type (extract or whole) and the amount of garlic used. Overall, garlic and other members of the onion family of plants may exert benefits in reducing blood cholesterol; and in some cases they may help balance blood glucose.

COROSOLIC ACID (LAGERSTROEMIA SPECIOSA OR PUNICA GRANATUM)

Corosolic acid is most often used as an extract of Punica granatum, due to the protection afforded the other sources of this compound, namely the pretty, endangered, flowering plant Lagerstroemia which grows in China and the Philippines. Corosolic acid is a botanical extract that has an inconsistent effect on lowering blood glucose levels and optimum doses have not been established.

STEVIA (STEVIA REBAUDIANA)

Stevia is used as a "non-approved" artificial sweetener, but it is worthy of special consideration for use in individuals with Syndrome X. The sweetness of stevia is valuable in "functional" beverages, but this herb may have an added advantage of reducing blood glucose. The dried leaf of the stevia plant taken in large doses (5 grams, three or four times a day) has been shown to lower blood glucose in healthy individuals by uncertain mechanisms. Stevia used at very high doses has an uncertain safety profile.

Much more research is required to assess this apparent combination of benefits of Stevia as an alternative sweetener and blood glucose "balancer." Stevia is not classified as Generally Recognized As Safe (GRAS), as a food ingredient. Stevia has become a very contentious issue with regulatory agencies who do not consider it to be a safe sweetener, based on some animal toxicity studies. The evidence that Stevia can regulate blood sugar is relatively weak.

MISCELLANEOUS BOTANICALS (HERBAL EDUCATION SECTION)

Many other herbs and botanicals have been proposed as potential nutritional support for glucose intolerance and some possess the added advantage of cholesterol control. Table 28 summarizes the potential benefits of some of these agents.

Herb/Botanical	Actions/Benefit
Tinospora cordifolia	Inhibits conversion of glycogen to glucose and may reduce cholesterol.
Pterocarpus marsupium	May provide inconsistent glucose balance and improve symptoms in Type II diabetes. May have an effect on regenerating beta cell (pancreas) activity due to catechin content.
Azadirachta indica	An adaptogen with variable benefit on sugar control.
Ficus racemosa	May be valuable for weight loss, variable glucose control.

Aegle marmelose	Of questionable benefit.
Syzygium cumini	Antioxidant components may help diabetes by AGE prevention.
Atriplex halimu	Reports of improved glucose tolerance in Israeli studies.
Vaccinium myrtillus	Benefits due to anthocyandin contents with particular antioxidant benefits on the eye, perhaps preventing eye complications of diabetes.
Korean Ginseng	May help energize and questionable effect on reducing blood sugar.
Opuntia ficus	Nopal is a Mexican botanical remedy for type 2 diabetes mellitus, but uncertain benefits may only be apparent with high dosage.
Ocimum sanctum	Holy basil has been reported to balance blood glucose and lower cholesterol in very limited studies.
Silybum marianum	The silymarin component of milk thistle is very versatile, offering liver protection, "detoxification", antioxidant effects and indications that it may improve blood sugar control, by unknown mechanisms.
Miscellaneous	There are many beneficial phytonutrients that can be advantageous in Syndrome X. These include antioxidants and specific botanical derivatives such as "natural" methyl inositol (pinitol) and flax seed meal which may work by its content of omega 3 fatty acid precursors.

Table 28: Herbs and botanicals with potential nutritional benefits for circumstances of abnormal glucose metabolism, perhaps Type II diabetes and the metabolic Syndrome X. These agents should be used with the advice of an expert healthcare giver. The safety, effectiveness and optimal dosage of these agents are not entirely clear and general use is not recommended in blood sugar control.

MANY NATURAL SUBSTANCES OF NUTRITIONAL VALUE IN DIABETES MELLITUS

I mentioned that the Greek word "diabetes" means "siphon." Water-soluble vitamins and several minerals are excreted in abundance by diabetic individuals. I can argue strongly that most diabetics should consider vitamin and mineral supplementation of their diet (Diabetic Multivitamins™). An adequate intake of vitamins and minerals is mandatory in the management of diabetes (Diabetic Multiminerals™). The powerful benefits of fish oil as nutritional support for people with abnormalities with sugar handling by the body means that many people with diabetes mellitus may want to consider the value of high concentrations of EPA in fish oil (Diabetic Fish Oil™, see Chapter 18).

While elements such as chromium and vanadium are known to assist the function of insulin, emerging research shows that the adequate dietary intake of calcium and magnesium is important for control of blood glucose and insulin receptor function (Diabetic Multiminerals™). The role of adequate mineral intake in the management of diabetes is underutilized, underexplored and grossly underestimated.

Soy foods are very valuable in the management of diabetes mellitus, but their value has been challenged by the "meat and dairy lobby." Soy has a low glycemic index, soy protein lowers blood cholesterol and soy isoflavones are powerful antioxidants. Soy protein is handled efficiently by the kidneys, which are commonly diseased in people with diabetes mellitus (Holt S, The Soy Revolution, Dell Publishing, NY, 2000). The anti-soy crowd remains often misguided.

DIABETES PREVENTION

In recent times, the American Diabetes Association has revised its guidelines on the management of Type II diabetes by stressing the role of diet and exercise as first-line options in management. Drug therapy for Type II diabetes, including oral hypoglycemic drugs and insulin-sensitizing drugs, is regarded increasingly as a "back-up plan," but drug treatment or insulin administration is often mandatory in established diabetes mellitus. No person should stop diabetic drug treatment or insulin administration without the advice of a medical practitioner.

KEYNOTE SUMMARY: BLOOD SUGAR

Medical historians have referred to physicians who claim that diabetes mellitus is curable as "quacks." Let the duck quack because pre-diabetes and early diabetes are reversible, at least for a period of time. I have encouraged many physicians, healthcare givers, and retailers of dietary supplements to consider the role of insulin resistance in propagation of obesity, high blood pressure, abnormal blood cholesterol, depression of immunity, cancer, inflammation, menstrual irregularities and infertility, or progression to type II diabetes mellitus… to name a few disorders.

A synergistic blend of botanical and nutritional factors that will assist in the combat against insulin resistance and assist in the promotion of a healthy blood sugar level includes the following: Cinnamon Bark, Fenugreek Seeds, Mulberry Fruit, Gymnema Sylvestre, Chromium, Momordica Charantia, Oat Bran, Alpha Lipoic Acid and Biotin.

The nutritional support of people with diabetes mellitus remains sometimes poorly managed by medical practitioners and patients themselves. There are several baseline supplements that are useful in individuals with diabetes. First, diabetics have to adjust their diet and they run a high risk of vitamin deficiency. This potential deficiency is compounded by extra needs for vitamins and minerals, which may be lost in the urine. The loss of minerals or water soluble vitamins is common when excessive urination is present for any reason.

Several studies show selective vitamin or mineral deficiencies in certain groups of individuals with diabetes. One of many examples is the urinary loss of zinc and this element is required for insulin function. Many of the complications of diabetes are due to oxidative stress in the body, which may be addressed by the administration of well balanced antioxidant supplements, especially berries and greens (Chapter 4). Finally, the use of fish oil has been underestimated in value in individuals with diabetes. Much disability and early death in the diabetic individual are due to cardiovascular disease and fish oil plays a major role in supporting cardiovascular health. In addition, EPA in fish oil may assist in insulin function. Optimal diet in diabetes is all important; and it is the most important first line option to apply for the maintenance of health and wellbeing in the diabetic individual. The optimal diabetic diet is restricted in simple sugar intake while being balanced and nutrient dense in other ways.

CHAPTER 18

FISH OIL

GOOD, BAD, UGLY AND VERY UGLY FATS

FOR many years fat was considered to be a "four-letter word" in nutrition. Over the past fifty years, nutritional science has identified healthy and unhealthy types of fat in the diet. There are two main types of fat. One type is referred to as saturated fat which is present in a solid form, found in "lard" or attached to red meat or chicken, or found within whole dairy products and eggs. Saturated fat should not be taken in excess because it is linked to the causation of cardiovascular disease and cancer. One of the biggest problems with much fast food is its content of saturated fat.

The second type of dietary fat is found in oils that come from fish or plants or seeds or nuts. Liquid types of fats are called unsaturated fats and they are most often found in our diet in vegetable oils (abundant in omega-6 fatty acids). The terms saturated and unsaturated refer to the chemical structures of the fats, where solid (saturated) fat has more hydrogen in its chemical structure.

It is possible to take liquid unsaturated fat and treat it commercially by passing hydrogen gas into these oils. This changes oils into a solid form. This is how a bar or tub of common margarine is often made. However, this chemical process of hydrogenation of oils can create byproducts of fat constituents called trans-fatty acids. Hydrogenated oils are cheap and they have excellent taste or mouth feel. It is a "rule of thumb" that delicious foods are sometimes iniquitous.

Hydrogenation makes liquid oils into convenient foods and these artificial fats are very ideal for baking and easy eating. That said, many of these hydrogenated fats are not healthy and trans-fatty acids may be quite damaging to the body. Unfortunately, many delicious snack foods are loaded with trans-fatty acids. This circumstance should make people think twice before they eat cookies, pies, some chips and other popular baked goods, without reading labels about their trans-fatty acid content.

After decades of research that has shown the potentially damaging effects of trans-fatty acids, the American government has recently placed (2006) labeling controls on food that may contain trans-fatty acids, because of their danger to health. The biggest risk of trans-fatty acids in the diet is cardiovascular disease which remains the number one cause of death. Therefore, new concepts in nutrition have started to define good fats (oils and liquid fat), bad fats (saturated fats) and ugly or very ugly fats (trans-fatty acids).

Please pause and think how much trans-fatty acids may have been consumed by American children or adults over their lifetime. I add one "ugly type of fat" to the mix, namely peroxidated or deteriorated fish oil. I have rejected fish oil liquid as obsolete for routine supplementation of active omega-3 fatty acids. The moment that a bottle of liquid fish oil is opened, deterioration of the contents proceeds rapidly, especially if the oil is not stored correctly. Denatured fish oil contains peroxides and altered fats. Some of these deteriorated fish oils may exhibit toxicity, known or otherwise. The way to take fish oil is in enteric coated delivery systems, to improve compliance, absorption and effectiveness.

Of course, my statements are over-simplifications. In recent years, there has been a global change in the types of "healthy fats" taken in the diet, where omega 6 fatty acids (vegetable and some nut oils) are abundant and taken in disproportionately large amounts in comparison to omega 3 fatty acids (found in precursor forms in some plants, but most abundant in cold water fish, fish oil). This means that the most simple, important message about fats is that many people do not have enough healthy, omega 3 types of fat in their diet. Dietary supplement products that combine omega 6 and omega 3 oils may be quite redundant because the real need is to correct the wide spread deficiency of omega 3 fatty acids that exists in many Western Nations. The healthiest type of fat to supplement routinely appears to be fish oil, taken in the correct form (enteric-coated).

THE ESSENTIAL NATURE OF FATTY ACIDS

Essential fatty acids (found in oils) cannot be synthesized by the human body. This makes some of these fatty acids just as important for health as vitamins in the diet. There are many different kinds of fatty acids, but most discussions in nutrition refer to the essential nature of the omega-3 fatty acids and omega-6 fatty acids. I repeat that there is a widespread deficiency of omega-3 fatty acids in the diet of Western nations, especially among children and, often, among many pregnant women. Omega 9 fatty acids are healthy (olive oil) and they are a mainstay of the Mediterranean diet.

Modern research has highlighted the importance of the ratio of omega-6 to omega-3 fatty acids in the diet. A disturbance in this balance has major effects on health. Omega-6 fatty acids are abundant in Western diets and the alteration of the dietary intake of omega-6 and 3 fatty acids has led to an over abundance of omega-6 fatty acids in a ratio of about 10 to 1, or more (omega-6 to omega-3 ratios), in many people. A consensus opinion has emerged among leading nutritionists that the best ratio of the dietary intake of omega-6 and omega-3 fatty acids should be as close to 1 to 1 as possible. There are very few people who approach this suggested, optimal ratio of omega-6 to omega-3 fatty acids in their diet. Omega-6 fatty acids are often not required to be supplemented in many people, but omega-3 fatty acids are!

WHERE DO WE FIND OMEGA-3 FATTY ACIDS IN OUR DIET?

Omega-3 fatty acids occur in nature in precursor forms in some plant oils, but active forms of these fats are abundant in fish oil. Too much emphasis has been placed on Omega-3 sources in plant oils, (e.g. flax seed oil, soy bean oil, walnut oil, and oils in dark green vegetables etc). These precursor plant oils are not a reliable source of active omega-3 fatty acids. These plant oils contain alpha-linolenic acid (LNA) which must be converted in the body to more active forms of omega-3 fatty acids such as eicosapentaenoic acid (EPA) and docosahexaenoic acid (DHA). Unfortunately, many people have deficiencies in their ability to convert the precursor forms of omega-3 fatty acids (LNA) to active forms of omega-3 fatty acids (EPA and DHA).

While the terminology describing these health-giving, essential types of fat is complex, it is important to realize that the most efficient source of omega-3 fatty acids is cold water fish or fish oil supplements. It is very difficult for many people to get enough fish in their diet and concerns exist about contamination of fish with heavy metals and other toxins. These circumstances have made pure fish oil supplements extremely important in the health maintenance of many people. A large proportion of the population is now appropriately taking fish oil supplements, at least on an intermittent basis.

The world faces a big problem with its contaminated fish supply because modern research shows a very important need for babies in the womb to receive omega 3 fatty acids, especially to build their nervous system. However, the fetus is very vulnerable to heavy metals that may contaminate some fish (large predatory fish or "bottom" dwellers).

DRIVING BODY METABOLISM AND PATHWAYS
OF INFLAMMATION WITH FATTY ACIDS

Certain types of essential fatty acids taken in the diet will drive body chemistry and chemical messengers in the body in various directions, some healthy directions and some unhealthy directions. Perhaps the most important influence of the omega series of fatty acids is their effects on inflammatory pathways in the body. I shall now discuss a very simplified view of the biochemistry of essential fatty acids.

Understanding the cascade of compounds that are synthesized from essential fatty acids (omega-3 and -6 fatty acids) is a task for even the most informed healthcare giver. The most common dietary types of essential fats are omega-6 fatty acids, found in large amounts in many vegetable oils. Omega-6 fatty acids include the precursor molecules linoleic acid (LA) and its end products of arachidonic acid and adrenic acid.

The intermediary omega-6 fatty acid called gamma-linolenic acid (GLA) is often mentioned for its positive health benefits and it is commonly found in Evening primrose and borage oils. Arachidonic acid (omega-6) and EPA (omega-3) are the main "intermediary" precursors of hormones and complex compounds called eicosanoids of which prostaglandins and leukotrienes are common examples.

Please recall that there is an over abundance of omega-6 fatty acids in many diets and the advantage of GLA in dietary supplements may have been overestimated in some circumstances. Also, I believe that combined formulations of omega-6 and omega-3 fatty acids are not ideal supplements because most people may not need to supplement omega-6 fatty acids.

There is no doubt that our modern diet is highly processed. Many foods rely too much on the inclusion of omega-6 fatty acids which are found in food items such as: baked goods, margarines, frozen dinners, sauces, and salad dressings. While omega-6 fatty acids are essential for health, they may play an overall, but poorly understood, role in increasing the occurrence of heart disease, inflammatory disease, and perhaps cancer. This circumstance may occur when omega 6 fatty acids are taken in excessive amounts in the diet and not balanced with the correct dietary intake of omega-3 fatty acids (found mainly in fish oil). I believe strongly that the many adults and children in Western nations can benefit from supplemental intake of fish oil in their diet, providing that they take the correct form of fish oil supplements (enteric-coated).

EICOSANOIDS AND LEUKOTRIENES DRIVE
INFLAMMATION AND BODY FUNCTIONS

The eicosanoids are compounds that are produced from essential fatty acids, including omega 6 and omega 3 types of fats. These eicosanoids signal a wide variety of body functions including: blood clotting, inflammation and blood pressure regulation. Linolenate (linolenic acid, LNA) is the omega-3 fatty acid precursor found in some plants and it can be used by mammalian tissues to generate the eicosanoid EPA (found in its active form in fish oil). EPA is readily convertible to DHA, but DHA is not able to be converted to EPA.

Eicosapentanoic acid (EPA) tends to result in the production of prostaglandins of types that are anti-inflammatory and anti-clotting in their actions. In simplified terms, EPA (an active omega-3 fatty acid) pushes the balance of production of lipid mediators (eicosanoids and prostaglandins) towards more "friendly" or "healthy" types of eicosanoids and resulting prostaglandins.

Prostaglandins are another example of hormonal or chemical messengers that affect many different body functions, including: blood pressure, inflammation, blood clotting etc. In contrast, arachidonic acid or other omega-6 fatty acids may sometimes have an overall "pro-inflammatory" effect (causing inflammation or other unwanted body responses). In simple terms, EPA exerts significant anti-inflammatory effects in the body. This is why I have referred to EPA as the Emperor of fatty acids... a well-deserved title. Please note: these comments are over-simplifications of very complex biochemistry.

OMEGA-3 FATTY ACIDS (FISH OIL)

Omega-3 fatty acids have many potent and versatile health benefits. Many books have been written about the use of fish oil in disease management. Omega-3 fatty acids are a principle component of cell membranes. This means that cellular health in all parts of the body is dependent upon the presence of omega-3 fats. The health benefits of omega 3 fatty acids in fish oils were extensively researched by looking at disease profiles in certain races that eat large quantities of omega-3 fatty acids, e.g. Eskimos. Overall, Eskimos, living under traditional circumstances, have a high consumption of fat that is rich in omega 3 fatty acids, but Eskimos have a low occurrence of heart disease, unless they embrace "western" or adverse lifestyle.

MULTIPLE HEALTH BENEFITS OF OMEGA-3 FATTY ACIDS (FISH OIL)

There are many cardiovascular health benefits of fish oil including: a reduction of total blood cholesterol, LDL (Low Density Lipoprotein) cholesterol and triglycerides. In addition, they cause inhibition of platelet slickness, variable lowering of blood pressure, variable reversal of anginal pain, and protection against sudden death from heart attack.

Several scientists and clinical practitioners have drawn attention to the benefit of fish oils in the treatment of neurological disease, rheumatoid arthritis, ulcerative colitis, Crohn's disease, psoriasis, migraine headaches, visual disturbance and even yeast infections. In general, components of fish oil, most notably EPA, have anti-inflammatory and indirect antioxidant actions.

Recent research has shown that omega-3 fatty acids are effective antidepressants; and they may provide nutritional benefit in children and adults with attention deficit disorder (ADD). A remarkable recent finding is the ability of omega-3 fatty acids to assist the function of genes that control insulin actions (vide infra). This finding has major implications for the use of fish oil in overcoming insulin resistance which is at the root of the cause of the metabolic Syndrome X. Fish oil is beneficial in diabetes mellitus.

The potential health benefits of omega-3 fatty acids are legion. Given an overall deficiency of omega 3 fatty acid intake in the diet, many healthcare practitioners are recommending fish oil supplements, but they may not be recommending fish oil to be taken in its most ideal formulation as a dietary supplement... namely enteric coated and targeted delivery formats (intentional echolalia).

OMEGA-3 FATTY ACIDS: TOO GOOD TO BE TRUE?

The beneficial effects of omega-3 fatty acids are so wide ranging that they seem like a health panacea. In fact, they may appear "almost too good to be true." I have a very strong opinion that fish oil supplements make a real difference to health and well being. This short overview of the health benefits of fish oil that I have presented is well documented in peer-reviewed medical literature, but many conventional physicians are still strangers to the routine use or recommendation of fish oil for general health.

TRUST IN GRANDMOTHER

Grandmother was correct when she had us all "choking on a spoon of fish oil." Why fish oil is not more applied in disease prevention or treatment is a mystery.

Consumers believe that fish oil tastes terrible, but they have not been introduced to fish oils that are deodorized, pure, and available in capsules that are enteric coated for better tolerability, absorption of their contents and convenient use. These enteric-coated capsules provide targeted delivery of active omega-3 fatty acids. This special form of fish oil capsules puts the active omega-3 fatty acids at their site of maximal absorption in the small intestine. Ideal fish oil supplements achieve their advantages by having a special surface coating that delays the release of the fish oil, so that the important omega 3 fatty acids are not destroyed by stomach acid. This enhances the amount of active omega-3 fatty acids that are absorbed (enhanced bioavailability). In this supplement form, the active EPA and DHA components of fish oil do not "hang around" in the stomach to cause "fishy burping" or bad breath or simple stomach upset.

The amount of fish oil required to exert documented health benefits has been shown in some studies to be quite high. Using "regular" fish oil in ordinary fish oil capsules or liquid fish oil preparations cannot result in a high degree of acceptability to many people. In fact, this is a huge problem in trying to encourage people to take fish oil. The advantages of enteric-coated fish oil capsules include an ability to tolerate high dosages of fish oil, improved absorption, convenience of dosage, better absorption of active omega 3 fatty acids and distinct cost advantages.

In the early 1990s, I developed what became one of the best-selling fish oil capsules in the US dietary supplement market. In fact, marketing material used to promote this product bears my endorsement and likeness. My new generation of enteric-coated fish oil capsules is designed to be an improved version of this earlier product that has gained much popularity.

High dosages of fish oil that has been flavored or partially deodorized can taste terrible and cause much digestive upset. Large dosages of liquid fish oil can cause diarrhea, belching, and rotten halitosis. Therefore, fish oil liquids are often redundant and have been largely replaced by new formulations of highly concentrated fish oils contained within special capsules that have a targeted delivery mechanism. In summary, enteric-coated fish oil capsules could be considered to be an optimal way to take fish oil because it is present in gel capsules that are coated in a manner that enhances the absorption of the active fatty acids from fish oil. To reiterate, this improves the acceptance and compliance with fish oil supplement consumption.

Taking fish oil in special, enteric-coated, capsules can result in up to a three times greater amount of fish oil being absorbed by the body. Therefore, less fish oil can be taken in this manner because of the enhanced absorption of the essential omega-3 fatty acids.

SPECIAL NOTES ON FISH OIL

I stress that the beneficial use of omega-3 fatty acids for health may involve the use of dosages of omega 3 fatty acids that are much higher than are available in most regular fish oil capsules or fish oil liquids. I have concerns about people using liquid fish oil because the omega 3 fatty acids are not stable compounds and as soon as regular fish oil is exposed to the atmosphere, decomposition of the oil may occur (spontaneous oxidation).

Liquid fish oil that is decomposed can contain peroxides of certain fats and these damaged fats may be quite unhealthy. Therefore, I think that liquid fish oils are now redundant, given the availability of high quality, highly concentrated, omega 3 fatty acids found in stabilized formulations in capsules that have special delivery systems. Enteric-coated capsules may cost a little more than a regular fish oil capsule or liquid, but the healthcare consumer may get more potent and versatile effects from fish oil capsules that are specially designed. This is why I developed a new generation, fish oil delivery system, which are 1000 or 500 milligram enteric coated capsules of fish oil, containing approximately 300 milligrams of eicosapentaenoic acid (EPA) and 200 milligrams of docosahexaenoic acid (DHA). While modest doses of fish oil are healthy, certain effects of fish oil such as potent anti-inflammatory effects or a reasonable effect on elevating mood (antidepressant), require gram amounts of standard fish oils. Ask a knowledgeable pharmacist or healthcare practitioner about the benefits of fish oil.

In some research circumstances, up to 10 grams of regular fish oil liquids or gel capsules have been given as a daily dosage, especially for an anti-depressant or anti-inflammatory effect. This kind of high dosing with fish oil is not safe for self management. It is important that very high intakes of fish oil be monitored by a skilled health care practitioner. For the average adult, I recommend 2 grams of enteric coated fish oil (600 mg EPA with 400 mg DHA) be taken. If the enteric coating on some fish oils resulted in 3 times greater absorption, then two, 1000 mg capsules (30:20) would be similar to taking up to several grams of regular fish oil per day (18:12 concentrate). One may now see the clear advantage of enteric coated fish oils.

Nutritional literature discusses frequently the possibility of an individual developing an increased bleeding tendency with fish oil usage. While this circumstance is theoretically possible and critical for people on blood-thinning medications (anticoagulants) or people with a bleeding tendency, there are few reports of significant episodes of excessive bleeding from the average use of fish oil supplements. However, fish oil must be considered a weak, blood thinner.

EPA: THE EMPEROR OF FATTY ACIDS (SOME TECHNICAL NOTES) (REVISION)

Much interest has focused on the omega-3 fatty acid EPA (eicosapentaenoic acid) because of its vital role in balancing favorable eicosanoid production. The acid EPA is readily converted to DHA, which is found in large amounts in cell membranes, especially membranes in the central nervous system. EPA is an effective inhibitor of the genesis of "undesirable" forms of eicosanoids from arachidonic acid. Eicosapentaenoic acid (EPA) is an anti-inflammatory principle, whereas docosahexaenoic acid (DHA) is not anti-inflammatory to a significant degree. The importance of DHA as a stand-alone, omega-3 fatty acid has been over-emphasized.

There are many genes involved in the body chemistry of fats (lipid metabolism) and sugars (carbohydrates metabolism). The active omega-6 and -3 types of fatty acids (not linoleic and linolenic acid precursors) control the expression of genes that alter body lipids. Active types of omega-3 and -6 fatty acids regulate more than 10 different types of genes involved in lipid metabolism or energy production.

Of major importance are a group of genetic controls related to specific receptors. (e.g. PPAR or peroxisome phospholipid-activated receptors that regulate the function of insulin) Evidence shows that EPA favorably affects the PPAR (receptor complex), which is involved in insulin action, carbohydrate metabolism and lipid chemistry. This is why I believe that fish oil supplementation is extremely important in weight control, pre-diabetes, the metabolic Syndrome X and diabetes.

The use of eicosapentaenoic acid (EPA) is emerging as an important way of countering insulin resistance, as a consequence of the regulation of certain components of PPAR receptors. Thus, EPA (found in fish oil) appears to be a natural antidote to insulin resistance and it is a first-line, nutritional option for the metabolic Syndrome X.

KEYNOTE SUMMARY: FISH OIL

In the early 1990's I developed one of the most popular fish oil capsules that was sold in the world market. This enteric-coating technology has now been widely applied and copied by other dietary supplement manufacturers. I developed this technology to improve patient tolerance to fish oil and increase the amount of active omega-3 fatty acids that can be absorbed from a fish oil capsule. The technology provided other advantages by decreasing gastrointestinal upset from fish oil and preventing bad breath and fishy burps. These adverse symptoms are often experienced with the use of fish oil liquids or standard capsules, even if deodorized fish oils are used.

There is a new generation of fish oil supplements that combine targeted delivery of the oils, with enteric coating in high dosage of active omega 3 fatty acids (Holt MD Technologies). These supplements provide enhanced absorption, increased bioactivity and better compliance; and they are rich in the most important active omega 3 fatty acids, EPA and DHA. Fish oil products should be cholesterol free and permit an individual to get higher dosages of fish oil in their diet to achieve the real health benefits of active omega 3 fatty acids. Standard fish oil capsules or liquids cannot meet the nutritional power or versatility of enteric-coated fish oil capsules.

Everyone should understand that there is a widespread deficiency of omega 3 fatty acids in many Western diets. Omega-3 fatty acids provide among the most potent and versatile nutritional support for health, among all dietary supplements. Scientific studies imply that taking omega-3 fatty acids will help prevent sudden death from heart attack, help prevent coronary heart disease, help reduce inflammation, help elevate mood and help improve central nervous system function or cognition. Omega-3 fatty acids support cellular health in many areas of vital body structures and functions. There are very few people on a typical Western diet who will not benefit from fish oil supplementation.

For further information you may read my books, "Natural Ways to a Healthy Heart", Evans Publishing Inc, New York, NY, 1999 or 'Combat Syndrome X, Y and Z…," or the book "Nutritional Factors for Syndrome X", Wellness Publishing, Little Falls, NJ, 2000 (available at www.wellnesspublishing.com).

CONCLUSION

The evidence for the beneficial nutritional effects of omega-3 fatty acids in cardiovascular disease (e.g. Syndrome X, atheroma, coronary heart disease), disordered immune function and nervous system disorders (e.g. depression and attention deficit disorder, ADD) is increasingly clear. Fish oil provides nutritional support for the heart, the brain, the nerves, the bowel, the blood vessels, and it lowers bad cholesterol and triglycerides. High concentrations of active omega-3 fatty acids, especially EPA, support overall cellular functions in the body and they are essential for health.

While optimal dosages or contents of fish oil concentrates (e.g. ratios of DHA to EPA) are still being defined, Holt MD Labs has pioneered the introduction of purified, concentrated fractions of fish oil contained within enteric coated capsules for targeted delivery and enhanced absorption of essential omega-3 fatty acids in the digestive tract.

CHAPTER 19

CHOLESTEROL: DON'T FORGET HOMOCYSTEINE!

BLOOD CHOLESTEROL BREAKS YOUR HEART

THE magnitude of the use of cholesterol lowering medications in Western society is staggering, but the first line option to control blood cholesterol is to alter diet, increase exercise, reduce stress and engage in positive lifestyle change. There are many nutrients, herbs and botanicals which carry evidence of "good scientific agreement" that they may promote a healthy blood cholesterol profile and level. In fact, natural substances may effectively lower blood cholesterol, but this is considered to be a "drug claim." The cost, disadvantages and limitations of popular drugs for cholesterol lowering are driving many people to consider natural ways to promote a healthy blood cholesterol (and blood homocysteine level). Cholesterol lowering drugs (statins) do not reduce elevated blood homocysteine levels which are an independent risk for heart disease. Many of these drugs do not raise good cholesterol (HDL).

An ever increasing number of scientific articles clearly document the relationship between high or abnormal blood cholesterol or triglycerides and heart, or generalized cardiovascular, disease. However, cholesterol is not the only type of blood fat (lipid) that influences health. There are good and bad types of cholesterol. In general, good cholesterol is high-density lipoprotein (HDL) and bad cholesterol is low density lipoprotein (LDL). Prevention of coronary artery disease is possible with interventions that lower specific types of blood lipids (fats). Overall, it is accepted that a high total blood cholesterol, a high LDL, a high very low-density lipoprotein level (VLDL), a high triglyceride level (TG), and a low HDL are all deleterious to health.

Low-density lipoproteins (LDL) carry cholesterol in the bloodstream. When LDL is oxidized, it is more likely to be deposited in the lining of arterial vessels leading to atheroma. Oxidized LDL and peroxidated polyunsaturated fats enhance atheroma formation (clogging of arteries). Trans-fatty acids do the same thing (Chapter 18). Natural ways to combat the oxidation of bad cholesterol (LDL) are very valuable in preventing heart disease. This can be achieved by taking dietary components that are rich in antioxidant components, e.g. fruits, vegetables, omega 3 fatty acids and certain minerals or vitamins.

GOOD CHOLESTEROL

In contrast to the characterization of LDL and VLDL as "bad types" of cholesterol, HDL is considered a "good type" of cholesterol. In simple terms, HDL draws cholesterol into the circulating blood and reduces the tendency for cholesterol to be deposited in arterial blood vessel walls. It is the deposition of blood fats (cholesterol) in blood vessel walls that causes "clogged arteries." Modern approaches to blood cholesterol management are emphasizing the importance of raising HDL. Many cholesterol-lowering drugs do not effectively raise HDL, but natural approaches often do!

OPTIMAL BLOOD LIPID LEVELS

The levels of blood cholesterol, triglycerides and other lipids that can be considered healthy for an individual cannot be determined precisely. In May 2001, new guidelines were issued for the definition, prevention and management of high blood cholesterol. These guidelines were proposed by the National Cholesterol Education Program, in conjunction with the National Heart, Lung and Blood Institute. Acceptable levels of blood fats (types of cholesterol) have been revised downwards. In fact, these new definitions have revised down optimal levels of bad cholesterol (LDL) and triglycerides, while revising recommendations for blood levels of good cholesterol (HDL) upwards (Table 29).

For sure, people with heart disease, or at high risk, must be meticulous about cholesterol control. It is the high risk patient that most often benefits from pharmaceutical control of blood cholesterol levels. Modern medical literature proposes some arguments that lowering blood cholesterol with "statin-type" drugs (e.g. Lipitor®, Zocor®, Crestor®, etc) in circumstances where cardiovascular risks are minor may not be cost beneficial or always safe.

Total cholesterol	Desirable: Less than 200 mg/dL Borderline high: 200 to 239 mg/dL High: Greater than 240 mg/dL
LDL cholesterol	Optimal: Less than 100 mg/dL Near optimal: 100 to 129 mg/dL Borderline high: 130 to 159 mg/dL High: 160 to 189 mg/dL Very high: 190 mg/dL and greater
HDL cholesterol	Low: Less than 40 mg/dL Optimal: 60 mg/dL High: greater than 60 mg/dL
LDL to HDL ratio	Less than 4:5
Triglycerides	50 to 150 mg/dL (more aggressive controls recommended)

Table 29: A guide to the levels of blood lipids that have been considered to be in healthy ranges. Please note: these guidelines were proposed by the National Institutes of Health in May 2001. These are new targets for blood lipids which are recommended with more holistic efforts to reduce cardiovascular risks. Opinion differs in some medical circles on ideal targets for blood lipids. In the presence of heart disease or high risks for cardiovascular disease attempts to control blood cholesterol are necessarily more stringent in medical practice. While the author accepts the standard management concepts in conventional medicine, blood cholesterol lowering drugs, especially of the "statin types" may be over-utilized or over-prescribed. The author questions the safety of "statin drugs" for use over the counter (OTC).

FIRST-LINE APPROACHES TO CHOLESTEROL LOWERING ARE NATURAL: NOT DRUGS!

One may reflect on pharmaceutical, TV advertisements for cholesterol lowering drugs. These adverts start by dismissing the correct first-line approaches of diet and exercise for health or cholesterol control. More than one of these TV commercials reflects or implies that diet and exercise "did not or does not work," while the message is to "peddle a drug prescription" for lowering blood cholesterol. Many physicians are not completely happy with TV advertising of drugs. These adverts place enormous pressure on US physicians to prescribe drugs. Furthermore, a "spot message" in a short-captioned commercial cannot give a healthcare consumer an accurate message or sufficient information to make an informed decision about whether or not to take a drug.

There are several natural ways to reduce blood cholesterol and, in turn, reduce risks of cardiovascular disease. Conventional medicine has not acknowledged or realized the power of these natural approaches. With well chosen combinations of dietary supplements, natural cholesterol-lowering strategies can often achieve what some drugs cannot. Lifestyle changes and natural substances have fewer side effects than drugs; and they may provide the added advantage of a less expensive, sustainable health outcome, with global health implications.

BLOOD HOMOCYSTEINE AND CARDIOVASCULAR DISEASE

High blood levels of homocysteine have been linked to cardiovascular disease and an increased risk of blood clotting. Elevations in blood homocysteine form an independent risk factor for heart disease and heart attack. Just like the high blood cholesterol, elevated blood homocysteine must be considered to be dangerous to health. This "homocysteine theory" in cardiovascular disease is not in opposition to the cholesterol theory of heart disease, but it helps to complete the picture of the link between diet and heart disease.

Not only does elevated blood homocysteine cause heart disease, it can be associated with an increased risk of stroke, poor circulation in the extremities, poor brain function (cognitive decline) and even osteoporosis (see Osteoporosis, Chapter 6). Several studies have shown that the important vitamins folic acid, vitamin B12 and vitamin B6 (pyridoxine), together with a supplement called betaine (trimethylglycine), can effectively lower homocysteine, in a potentially beneficial manner for cardiovascular and general health (see Chapter 31).

So important is the role of homocysteine in heart disease that it is shocking that many people do not consider lowering blood homocysteine at the same time as lowering blood cholesterol. This is why I propose synergistic products to address nutritional support for a healthy blood homocysteine level, as well as a healthy blood cholesterol level, at the same time.

I consider supplements for cholesterol control that do not also assist in blood homocysteine control to be quite inadequate in their formulation. Homocysteine control is a powerful component of my recommendations (again, the issue of synergy). The formulation strategy is used for educational purposes on supplement ingredients.

AN ULTIMATE COMBINED APPROACH TO CHOLESTEROL CONTROL

I have written extensively on natural ways to cardiovascular health (Holt S,

"Natural Ways to a Healthy Heart," M Evans Publishers, Inc, NY, 2000). In my writings, I have focused on the power of combining a number of positive lifestyle changes and dietary supplements to approach an effective control of blood cholesterol. These natural approaches are summarized in table 30. My nutritional recommendations form the basis of new, synergistic dietary supplements. Effective dietary supplements combine nutrients and botanicals for the nutritional support of healthy blood cholesterol and homocysteine levels.

ACTION	OUTCOME
Exercise	A panacea health effect, e.g. approx. 5% to 10% reduction in blood cholesterol
Reduce saturated fats and intake of trans-fatty acids in the diet (see Fish Oil, Chapter 18).	Approx., 15% reduction in total blood cholesterol with lowering of LDL and triglycerides
Increase fruit and vegetable intake	Approx., 10% cholesterol reduction with beneficial antioxidant effects and other health benefits
Moderate alcohol intake	New studies show reductions in occurrence of diabetes mellitus with moderate drinking and several studies show benefits of moderate alcohol intake on HDL and lowering of total blood cholesterol
Other dietary supplements for cholesterol control: oat bran, beta glucans (see Syndrome X, Chapter 16), phytosterol concentrates from soy, policosanol and red yeast rice	Ingredients cause a reduction in total blood cholesterol of up to approx. 20% plus
Reducing blood homocysteine levels	Vitamin B6 (pyridoxine), folic acid, vitamin B12 with or without trimethylglycine

Table 30: Combined natural strategies to promote healthy blood cholesterol. The author proposes the concept that natural interventions to promote a healthy blood cholesterol level are additive. Many healthcare givers or healthcare consumers may give up prematurely on the use of natural approaches to control blood cholesterol, before they have exhausted the additive benefits of exercise, lifestyle change and combinations of multiple nutritional agents to promote a healthy blood cholesterol level. The author emphasizes the need for multiple nutritional agents to support a healthy blood cholesterol level and the use of single agents alone may be somewhat redundant (courtesy Holt MD Technologies).

LIFESTYLE AND SUPPLEMENT SYNERGY FOR HEART HEALTH

I believe that combined natural strategies to lower blood cholesterol can work together in an additive manner (Table 30). The options provided in table 30 involve a change of lifestyle and the addition of nutritional agents. These provide a pathway for a highly significant reduction in total blood cholesterol. I would go as far as saying that compliance with this kind of natural program may be superior in some aspect, compared with the isolated use of some cholesterol-lowering drugs alone.

I am concerned that some people who take cholesterol lowering drugs may develop a false sense of security and continue to engage or lapse back into adverse lifestyle that promotes cardiovascular or other health problems. The idea that cholesterol lowering drugs are fool-proof insurance against cardiovascular risks is misguided.

There are individuals who claim that they are "non-responders" to combined natural strategies to control blood cholesterol. I believe that many of these people are not compliant with the types of "first-line," natural approaches that I propose (Table 30). While there are few if any direct comparisons of drug treatments with the combined natural approaches that I describe, much "corroborating science" exists to support my statements concerning the nutritional support of healthy blood cholesterol. There have been several advances in the definition of natural agents to control blood cholesterol profiles and these nutritional advances can be combined in dietary supplement formulations. Many people have to stop taking cholesterol-lowering drugs because of side effects, e.g. abnormal liver function. Natural approaches to lower blood cholesterol may be ideal to try in such people.

SPECIAL TYPES OF OAT FIBER AND HEALTH: BETA GLUCAN

While everyone recognizes the general health benefits of dietary fiber, modern research has started to pinpoint the active constituents of soluble fiber that make a real difference to cardiovascular health. Using special manufacturing processes, oat fiber can be concentrated; and the special health-giving fractions of fiber called "oat beta glucans" can be isolated in high concentrations (see Syndrome X, Chapter 16).

The described cardiovascular benefits of beta glucan-enriched types of oat soluble fiber include well recognized benefits in lowering blood cholesterol, with secondary, modest improvements in blood pressure. Furthermore, oat soluble fiber can assist with control of blood sugar and exert benefits in the nutritional management of diabetes mellitus. There are dozens of scientific studies which show the versatile and potent cardiovascular benefits of special types of soluble fiber.

Recently, food scientists have been able to make concentrates of beta glucan in excess of 50% and this provides the ability of giving the concentrated and active components of soluble fiber in a convenient form in a capsule or tablet. While many people are aware of TV ads with claims for cereals lowering blood cholesterol (e.g. Cheerios®), there is now an approved food claim that oat fiber in certain doses and concentrations may reduce the risk of heart disease.

PHYTOSTEROLS: PLANT EQUIVALENTS OF CHOLESTEROL

Scientists have recently clarified the biological effects of phytosterols. The complicated word phytosterol comes from "phyto" meaning plant and "sterols" meaning chemical similarity to cholesterol. Cholesterol itself does not occur in plants, but there are sterols that have a chemical structure rather like cholesterol. These compounds are found in many botanical extracts. Sterols help antagonize "cholesterol excesses" in the diet. It is clear that vegetarians have a higher intake of plant sterols and this may be one of several reasons why vegetarians tend have better cardiovascular health than people who eat large amounts of meat or poultry products. Remember, vegetable soy protein may lower blood cholesterol.

Much science shows the ability of phytosterols to lower blood cholesterol and they do this primarily by inhibiting the absorption of cholesterol from the diet. In addition, they work by stopping the re-absorption of cholesterol in the gastrointestinal tract. This is an interesting trick of nature where a compound that resembles the chemical structure of cholesterol tends to "cheat the body," by reducing cholesterol input and increasing cholesterol elimination in the digestive tract. Phytosterols have complicated chemical names and they are most often produced by processing soybeans.

Common types of phytosterols include beta-sitosterol, stigmasterol and campesterol. Not only are these sterols important in the promotion of cardiovascular health, they are also beneficial for prostate health. Phytosterols provide an excellent additive component for supplements aimed at cholesterol control and cardiovascular health.

RED YEAST RICE

Many people are taking "statin types" of cholesterol-lowering drugs. These drugs are highly effective at reducing blood cholesterol, but they have unfortunate adverse effects. Adverse drug effects with statin medications include liver toxicity and sometimes serious damage to muscle tissue. Statin drugs deplete the body of the important energizing compound called Co-enzyme Q10 (CoQ10). I believe that CoQ10 should be replaced in everyone taking a statin drug (see Syndrome X, Chapter 16).

Nature has provided us with its own natural types of "statin compounds." Red yeast rice contains a substance called mevinolin (lovistatin, about 2%), which acts like a "statin-type" drug. This mechanism of action may occur by blocking the enzymes involved in the synthesis of cholesterol in the body (HMG CoA reductase). Red yeast rice has been marketed in the US as a dietary supplement, but it has been the subject of much debate among lawmakers. No doubt, the manufacturers of statin drugs felt challenged by a "natural statin" effect in plants.

One may reflect that there are many natural substances from herbs or botanicals that act like a drug and many prescription drugs have a structure that can be found in plant extracts. Red yeast rice is known to be effective in promoting a healthy blood cholesterol level with good tolerance by its users. Red yeast rice is used in cholesterol-lowering formulations, in a form that is extracted for its content of active natural principles.

THE POWER OF POLICOSANOL

Policosanol is a mixture of compounds isolated from plant waxes. Plant waxes from sugar cane and yams are preferred sources of this important complex, natural product. Policosanol has been shown to inhibit blood clotting, have favorable effects on lining cells in blood vessels (endothelium) and have significant benefits for controlling blood cholesterol. These plant wax components are known to decrease the stickiness of blood platelets which are involved in unwanted blood clotting; and this valuable action is complemented by supporting the health of the lining cells of blood vessels. It is negative changes in blood clotting and lining cells of blood vessels that cause the buildup of plaque in arteries (atheroma) and tend to form clots that occlude arteries. Atheroma underlies the manifestations and progressions of heart disease, heart attack, stroke and poor circulation. This process is clogging of arteries.

It appears that policosanol inhibits the synthesis of cholesterol in the body and it may increase the breakdown of bad cholesterol (LDL) by the liver. Animal studies have shown that policosanol may even prevent, and in some cases, reverse athcroma and thrombosis in blood vessels. Moreover, it is a powerful antioxidant that helps to prevent the formation of damaging types of oxidized cholesterol. In addition, other benefits have been noted with policosanol supplementation including: favorable changes in blood pressure, improvements in symptoms of coronary heart disease and better blood circulation to the extremities.

Short-term studies have compared the effectiveness of policosanol versus a popular type of a "statin," cholesterol-lowering drug. These studies that compared policosanol with a statin-type drug show similar decreases in bad cholesterol with similar increases in good cholesterol with each "treatment" (Benitez M and colleagues, Curr Ther Res, 58, 859, 97). These favorable results may be dose dependant, but I do not recommend the use of policosanol alone for the nutritional support of a healthy blood cholesterol level. Policosanol is a valuable component of my concepts of synergistic formulations.

OTHER BOTANICALS FOR CHOLESTEROL CONTROL

Garlic extract, guggulsterones (or Guggulipids®, Sabinsa Corp., NJ), and artichoke leaf have been used widely as dietary supplements to promote healthy blood cholesterol. Good scientific agreement exists that these three botanicals are active by virtue of their content of allicin, guggulsterones and cyanarin, respectively. These natural substances can be used in the formulation of synergistic supplements because of the long-standing precedent that they have for benefits in cholesterol chemistry. Some of these botanical agents have anti-inflammatory properties and it is known that cardiovascular disorders are closely linked to states of inflammation in the body (e.g. elevated blood C-reactive protein, CRP, a marker of inflammation). Remember the concepts of **"obesitis"** and **"diabetitis"** (add **"cardiovascularitis"**).

OTHER INGREDIENTS OF SYNERGISTIC SUPPLEMENTS:

Within my recommendations for heart and cardiovascular health are vitamin B12, vitamin B6, niacin, folic acid and trymethylglycine in a form that will help to promote a healthy blood homocysteine level. A further addition to cholesterol lowering formulae is chromium polynicotinate. Chromium has much scientific backing to support its benefit for assistance in the function of insulin and the promotion of healthy blood cholesterol. I believe that there is little evidence to suggest polynicotinate forms of chromium are any more or less effective than picolinate forms.

KEYNOTE SUMMARY: CHOLESTEROL
(DO NOT FORGET HOMOCYSTEINE)

I have a strong opinion that consumers of dietary supplements are not served well by the recommendations for single component supplements to promote a healthy blood cholesterol level. This is why I formulated versatile supplements for cholesterol control. These formulations have been adopted by others. The promotion of healthy blood cholesterol has become an appropriate national obsession, resulting in the sale of billions of dollars worth of cholesterol lowering drugs, mainly of the statin type. Lowering blood cholesterol with statin drugs in groups of individuals that are at high risk for cardiovascular disease and stroke is documented to be cost effective and appropriate in medical practice. What may be questioned about these drugs is their use as first line options to lower blood cholesterol, without paying appropriate attention to lifestyle adjustments and nutritional interventions to promote a healthy blood cholesterol level.

The statin group of drugs causes common side effects and, on occasion, they cause serious adverse effects including skin rashes, liver problems and severe damage to muscles, with occasional, but infrequent deaths. I believe that the first line option to deal with cholesterol problems involves lifestyle change with specific dietary adjustments and the use of dietary supplements or healthy foods. The prime objectives are to lower bad forms of cholesterol (low density lipoproteins, LDL) and increase good forms of cholesterol (high density lipoproteins, HDL), preferably by natural means.

Drugs used to lower blood cholesterol exert most of their effects on lowering LDL only. Recently, drugs have been developed that may both lower LDL and increase HDL. That said, natural agents may often be more versatile at raising HDL, when combined with exercise, in comparison to some drugs. Furthermore, natural substances that provide nutritional support to promote healthy blood cholesterol have a high margin of safety and they do not share the adverse event profile of commonly used cholesterol-lowering drugs. Natural approaches to promote a healthy blood cholesterol level are often less expensive than prescription drugs and they can incorporate blood homocysteine-lowering strategies.

"Statin type" drugs are often prescribed to people with the metabolic Syndrome X for their disorders of blood cholesterol, but individuals with Syndrome X may often have underlying liver disease due to fatty liver. This means that a large proportion of the target population using "statin drugs" have pre-existing, disordered liver function, as a consequence of their disease. Furthermore, one must appreciate that the commonest reason for an individual to stop taking a statin drug is liver toxicity. Therefore, common sense would question the widespread use of some statin drugs in people with the metabolic Syndrome X. One may appreciate why so many people on statin drugs have to stop these medications because they develop laboratory abnormalities that signal the presence of liver damage (raised blood levels of liver enzymes). This information may have been "brushed under the carpet." Make sure you spot Syndrome X.

There are several compelling reasons why one would elect to take a safe, natural and simple approach to promoting a healthy blood cholesterol and homocysteine level. Please note that the author avoids direct statements about "lowering blood cholesterol" because such statements are reserved for drug treatments. The author emphasizes that cholesterol-lowering drugs have a real benefit and specific role when used correctly. Dietary supplement companies that completely deny the benefits of cholesterol-lowering drugs are not serving the best interests of the general public. Statin drugs are valuable when used correctly.

The risk of heart disease and stroke is not all about cholesterol alone. Elevated blood homocysteine and body inflammation are important independent risk factors for cardiovascular disease. Cholesterol lowering drugs do not address the problem of elevated blood homocysteine. Many of the 70 million Americans with the metabolic Syndrome X have elevated blood cholesterol related to insulin resistance and, again, drugs used to lower cholesterol do not address insulin resistance. However, some evidence exists that statin drugs may exert their benefits in cardiovascular disease prevention by an anti-inflammatory effect. Moreover, there are many natural substances which can provide nutritional support to alter the normal body function of an inflammatory response (see Chapters 4 and 18 on Antioxidants and Fish Oil).

My proposals involve the use of dietary supplements to promote healthy blood cholesterol and a healthy blood homocysteine level. Proposed supplement formulations contain a wide range of botanical agents that may promote healthy blood cholesterol and homocysteine levels; and some of the valuable supplements' ingredients may partially modify aspects of the normal body function of an inflammatory response. Fish oil (Chapter 18) is a "must" to consider for cardiovascular health.

CONCLUSION

Controlling high blood cholesterol and homocysteine are important issues in the promotion of cardiovascular health. First-line options to deal with lowering blood cholesterol and homocysteine do not include drugs, for many people. Lifestyle changes from negative to positive, together with well planned nutritional interventions can make a real difference to the cardiovascular and general health of the US nation. Furthermore, natural approaches to cholesterol control may complement conventional medical ways of dealing with high blood cholesterol!

CHAPTER 20

HEART

NATURAL WAYS TO HEALTHY CARDIOVASCULAR STRUCTURE AND FUNCTION

CARDIOVASCULAR disease remains the number one killer in industrialized societies. Ensuring cardiovascular health is much more complex than taking a single dietary supplement, a drug or a combination of supplements and drugs. The importance of positive lifestyle figures strongly in the prevention of cardiovascular disease. This issue requires reinforcement. Heart disease is closely linked to the increasing epidemics of obesity, metabolic Syndrome X and diabetes mellitus. In fact, the presence of diabetes mellitus may increase the risk of developing heart disease in some people by a factor up to several times.

The causes of cardiovascular disease are many and varied. Indeed, opinions change on the importance of certain factors in promoting heart disease. For half a century the role of cholesterol in the promotion of heart disease has been at the forefront of medical thinking. In recent times, the role of elevated blood homocysteine, oxidative stress, altered immune function and inflammatory responses in the body, (elevated blood C-reactive protein, CRP, etc) have attracted much attention as important risk factors for heart disease.

Much emphasis has been placed on controlling bad types of blood cholesterol (LDL) for the prevention of heart disease. Modern research implies that increasing blood levels of good cholesterol (HDL) may be as powerful as lowering total blood cholesterol. Heart disease cannot be approached from one single dimension. Programs that are designed to manage or prevent heart disease must be "holistic." Furthermore, intensive nutritional and lifestyle changes may reverse heart disease, to a variable degree.

Many people could ask an important but simple question: "Why do we still have such a stubborn presence of disability and premature death from heart disease, when we have had so many advances in the diagnosis and treatment of cardiovascular disorders, such as: new diagnostic testing, new drugs and new surgical procedures?" The answer to this question may be simpler than many people think.

I believe that medicine has focused too much attention on addressing one risk factor for heart disease, at the expense of considering the simultaneous management of multiple risk factors for heart disease. In other words, I am talking about "connecting the dots" among disorders that promote heart disease. This is why concepts such as the metabolic Syndrome X are so important. In these and other circumstances, several cardiovascular risk factors aggregate together in a very damaging manner (Syndrome X, Chapter 16).

I believe that the preferred approach to preventing heart disease is to tackle as many risk factors as possible at the same time. This philosophy underscores the importance of managing the metabolic Syndrome X, but the "penny is still waiting to drop" in modern medicine and even in the dietary supplement industry. In several public presentations, I have referred to the nutritional and lifestyle management of the metabolic Syndrome X as the most important initiative for natural medicine and the health food industry. Indeed, this initiative is the most important public health initiative for all healthcare givers in Western society (Appendix C).

Against this background, who could be so naïve enough to believe that "just" lowering blood cholesterol or "just" losing weight or "just" controlling blood pressure, in the absence of a comprehensive medical approach, could lead to a substantial reduction in the occurrence of heart disease? Few people could argue that the most important intervention for heart disease prevention includes public education and positive lifestyle change. These public health interventions will do more to improve the general health of the population than any new drug or new surgical procedure. This approach requires education ("edutherapics").

Perhaps some of our clear priorities in health care are ignored. "An ounce of prevention is definitely worth more than one pound of a cure." The reader may reflect on the fact that most money spent on healthcare in the US goes to cover the cost of established disease, where only "rehabilitation," rather than cure, may be possible. Certainly, disease should be avoided if it can be avoided.

FURTHER OBSERVATIONS ON CARDIOVASCULAR DISEASE

In recent times, physicians, patients and major bodies of medical opinion (e.g., American Heart Association) have drawn attention to the mismanagement and misdiagnosis of heart disease in mature women. Management of cardiovascular disease in women is associated with "red flags" and, these days, "red dresses."

The significance of menopause for cardiovascular health in women is the recognition that heart disease in the postmenopausal female occurs with a similar frequency to that of men of the equivalent age (see Chapter 3, Menopause and PMS). In other words, the heart protection afforded the pre-menopausal female does not survive the transition of the menopause. Thus, menopause can be seen to be a time in life where the occurrence of cardiovascular disease "equilibrates" in men and women.

It has been well-recognized that pre-menopausal females are relatively protected from cardiovascular disease, but the common nature of heart disease in postmenopausal females has only recently become a focus of public interest (see Chapter 3, Menopause and PMS). The presentation of heart disease in women may be quite atypical, in comparison with its presentation in mature men.

Signs of heart disease in women are often more subtle than they are in men; and this tests the diagnostic acumen of a treating physician. It is unfortunate that HRT or perhaps ERT affords no consistent protection against the occurrence of heart disease in mature women (Chapter 3). In some women with circumstances of cardiovascular risk, conventional HRT may compound the risk of heart disease (Holt S, Menopause and PMS Naturally, Wellness Publishing, Little Falls, NJ, 2008). It is not known if bio-identical hormones are any safer in this context.

DIETARY SUPPLEMENTS FOR HEART HEALTH

There is no simple dietary supplement or simple natural formula that could cover all aspects of the nutritional support of heart health. I stress the importance of controlling weight (Weight Management, see Chapter 15) and a combat against the metabolic Syndrome X (see Syndrome X, Chapter 16) in promoting heart health. Furthermore, one cannot underestimate the benefits of fish oil for heart health (see Fish Oil, Chapter 18). Of course, I must focus on the importance of healthy blood cholesterol and healthy blood homocysteine (see Cholesterol, Chapter 19).

Synergistic formulae for heart health contain a number of nutrients, herbs and botanicals that have beneficial effects of cardiovascular structure and function. In brief, Gingko biloba promotes blood flow and citrus bioflavanoids support small vessel structure in the body. Magnesium may be deficient in many people with heart disease, especially when water tablets (diuretics) are taken or if excessive urination, is present e.g. from alcohol intake or diabetes or pre-diabetes. The botanicals, garlic and Hawthorn berries have well-documented cardiovascular benefits and they may be included in dietary supplements that are "heart healthy." Isoflavones are included in my proposals because of their potent and versatile antioxidant effects and their ability to inhibit stickiness of platelets that may cause blood clotting. Resveratrol and selenium are important antioxidant compounds for heart health and extra B vitamins are included in the recommended formulae for their general nutritive and anti-stress properties that support cardiovascular health.

KEYNOTE SUMMARY: A HEALTHY HEART

Many things can "break" the human heart. The role of common depression in promoting heart disease is often overlooked. In spite of major advances in medical research, many people die of a heart attack or cardiovascular disease.

The author has proposed a "Cardio Plan" for maintenance of heart health which includes the obvious such as weight control, blood pressure control, exercise, and cessation of substance abuse, maintenance of psychological wellbeing and moderation of type A behavior. (Holt S. *Natural Way to a Healthy Heart*, M. Evans Publishers, NY, NY, 2000) The dietary supplement industry keeps focusing upon single agents for heart health, such as Vitamin E, co-enzyme Q10, ribose and the rest. Again, who would be so naïve enough to believe that a single agent is a solution to the problem of cardiovascular disease, with its multiple causes?

My supplement proposals are examples of synergistic dietary supplements that must not be used in the absence of positive lifestyle changes to promote cardiovascular health (edutherapies). Healthcare givers who minimize the importance of healthy blood cholesterol levels should join "the flat earth society" (see Cholesterol, Chapter 19), but prevention of heart disease involves much more than just lowering blood cholesterol. Please do not forget homocysteine.

Education in the prevention of heart disease is the most important issue in the promotion of cardiovascular health. Dietary supplements that provide nutritional support for heart health may be quite valuable for many people. Complex formulations of natural ingredients that support heart health are preferred.

The ingredients of optimal heart healthy supplements include synergistic blends of natural nutrients and botanicals that have an evidence base as nutritional support for cardiovascular health. These ingredients include: N-Acetyl-L-Carnitine, Gingko biloba, Magnesium, Citrus Bioflavanoids, Garlic Extract, Hawthorne Berries, Lecithin, Trimethylglycine, Isoflavones, Resveratrol, Vitamin B6, Folic Acid, Selenium, and Vitamin B12. The potent and versatile ability of omega-3 fatty acids (fish oil) to promote cardiovascular and general cellular health must be considered.

I deliver a simple message that heart disease is a legacy of bad diet, substance abuse, idleness and all of those factors that contribute to the cause of metabolic syndrome X. Modern research links depression and anxiety, with or without identifiable stress as primary factors that promote heart disease, with its stubborn negative outcomes for millions of people.

CHAPTER 21

PROSTATE

ENLARGEMENT of the prostate is so common that it effects every man if he lives long enough. Prostatic enlargement contributes to poor sexual function in mature males (Sex, Chapter 22). The modern man has learned to "love his prostate." This means that the use of appropriate diet, lifestyle and dietary supplements have emerged as valuable options for maintaining healthy structure and function of the prostate. Symptoms of prostatic enlargement include frequency of urination, poor urinary stream, and "dribbling." It is important to know if these symptoms are due to cancer of the prostate and any man with these symptoms should be screened to exclude prostate cancer.

Consumer surveys show that mature females are concerned increasingly about prostate health in their partners. A mature woman often contributes to the general maintenance of health and well-being of her husband and their family. There are several general nutritional principles that are to be considered for the promotion of prostatic health. These include the restriction of simple sugars in the diet, the drinking of alcohol in moderate amounts and the avoidance of smoking. The role of excessive protein and saturated fat intake in the diet as a cause of prostate cancer remains debatable, but much evidence has suggested that the enhancement of vegetable protein intake, e.g. soy, is highly benificial for prostate health (Holt S. "The Soy Revolution," Dell Publishing, NY. 2000).

Several specific vitamins and trace elements have value in the nutritional support of a healthy prostate. The evidence for supporting good prostatic structure and function with selected dietary substances has increased dramatically over the last ten years. There is good scientific agreement that several herbs or botanicals can benefit prostate health. This has resulted in the emergence of many different dietary supplements to support prostate health, but many of these dietary supplements do not contain a sufficient amount or range of beneficial natural substances for the support of prostatic structure and function.

Well formulated products for prostate health contain a complete and versatile combination of natural substances, including botanicals, herbs and nutrients that have a scientific basis for use as nutritional support for a healthy prostate (Table 30). These concepts are the basis of the complex formula that I propose for a healthy prostate.

A RANGE OF NATURAL SUBSTANCES TO PROVIDE NUTRITIONAL SUPPORT FOR PROSTATE STRUCTURE AND FUNCTION

Saw Palmetto	Stinging Nettle Leaves
Pygeum Africanum	Pumpkin Seed
Beta Sitosterol Complex	Lycopene
L-Alanine	L-Glycine
L-Glutamic Acid	Soy Isoflavones
Vitamin E	Zinc
Vitamin A (Acetate)	Vitamin C
Vitamin D3	Vitamin K1
Vitamin B Series	Pantothenic Acid
Niacinamide	Iron
Folic Acid	Potassium
Calcium	Copper
Magnesium	Boron
Iodine	Chromium
Selenium	Vanadium
Molybdenum	

Table 30: Natural substances that provide nutritional support for prostate structure and function (Holt MD Technologies).

KEYNOTE SUMMARY: PROSTATE HEALTH

The common occurrence of negative changes in the structure and function of the prostate with age means that every mature man must focus attention on a healthy prostate. There are several general lifestyle and nutritional principles that are to be considered for the promotion of a healthy prostate. There is good scientific agreement that several nutrients, herbs or botanicals can benefit prostate health.

MOST PROSTATE SUPPLEMENTS ARE INADEQUATE IN THEIR RANGE OF CONTENTS. NEW INFORMATION EXISTS ON THE BENEFIT OF NATURAL MEDICINE FOR PROSTATE HEALTH.

CHAPTER 22

SEX NATURALLY

BACKGROUND

ERECTILE dysfunction (ED) is the inability to achieve or sustain a penile (or clitorine) erection. It is treated often by Viagra® and related drugs (Cialis® and Levitra®). The sexual response cycle involves more than just "woody" appendages. There are dietary supplements which may act favorably on the sexual response cycle. The effectiveness of drugs in the immediate reversal of ED may exceed that of many dietary supplements that are used to support sexual function. However, I reiterate that there is much more involved in sexual union than the rapid achievement of penile hardness (tumescence). Many people believe that the management of ED is by no means a medical emergency. On this basis, many people are exploring the use of natural options as first-line approaches for sexual wellbeing (Holt S, "Sex Naturally," Wellness Publishing Inc, Little Falls, NJ, 2008).

Drugs that are approved for the treatment of ED go to only a limited part of the sexual response cycle. This complex cycle of sexual function involves foreplay, plateaus of excitement and orgasm. It is well recognized that good cardiovascular function is a key factor in promoting good sexual function. Positive lifestyle changes and good nutrition can help the structure and function of the genital organs in both women and men. In particular, nutritional support with the nutrient Arginine may assist blood flow to the pelvis and sexual organs. Arginine is heart healthy and it is a precursor of nitric oxide. In contrast, drugs used in erectile dysfunction have been associated with adverse cardiac events.

ARGININE: A NITRIC OXIDE TOOL FOR SEXUAL FUNCTION

Who would think that Arginine, a common amino acid found in dietary proteins, could help in the promotion of sexual function? The amino acid L-Arginine has been proposed as a component of nutritional supplements that represent a gradual, simple, gentle and natural approach to supporting cardiovascular health and blood flow to the penis or female genital organs.

L-Arginine is a nutrient that is a precursor of nitric oxide (NO) in the body. It provides nutritional support to generate chemicals that relax smooth muscle in the penis or perhaps the clitoris. This process of relaxation of smooth muscles initiates and maintains penile or clitorine erections. Relaxation of muscles in blood vessels permits bloodflow. It is the engorgement of tissues in the penis or clitoris that causes erections of these body appendages. L-Arginine has been proposed for many years and featured as nutritional support for cardiovascular health in two important books entitled "The Arginine Solution" by Robert Fried, PhD, and Woodson Merrell, M.D., (Warner Books, N.Y., 1999) and "The Amino Revolution" by Robert Erdmann, Ph.D., (Simon and Schuster, N.Y., 1987).

An understanding of the benefits of L-Arginine as a dietary supplement involves an understanding of the role of nitric oxide (NO) in driving several healthy body functions. The role that nitric oxide plays in body functions was elucidated by American researchers in the 1990s. These researchers were awarded the Nobel Prize for Medicine in 1998. In brief, L-Arginine is converted by the body into nitric oxide.

FUNCTIONS OF NITRIC OXIDE (NO)

Nitric oxide works as a chemical messenger which affects communications that control several body functions such as:

- It is used by the brain itself to store memory and regulate blood flow to the brain.
- It helps to maintain normal blood pressure, the opening of arteries supplying the heart, antioxidant functions, actions on body immunity, assistance with function of the lungs, and the release of vital hormones that are required for well-being.
- It enhances blood flow to the penis or female sexual organs and helps boost penile or clitorine erections.

While L-Arginine is nutritional support for blood flow, it needs to be taken at least an hour or two before sexual intercourse and preferably taken in a consistent daily manner over a period of several weeks. There is no clear recommendation on the ideal dose of L-Arginine to support sexual functions, but observations indicate that at least one gram per day of L-Arginine must be taken to load the body over a period of a couple of weeks or so and it should be continued thereafter, when required. Thus, regular Arginine use is required for an effect.

L-Arginine has a good safety margin and there is no problem in taking larger doses of L-Arginine, as required, e.g. up to six grams per day. There are some ways of potentiating the benefits of the use of the nutrient L Arginine by using certain herbs or botanicals that may also improve sexual function. The use of L-Arginine in this form, combined with other natural supplements, can form a dietary supplement to promote healthy sexual activity. L-Arginine must not be taken with Viagra or related drugs, because it increases NO levels in the body and so does Viagra and related drugs. There are no conclusive, comparative, scientific studies that compare the effectiveness of L-Arginine supplementation with Viagra or related drugs for the management of disordered sexual function.

SYNERGISTIC FORMULATIONS FOR SEXUAL FUNCTION

I propose the combination of L-Arginine with the variable addition of standardized extracts of Ginkgo biloba (24% extract), Tribulus terrestris (40% extract), Maca root (0.6% extract), Panax ginseng (5% extract), Muira puama (variable strength), together with niacin, in variable amounts. This combination is the basis of a dietary supplement. This dietary supplement has to be taken on a continuous basis in order to have nutritional benefits. Individuals are strongly advised to not mix drugs and supplements without advice. Holt MD Technologies has produced more amplified versions of nitric oxide generators by dosage adjustments in formulations.

KEYNOTE SUMMARY: SEX

Healthy sexual activity prevents and heals disease and it promotes enormous wellbeing. It is a key anti-aging strategy. Supporting the structures and functions of the reproductive tract is possible with several herbs and nutrients. A new area of science has emerged in the nutritional support of sexual function in men and women. ("Sex Naturally," Wellness Publishing Inc., Little Falls, NJ, 2008)

Healthy and gratifying sexual encounters involve more than a focused approach with drugs that correct erectile dysfunction in men or poor pelvic blood flow in women. A common underlying cause for poor sexual function in men and women is poor cardiovascular function. Drugs for erectile dysfunction work by increasing levels of nitric oxide which is a chemical messenger that promotes blood flow. Dietary supplements are available that contain L-Arginine with the addition of several other nutrients or herbs that have a variable evidence base to support sexual function. L-Arginine is the origin of the nitric oxide in the human body and its administration drives the production of this chemical messenger to promote blood flow in several regions of the body. Furthermore, L-Arginine is heart healthy.

In addition to the precursor technology of L-Arginine, proposed sex supporting supplement formulae contain Tribulus terrestris, Maca root, Muira puama, Horny goat weed, Gingko biloba, Ginseng panax, Grape seed and Niacinamide. These dietary supplements provide added health advantages because of their antioxidant content and potential energizing benefits. Some of the adaptogenic herbal components of synergistic, sex-enhancing formulae may promote "feelings" or drives toward sexual activity, but these outcomes are difficult to measure. Dietary supplements of this type must be taken on a regular basis for best nutritional effects. Healthy sex is part of a healthy lifestyle program.

CHAPTER 23

MEMORY: BRAIN FUNCTION

POOR BRAIN FUNCTION: ROBBING QUALITY OF LIFE

POOR mental functioning often affects the quality of life of our cherished elderly population. Temporary changes in cognition (brain function) are noted in women with PMS, menopause and post-menopause. Women with PMS describe forgetfulness, poor concentration, clumsiness and even the "jitters"; and those in the menopausal transition often develop episodes of poor mental function, compounded by anxiety and emotional disturbance. Temporary upsets of cognition also affect men commonly, especially during stressful life events.

The menopause may herald a slow decline in overall brain function in some women. Elderly women may develop significant loss of brain function and even dementia, from diseases such as Alzheimer's disease or cerebrovascular disease. Declining brain function many have several different causes, but common temporary upsets in cognitive activity (general brain function) should not be seen as symptoms of serious brain disease. These temporary upsets in the workings of the brain seem to go away often (spontaneous resolution or healing). A common cause of short-lived episodes of poor brain function is sleeplessness. This circumstance is reversed readily with restoration of healthy sleep. However, this is not the situation in serious forms of dementia that can occur in a progressive manner in the mature man or women.

Few people realize that chronic brain damage from cardiovascular disease or Alzheimer's disease begins many years before declining brain function becomes obvious. In the case of Alzheimer's disease, changes in the brain that cause this disorder may occur in the age group 40-50 years. However, the diagnosis of Alzheimer's disease does not usually become apparent until an individual is about 60 or more years of age. These days, many people are taking early steps to try and prevent common deteriorations in the structure and the function of the brain. Prevention of deterioration of brain function can be approached by positive lifestyle changes, including good nutrition and restful sleep. During sleep the brain creates new connections (synapses) and it "orders" thoughts. Sleep deprivation results invariably in poor psychomotor body function (Sleep, Chapter 3).

MAINTAINING BRAIN HEALTH

There are many new treatments or interventions that have been proposed to prevent or reduce age-related declines in brain function. Impairment of brain function is often called "cognitive" decline or deficit. Cognitive decline has been perceived, perhaps incorrectly, as an inevitable consequence of growing old. I reject this idea and I propose that there are many natural first-line options that can be exercised to maintain "cognitive vitality" (good brain function).

While memory is seen as a primary function of the brain, an individual's conscious awareness comes from outside the body; and memory is probably a function of the whole body itself. For example, the gastrointestinal tract and the immune system function with their own cognitive skills and the organs of the digestive tract have both memories and learning skills! This modern concept credits the gastrointestinal tract with its own series of small brains and an ability to engage in what has been called "visceral learning." These concepts are some of the many details of mind-body interactions. Without a healthy mind, there cannot be health of the body and vice versa.

We know that a decline in brain function occurs for many reasons. Impairments in mental agility vary greatly from episodes of simple forgetfulness or "blocking of thoughts," through to complete states of mental vegetation or dementia. The elderly population is rapidly expanding in Western society. Up to one in four of these elite citizens suffer from significant degrees of poor brain function.

A common cause of cognitive decline is Alzheimer's disease. Alzheimer's disease has an inflammatory component and it is linked with Syndrome X. Early promises that HRT and ERT would prevent declines in brain function in women have been replaced by findings that some women who have taken HRT are found to be at greater risk of dementia (see Menopause and PMS, Chapter 3). This observation may be related to the timing of taking HRT and it is a complex issue.

WHAT CAUSES COGNITIVE DECLINE?

There are many risk factors for poor brain function. The risks include: cardiovascular disease, chronic stress, poor diet, lack of both physical and "brain" exercises and head injury of various types. "Mental cloudiness" is experienced often by people who severely restrict dietary carbohydrate intake in order to lose weight. Mental fuzziness occurs during low-carb diets because the simple sugar (glucose) is the principal source of fuel for the brain cells.

Some people with poor cognitive function get a temporary improvement in their memory with glucose intake, but this is not a reason to use excessive amounts of simple sugars in the diet (Syndrome X, Chapter 16). Several studies have linked cognitive decline and dementia with the metabolic Syndrome X. I restate that every woman should now understand how important a combat against Syndrome X is for their general well-being (Syndrome X, Chapter 16 and Blood Sugar, Chapter 17). Remember, Syndrome X "loads the gun" of disability often and menopause "pulls the trigger."

Population studies show that diets high in saturated fats and low in Omega-3 fatty acids (fish oil) may contribute to cognitive decline. I advise everyone who is seeking cardiovascular and brain health to consider increasing the amount of Omega-3 fatty acids in their diets by eating fish and/or by taking high quality fish oil supplements, preferably in enteric-coated gels. (see Fish Oil, Chapter 18).

Omega-3 fatty acids (DHA) are principal building blocks in the brain and there is a widespread deficiency of omega 3 fatty acid intake in Western diets. Blood cholesterol and homocysteine control is very important for the maintenance of brain function. These can be achieved with the use of lifestyle change combined with optimal diet and the use of selected dietary supplements (Cholesterol, Chapter 19).

I must emphasize that cardiovascular health goes hand in hand with brain health. Diseases of the cardiovascular system such as stroke and hardening of the arteries (atherosclerosis) can cause irreparable damage to brain tissue (Cholesterol, Chapter 19).

LIFESTYLE AND NUTRITIONAL ADVICE FOR GOOD BRAIN FUNCTION

While some interventions for improving brain function are obvious, others are so obvious that they are often overlooked. Much evidence has emerged that there is a growing epidemic of sleeplessness. Sleep deprivation causes both physical and mental disability, largely because it disturbs biological rhythms, affects cognitive function and causes hormone imbalances. Good sleep hygiene and well selected nutritional support for sleep are important antidotes to poor mental function. I have discussed these matters in detail in the book entitled "Sleep Naturally" (Sleep, Chapter 2).

Physical exercise confers benefits on general body health and mental function. The type and amount of exercise required for health in mature people does not have to be strenuous, but it should be undertaken on a regular basis. Regular exercise in any age group consistently improves general health. While the body needs to be exercised and kept in peak condition, the brain requires "exercise" by activity that challenges thought processes.

Anyone who is troubled by declining mental function can benefit from hobbies or pleasurable games such as chess, crossword puzzles or simple arts and crafts. In fact, there are studies showing that people who engage in "mind exercises" were more than two and one half times less likely to develop Alzheimer's disease.

Scientists and physicians have described the "disuse syndrome". In this condition, inactive people who do not motivate themselves to "move or think" can age more rapidly than the active individual. There is no doubt that modern lifestyle has encouraged mental and physical idleness (Antiaging, Chapter 31).

It may seem that my comments are more relevant to the elderly, but modern medicine has not emphasized the need to use lifestyle changes in younger people to prevent later declines in brain function. What I recommend in lifestyle changes is just as relevant to mature adults or middle-aged individuals as it is to the elderly.

STRESS BUSTING AND GOOD BRAIN FUNCTION

Stress is a great mimic of disease. When one is placed under excessive stress, mental function can decline. This leads to the obvious conclusion that "stress busting" is very valuable in reversing temporary upsets with memory, mental focus and general body skills. Relaxation exercises or healthy interventions, such as yoga or music therapy, can help the mind and brain to restore balance.

Stress hormones produced by the body may be somewhat "toxic" to the nervous system and high levels of these hormones have been associated with poor memory. Therefore, many physicians are recommending techniques to cope with psychological problems. Some psychological stresses can adversely affect brain function in a profound manner e.g. bereavement, divorce etc.

MEMORY-PROTECTIVE DIETS AND PSYCHO-NUTRITION

Of all interventions, good nutrition affords great promise for the protection of memory and efficient thought processing by the brain. I restate that general nutritional recommendations for memory protection include controlled calorie intake, limitation of saturated fat intake in the diet and other positive dietary changes, such as increased consumption of Omega 3 fatty acids, increased dietary fiber intake, increased fruit and vegetable consumption, reduced meat intake and the avoidance of chemical pollutants in the environment.

Beyond these general recommendations are a number of specific nutrients or botanicals that have a basis in science for the nutritional support of brain function. Combinations of these brain specific natural agents can be used to make valuable dietary supplements to promote cognitive function. I am a great supporter of fruit, berry, vegetable and greens powders that can provide "missing-links" of antioxidants for good brain health. Hormonal deficiencies can affect brain function profoundly, e.g. hypothyroid states and adrenal gland compromise (Chapter 32).

THE POWER OF PHOSPHOLIPIDS FOR BRAIN STRUCTURE AND FUNCTION

Phospholipids are naturally occurring chemical compounds that form a key structural component of all membranes that surround cells. The function of the brain is highly dependent upon the health of membranes around nerve cells. Thus, a good dietary source of phospholipids can have major benefits on the structure and function of the brain. Important types of phospholipids that have specific nutritional benefits for the function of the central nervous system include: phosphatidylserine (PS), phosphatidylcholine (PC), phosphatidylthenolamine (PE) and phosphatidylinositol (PI) … don't get "bogged down" in names!

In nervous tissue, PS plays a major role in the conduction of nerve impulses. This conduction of messages through the brain involves the release of chemical substances that are involved in the transmission of nervous signals. Scientific studies have shown that PS can improve measures of brain function in people with cognitive impairment (poor memory or lack of mental alertness); and PS has been shown to be valuable in the nutritional support of certain brain functions in people with early Alzheimer's disease.

Not only has PS been shown to have this usefulness in helping to improve cognitive deficit, it seems to improve loss of memory associated with aging and poor mental function in dementia from causes other than Alzheimer's disease.

Added benefits of PS are its positive effects on immune function and even its ability to reduce "stress" to the body that is caused by exercise (adaptogenic formulations). In other words, phospholipids can counter oxidative stress to brain tissues.

The evidence of the benefits of PS has been shown in double-blind clinical studies and in many animal experiments. In one large study in humans, performed in different medical centers of excellence, improvements on several measures of brain function were recorded in people with Alzheimer's disease and these results were found to be significant. Therefore, phospholipids are evidence-based for the support of brain function and they form an important part of the formulation of the dietary supplements, used to support brain function. Phospholipids are "adaptogenic nutrients."

The other types of phospholipids that have emerged with value for their nutritional support for brain function and structure include: phosphatidylcholine (PC), phosphatidylthenolamine (PE), and phosphatidylinositol (PI). These phospholipids have very complicated names but they all share in common an ability to improve the membrane structures of the central nervous system. Each of these phospholipids have added, unique health benefits. For example, PC (phosphatidylcholine) has an ability to provide constituents of the chemical transmitters that are used by the brain (e.g., the neurotransmitter acetylcholine). Furthermore, PC (phosphatidylcholine) may have protective effects on the liver and it alters blood lipids (cholesterol) in favorable ways.

ENERGY CONVERSION FOR BRAIN FUNCTION: ACETY-L-CARNITINE

Acety-L-Carnitine [ALC] provides versatile and potent support for the function of nervous tissue. On the one hand, ALC assists in the burning of fuel inside energy factories (mitochondria) in nerve cells, whereas, on the other, it involves itself in the manufacture of chemicals that transmit messages in the brain (neurotransmitters). ALC has a rich history of scientific study in the nutritional management of declines in cognitive function.

In some disorders of cognition, there is a deficit in the neurotransmitter acetylcholine and ALC may help reverse this deficit. ALC has been shown to improve the action of phospholipids in nerve cell membranes by favorably altering chemistry in the brain. These properties of ALC mean that it has an additive benefit when used with other phospholipids. This is a clear example of producing nutritional synergy.

Of major importance, is the potential anti-aging activity of ALC, where it may alter cross-linking between sugar and protein (AGES). This activity of

ALC makes it a very desirable supplement for use in people with Syndrome X, prediabetes or diabetes mellitus. In summary, ALC shows protective effects on the structure and function of nervous tissue and it may increase blood flow to the brain. Research indicates that ALC plays a role in the nutritional management of neuropathies. These are disorders of the nerves supplying various parts of the body, especially the feet and hands e.g. diabetic neuropathy. ALC has important antiaging actions (Chapter 31).

VINPOCETINE: A MEMORY SECRET

Vinpocetine is derived from a plant that is a member of the periwinkle family (Vinca minor). While vinpocetine is widely used in Europe and Japan as a drug for the treatment of cognitive disorders, in the U.S. vinpocetine is available as a valuable dietary supplement.

This extract of periwinkle plant increases blood flow to the brain and has a positive effect on the overall chemistry of the brain. It is an antioxidant which seems to protect nervous tissue against free radical damage and enhance brain function in a general manner. Antioxidants generally have anti-aging properties on many body tissues (Chapters 4 and 31). Vinpocetine may exert some effects on dilating blood vessels that supply the brain. It appears that vinpocetine has special nutritional properties in circumstances of problems with vascular structure and function of the brain. This clumsy way of saying things is related to regulatory constraints that govern claims about supplements. I speak the forced language of "neologisms."

Some studies support the nutritional value of vinpocetine in people with dementia. The nutritional power of vinpocetine is more apparent in cases of cerebrovascular disease. Added benefits of vinpocetine include a protective effect on the stomach, reduction in motion sickness, and some protective actions for good sight and hearing.

A SOY TREASURE: L-ALPHA-GLYCERYLPHOSPHORYLCHOLINE (ALPHA-GPC)

Alpha-GPC is a natural substance that originates from lecithin, a major component of soybeans. Lecithin is quite valuable for cardiovascular and central nervous system structure and function. There have been many proposals about the health benefits of Alpha-GPC. This potent and versatile supplement can enhance the actions of the neurotransmitter acetylcholine. It is recognized that people with Alzheimer's disease can suffer from a relative deficiency of acetylcholine and

Alpha-GPC may partially compensate for this deficiency. Studies show that Alpha-GPC provides valuable nutritional support in people with Alzheimer's disease.

An interesting effect of Alpha-GPC is its ability to enhance the overall actions of growth hormone. Growth hormone is commonly used in anti-aging medicine. It is speculated that Alpha-GPC may enhance growth hormone secretion from the pituitary gland. The complex actions of Alpha-GPC have led to its use as "an anti-aging supplement" that can enhance the availability of human growth hormone in the body. Alpha-GPC is gaining increasing acceptance in alternative medicine as valuable nutritional support for cognitive disorders (Antiaging, Chapter 31).

SUMMING UP ON BRAIN FUNCTION

Dementia, in mature men and women, is on the rise. My messages are not just for those who have experienced declines in cognitive ability. Mature individuals are advised to think far in advance to support their brain function. People must not let the "misplaced keys of today" become the "cognitive decline of tomorrow." An ounce of prevention is certainly worth more than a pound of cure to promote health, longevity and quality of life in society. Contrary to legal mandates, people are using supplements increasingly to prevent disease.

KEYNOTE SUMMARY: MEMORY

The reduction of age-related decline in brain function is a key health initiative for Western society. Sometimes referred to as cognitive decline or deficit, this group of disorders is feared by a large proportion of the middle-aged or elderly population who wonder about the presence of early Alzheimer's disease.

Elegant things are often simple. Without good basic structure and function of the brain, there cannot be good memory and cognitive activity. Combination or synergistic dietary supplements can be designed to support the general structure and function of the central nervous system, so that individuals may maintain mental agility. Synergistic blends of nutrients may support brain structure and function, in a manner that can provide a nutritional complement to conventional medical treatments for declines in brain function. This approach assists in promoting a good structural basis for the central nervous system to exert its normal functions. Overall, the conventional drug treatments for dementia have been disappointing and associated with frequent adverse effects.

Promises that drug X or supplement Y can reverse established and serious declines in brain function are often shallow promises. Individuals must take preventative actions to combat the many risk factors for the development of poor brain function.

There have been a whole host of memory protective diets proposed to be of value. Many principles of "psycho-nutrition" have benefit. Obtaining all brain supporting nutrients from a standard Western diet (SAD) is not feasible for many people. For these reasons, scientists have researched brain-specific, supporting nutrients and botanicals that may exert beneficial effects on thinking, memory and overall mental agility. Forgetfulness and blocking of thoughts are the most embarrassing events for mature individuals. I must emphasize the importance of taking adequate amounts of Omega 3 fatty acids to support brain function (see Fish Oil, Chapter 18). Depression sometimes masquerades as mild dementia, especially in the elderly. Elevated blood homocysteine is associated often with poor brain function. Many supplements are proposed for memory but only evidence-based approaches should be considered.

The idea that single supplements or natural substances can support the complex structures and functions of the brain is quite naive. A complex combination of brain supporting nutrients that have an evidence base for nutritional support of the central nervous system is most desirable. My formulation proposals support brain function with: N-Acetyl-L-Carnitine, Lecithin, Alpha GPC, Turmeric Root, Green Tea, Ginkgo Biloba, Phosphatidyl Serine, DHA, Vinpocetine, Vitamin B6, Vitamin B1, Folic Acid and Vitamin B12. This formulation is proposed with the added advantage of promoting a healthy blood homocysteine level. Please review memory formulations and understand their inadequacies or advantages.

PSYCHONUTRITION WITH POSITIVE LIFESTYLE PROTECTS COGNITION. SYNERGISTIC FORMULATIONS OF SUPPLEMENTS HAVE CLEAR ADVANTAGES FOR HEALTHY COGNITION.

CHAPTER 24

SKIN, NAILS AND HAIR SUPPORT

COSMETICS AND COSMECEUTICALS

COSMETICS are a big part of the modern woman's life and they are increasingly important to men. Medical literature estimates that many Americans have side effects or adverse health outcomes from the topical use of synthetic chemicals that are often present in cosmetic products. While people discontinue cosmetics that are disagreeable, side effects are often unreported. Therefore, the damage caused by some of the toxic compounds found in cosmetics often passes unrecognized. Toxic chemicals can be absorbed readily through the skin and they can pass into the body with undetected consequences. Some topical poisons are absorbed and stored in body fat where they cause abnormal body chemistry.

Many individuals have an inappropriate opinion that the skin is a totally effective barrier to toxins. This mistaken assumption ignores the massive absorptive capacity of the human skin. The skin is the largest organ of the body and its appearance is a reflection of inner health. Like a plant, the skin receives incomplete nourishment from things applied externally, but the skin and a healthy plant, are nurtured from within their bodies. This is the concept of beauty from "within" rather than from "without" the body. Dermatologists, estheticians and cosmetologists are becoming very focused on "inner beauty" supported by good nutrition. Your beauty lies within©.

The growth of the "cosmeceutical industry" (natural skin-care products) is based on the idea that many natural substances provide effective alternatives to the man-made chemicals found in popular cosmetics. At least 500 harmful ingredients are found in commonly used makeup, hair products and skin creams. In his book, "Health Risks in Today's Cosmetics," (Alliance publishing, Va., 1994), my friend, Nikolaus J. Smeh, describes how to substitute many toxic chemicals found in cosmetics with natural extracts of herbs, botanicals and food substances. The list of side effects of some artificial cosmetic ingredients is horrifying, ranging from acne to cancer.

Modern cosmetologists have started to finally recognize the power of dietary supplements to support skin health. Antioxidants have found a great role in skin anti-aging, but they are probably more effective when given by mouth, compared with topical application. These are concepts that can be used in the ultimate care of the skin, where lifestyle issues are important. Cosmetics can hide a lot, but continuing to smoke, worshipping the sun and the adoption of a poor diet are the enemies of beautiful skin. Ordering fast food during a "cosmetic pampering" at a spa facility destroys the whole essence of a quest for beauty.

KEYNOTE SUMMARY: SKIN, NAIL AND HAIR SUPPORT

Anyone can "slap" cosmetics or other topical beauty aids on their skin and hair and get a temporary beneficial effect, but the appearance of the skin, nails and hair is a complete reflection of inner health. Healthy looking skin, nails and hair is always present in an individual who has a healthy body. This is what I refer to, again, as the concept of beauty from within the body, not beauty from the outside of the body, using "cosmetic cover-ups."

Antioxidant compounds have found a great role in topical products but antioxidants are most effective when given in the correct formulation by mouth as a dietary supplement. Dietary supplements of particular value in the support of skin, nail and hair structures include substances that will help build skin-supporting tissues that contain collagen, natural anti-wrinkling agents and antioxidants. Skin, nail and hair support products involve the use of a complex combination of nutrients and botanicals that will provide nutritional support to skin, nail and hair structure and function.

Skin and hair support formulations should contain innovative ingredients that have come to the forefront of nutritional sciences, as applied to skin care. Apart from the powerful antioxidant profile within these products, there are collagen-building substances and connective-tissue-supporting substances such as hyaluronate. The formulation possibilities are mentioned to provide examples of the many nutrients and botanicals that can provide nutritional support for skin health. The contents of proposals for skin, nail and hair support include the most complete array of skin-supporting natural substances in combined formulation and they include: Calcium (Eggshell), Horsetail, Olive Leaf, Vitamin C, Alpha Lipoic Acid, Fish Oil, DMAE, Grape Seed, Green Tea, Lecithin, MSM, Collagen, Aloe Vera, Vitamin E and Hyaluronate Sodium. The science of supplement support for "inner beauty" is expanding.

BEAUTYCEUTICALS

The concept that the perception of beauty is governed by inner health of the body has been grossly underestimated in medical sciences. There are several approaches, using herbs, botanicals and nutrients, to support the structure and function of the skin. A key factor in premature aging of the skin is excessive exposure over prolonged periods of time, to sunlight. This has led to the use of many topical agents that have variable degrees of ability to protect the skin and subdermal areas from solar radiation. This protection is recorded on lotions or creams etc. as an SPF factor. It is possible to protect the skin from sun damage by the use of certain botanicals and nutrients. This is the concept of oral photoprotection. Observations in experimental animals and humans show the ability of the herb Polypodium leucotomas to protect the skin from sun damage. This botanical has been used as an anti-inflammatory agent for arthritis and inflammatory skin disease, such as psoriasis. The addition of vitamin D to oral photoprotective agents is considered to be a healthy approach because there is a theoretical risk of diminishing vitamin D synthesis in the body, which occurs as a direct response to sunlight exposure. The requirements for sun protection are clear, given the increasing incidence of skin cancer in the US and its alarming increase in prevalence in certain countries, e.g. Australia.

Other innovative approaches to promoting beauty by oral supplements include: substances that will assist in renewal of collagen in the skin (e.g. hyaluronic acid), potent oral antioxidants, multivitamins, minerals and mixed anti-aging formulae (Chapter 31). It is surprising that few effective natural supplements have been proposed for the management of common acne. The role of excessive androgenic hormonal drive may be counteracted by soy isoflavones and medical literature supports the use of natural anti-inflammatory substances such as Boswellia serrata, guggulsterones and curcuminoids. The technology to support the concept of physical attraction determined by inner health is emerging, but its applications are slow to surface and underestimated. There is too much emphasis placed on topical approaches to beauty, at the expense of considerations of inner health.

CHAPTER 25

EYE CARE

HEALTHY EYES

AGE-RELATED declines in visual function affect everyone to a variable degree. There are several common causes of blindness or lack of visual acuity in the elderly. With age, changes in the function and structure of eyes may cause a common condition called "presbyopia". This condition is manifest by short- or long-sightedness. Other common causes of loss of vision include glaucoma (excess pressure in the eyeball), age-related macular degeneration (AMD), cataracts and ocular complications of diabetes mellitus. There are thirteen million adults in the US with AMD.

There are two types of AMD, one called "dry" and one called "wet." The dry form of AMD accounts for about nine out of ten of all cases of AMD. This disorder is caused to a major degree by oxidative tissue damage and poor circulation in the special light-sensing area of the back of the eye (retina). This area of the retina is called the macula. In dry AMD, spots of damaged tissue accumulate below the macula and cause distorted vision by damaging special cells that receive and process light. Oxidative damage also plays a major role in the progression of cataracts and retinal damage that occurs in diabetes mellitus.

The clear approach to visual health is to engage in positive lifestyle and to have good nutrition. There are several specific nutrients or botanicals that play a special role in the nutritional support of the healthy structure and function of the eyes. These include lutein, zeaxanthin, spinach, bilberry and other natural agents. Each of these natural substances has a good evidence base for the support of eye health. There are many reports of the benefit of these antioxidants for ocular health in the scientific literature and their combined administration makes most sense (synergy).

KEYNOTE SUMMARY: EYE CARE

The use of nutritional supplements to support the structure and function of the eyes has become very popular. Many supplements used for eye care are incomplete in their content of health giving nutrient compounds. More comprehensive supplements are available in synergistic formulations. These supplements contain a comprehensive array of nutrients and botanicals that have major antioxidant functions with examples of specific actions on eye health.

Modern medicine has focused attention on the correction of damaged structures in the eye. Far more attention should be paid to the prevention of eye damage by simple, gentle and natural means. Damage to the eyes can be expected in many individuals with diabetes mellitus and evidence exists that damage to the retina or lens of the eye is caused to a major degree by oxidative damage. Given the epidemic of type II diabetes and the forerunner disorders of pre-diabetes and metabolic syndrome X, many more individuals should consider nutritional support for eye health at an earlier age. It is never too early or too late to take steps to protect the precious gift of vision.

Natural substances that have a defined role in the nutritional support of the structure and function of the eye include: beta carotene, spinach leaves, vitamin C, bilberry fruit, vitamin E, zinc, copper, lutein, lycopene, zeaxanthin and selenium. These substances are best used in combination.

**SEEK COMPREHENSIVE NUTRITIONAL
SYNERGY FOR EYE CARE.**

CHAPTER 26

HIGH ENERGY

WHERE IS MY ENERGY?

EPISODES of feeling "drained of energy" affect almost every active adult. When lack of energy exists, it is important to exclude medical disorders that cause fatigue, such as inflammation, cancer, pre-diabetes, the metabolic Syndrome X or diabetes mellitus. The most common cause of temporary lack of energy is simple body fatigue, often aggravated by sleeplessness.

Cycles of loss of energy are often associated with sleep deprivation. Sleeplessness is an almost universal event at times of stress (Sleep, Chapter 2). This kind of stress is most apparent during the transition of menopause and with PMS. Apart from this obvious dialogue on rest and relaxation, there are several causes of lack of energy that must be defined.

The metabolic Syndrome X or pre-diabetes or diabetes often present with non-specific signs of tiredness or loss of energy (see Chapters 16 and 17.) Poorly defined nutritional deficiencies may contribute to fatigue. Recurrent bouts of hypoglycemia (low blood sugar), aggravated by excessive intake of simple sugars is a common cause of dramatic changes in energy levels (Chapter 16). A common "dynamo" to correct lack of energy in many people is optimal mineral intake. Individuals who take mineral supplements or coral calcium often describe "energy boosts" as an anecdotal benefit. Chronic viral disease robs energy from the body.

CHRONIC FATIGUE SYNDROME

The chronic fatigue syndrome may be over-diagnosed in modern society, but in its full-blown circumstances it causes:

- Feelings of apathy and recurrent depression.
- Poor brain function and memory loss.
- Muscle pain, low-grade fever, general aches and pains, glandular swelling.
- Worsening of any existing illness and a greater risk of illness.
- A host of other non-specific complaints … and more.

Many books have been written on chronic fatigue syndrome. This disorder comes with "different labels," such as "Raggedy-Ann Syndrome," "Yuppie disease," "Chronic Viral Debility" and many more. The most researched cause of chronic fatigue syndrome is chronic viral infection with Epstein-Barr virus and other viruses (e.g., Hepatitis B or C virus infection, cytomegalovirus (CMV) and several types of Herpes virus). However, not all sufferers with chronic fatigue syndrome have evidence of past or present viral infections. It should be remembered that human immunodeficiency virus (HIV) infection can present like a chronic fatigue syndrome. Moreover, many cases of exposures to various toxins, toxicants and synthetic chemicals cause a chronic fatigue syndrome. These circumstances are highlighted by symptoms in Gulf War veterans and rescue workers who attended the 9/11 collapse of the World Trade Center.

Many nutritional approaches have been applied to chronic fatigue syndrome, including drastic, dietary changes, detoxification programs, and a host of nutrient substances, including multivitamins, minerals, immune-boosting or balancing substances and energizing herbs or botanicals. General advice for anyone with "energy problems," is summarized in Table 31.

- Laugh, play, relax, and maintain psychological well-being.
- Good, balanced diet, three meals per day, always have breakfast.
- Consider weight control and management of Syndrome X.
- Engage positive lifestyle, smoking cessation.
- Exercise at least one hour three times a week—or just walk!
- Consider a multivitamin, multiminerals, antioxidants and berries and greens.
- Detect and combat Syndrome X.
- Avoid energy-draining activities, e.g., drinking alcohol, smoking, excessive caffeine or cola consumption and stay away from junk food.
- Get toxins out of your environment and your body.
- Restore normal sleep patterns.

- Try to drink eight 8-oz. cups of pure water daily.
- Consider detoxification methods.
- Consider an immune-boosting supplement.

Table 31: Energizing strategies using natural options

KEYNOTE SUMMARY: HIGH ENERGY SUPPLEMENTS

A variety of botanicals or nutrients may revive energy (Table 32). Important antidotes to recurrent episodes of loss of energy are well planned aerobic exercise and restoration of the biorhythm of restful sleep.

Supplement	Comment
Green tea	Very valuable in liquid concentrates, balanced with other antioxidants (see Chapter 4). The "perk" with green tea is not completely related to caffeine.
Combat Syndrome X	Syndrome X combined nutrient approach (Chapters 15, 16 and 17).
Restoring sleep	Lifestyle: "The Sleep Naturally Plan" with nutritional support (Chapter 2).
Ultimate energy formulas	Avoid strong stimulants for a temporary "pep." Use balanced energy formulas.
Multivitamins/multiminerals, antioxidants	Underlying energizing effects (see Chapters 1 and 4).
Addiction, withdrawal of substances of abuse	Kudzu (alcohol) (Chapter 28).
Healthy weight-control supplements, not to be used alone for weight control	Hoodia from South Africa has shown great promise as a non-stimulant appetite suppressant, Seaweeds e.g. Fucose vesiculosis, Dietary Fiber etc. (Chapters 15 and 32).
Miscellaneous	Fish Oil (see Chapter 18), Astragalus, Co-enzyme Q 10, Sarsaparilla, Schizandra, Ginseng, Spirulina (Chapter 32).

Table 32: Dietary supplements that energize directly or indirectly (see text).

A complex, but synergistic (additive) formulation of many herbs and botanicals can promote a wide range of energizing properties for the body. Anti-stress or adaptogenic natural substances are valuable in managing fatigue. Certain natural substances have a long history of safe use by a variety of cultures and most ingredients provide antioxidant functions and others contain specific valuable phytonutrients.

Single botanical agents that give a "kick" (e.g. ephedra) have been misused by consumers of dietary supplements. Strong stimulants are best avoided because they may alter blood pressure; provoke anxious feelings, cause the heart to race and compound cardiovascular risk factors. Safer energy promoting supplements involve the selection of natural agents that work in an additive manner on many aspects of body metabolism. Not only should the ingredients in energy-boosting supplements be designed to promote positive energy, they should be adaptogenic, meaning that they balance body function, with anti-stress actions.

Energizing supplements should not be taken in the evening to avoid interference with sleep. The recommended dose of energizing supplements should not be exceeded. These supplements are not suitable for use by children or pregnant women. Selected contents of energy formulae include: Guarana seeds, Gotu kola, Ginseng panax, Eleutherococcus senticosus, Green tea, Peppermint leaves, Bee pollen, Green coffee bean extract, Royal jelly, spirulina, chlorella, kelp, and Cayenne peppers. I have formulated several of these ingredients in a synergistic manner for non-specific, energy-boosting supplements, but defining the cause of lethargy, and correcting the cause, is the best approach to wellbeing.

CHAPTER 27

NATURES CALCIUM®
AND CALCIUM SUPPLEMENTS

BACKGROUND

MANY practitioners of Integrative Healthcare believe that calcium supplements of natural origin are preferred. There are several clear advantages of Natures Calcium®. Natures Calcium® is eco-friendly, eggshell calcium that is produced by a special recycling process. Scientific studies have shown clear nutritional benefits of the administration of eggshell calcium, including the promotion of bone strength. Natures Calcium® contains high concentrations (up to 46%) of naturally-chelated calcium that is well assimilated and absorbed by the human body. The calcium from eggshells is processed to be presented in a special small-particle size and it has a valuable, naturally occurring, mineral profile.

Natures Calcium® provides a highly concentrated source of calcium that guarantees purity, quality and real cost advantage. Added to the benefits of eggshell calcium is the excellent micro-nutrient mineral profile that occurs in Natures Calcium®. This profile includes at least 17 different trace elements, in addition to calcium. These extra micronutrients include: magnesium, sulfur, boron, phosphorus, silicon, chromium, potassium, copper, cobalt, iodine, iron, manganese, molybdenum, selenium, strontium, vanadium and zinc, in variable or trace amounts.

Many consumers have become aware of the problem of heavy metal contamination in many forms of natural calcium. For example, marine sources of calcium may be contaminated with heavy metals such as mercury or lead, and mercury contamination has been an intermittent problem with some calcium supplements that are derived from hydroxyapatite or "cow bone." Natures Calcium® does not contain any significant levels of heavy metals.

One of the most appealing characteristics of Natures Calcium® is its ultimate eco-friendly status where recycled eggshells are used to produce a quality dietary supplement. Natures Calcium® is one of the most ideal sources of natural calcium in the diet.

SUMMARY

Natures Calcium® is an exceptionally high quality, natural form of calcium with more than 17 nutrient micro-minerals all sourced from eggshells. It is of note that eggs have been through the ultimate biological system in the birth canal of a chicken; and, as such, they have been protected from many environmental pollutants in the formation of this treasured source (eggshell) of nutrients. Table 33 lists some of the advantages of eggshell calcium found in the supplement Natures Calcium®.

- Scientific studies show clear nutritional benefits of eggshell calcium.
- Calcium is assimilated well in micronized form in Natures Calcium®.
- Factors have been identified in egg shell calcium that facilitate calcium absorption.
- Purity, quality and real cost advantage.
- Excellent micronutrient mineral profile with at least 17 trace elements in addition to calcium.
- No heavy metal contaminants in comparison with some types of marine calcium and hydroxyapatite.
- Eco-friendly status from recycled eggshells.
- Produced by a special process.

Table 33: Advantages of Natures Calcium®.

Natures Calcium® is available with the addition of vitamin D3. Vitamin D3 is valuable in helping the body utilize and absorb calcium and it has other benefits for health. Readers should be aware of the emerging importance of calcium in the support of many body structures and functions, other than healthy bones or teeth. Calcium is believed to play a role in weight control, colon cancer prevention and it has versatile effects on muscle and nerve function.

It is very difficult for many people to reach recommended daily intakes of calcium in their diet and some foods that are considered rich sources of calcium, such as green vegetables, may contain naturally occurring compounds that block calcium absorption. Eggshell calcium has specific, naturally occurring components that help to promote calcium absorption. Modern nutritional principles highlight the benefits of taking calcium with other minerals, especially magnesium. A real advantage of Natures Calcium® is its naturally occurring micromineral profile.

There is mounting concern that teenagers, especially females, who are often on diets for weight control, have very poor calcium intake. I have stressed that the prevention of osteoporosis is more than taking calcium alone, but lifelong calcium deficiency is an important contributory factor to osteoporosis. These circumstances have led to proposals that many teenagers may benefit from calcium supplements, not just mature adults!

A review of Natures Calcium® precipitates a need to fully understand the advantages, disadvantages or limitations of different forms of natural calcium supplements.

A CLEAR UNDERSTANDING OF THE LIMITATIONS OF CALCIUM SUPPLEMENTS ALONE FOR OSTEOPOROSIS IS REQUIRED. DISCUSSIONS OF ABSORPTION OF DIFFERENT FORMS OF CALCIUM ARE OVEREMPHASIZED IN MARKETING. LIMITATIONS OF CALCIUM ABSORPTION MAY BE LARGELY OVERCOME BY GIVING MORE CALCIUM. THERE ARE CIRCUMSTANCES WHERE EXCESSIVE CALCIUM INTAKE IS BEST AVOIDED E.G. RENAL FAILURE OR RISKS FOR "MILK-ALKALI SYNDROME."

CHAPTER 28

ANTI-DEPENDENCE

ADDICTIONS AND DEPENDENCE ON SUBSTANCES: GROWING PUBLIC HEALTH PROBLEMS

THE word "addiction" has its roots in the Latin term, *addictus*. This term implies "great devotion." Modern scientists in socio-behavioral medicine prefer to use the term "dependence." In essence, the addict devotes him or herself to an act in a habitual manner. The basis of addiction implies intemperance. In modern society, dependence often involves the use of a drug (prescription or illicit), but nutrients (sugar) may induce dependence.

A large proportion of the American population has become devoted to, prone to use, accustomed to, attached to, inclined to use or habituated to a variety of substances. Individuals with addictive personalities are usually dependent on more than one substance of abuse. For example, heavy smokers are often heavy drinkers and vice versa. Individuals who become addicted to "street drugs" usually have other addictive habits.

Addictions to substances have extremely damaging effects on society. America's love affair with simple sugars has contributed to the promotion of obesity, the metabolic Syndrome X and type II diabetes mellitus. Alcohol and drug dependence are so common that they may pass unrecognized in society. Many people may be surprised that excessive alcohol consumption requires early identification and intervention, before the prognosis for alcohol dependence becomes poor. However, it is not often remembered that about 45% of all men between the ages of 18 and 45 years have a history of problem drinking. Early signs of substance abuse, such as excessive drinking, present as socio-behavioral problems that result often in strained interpersonal relationships, loss of jobs, marital problems and inappropriate, tragic divorce.

One may be unimpressed with the use of pharmaceuticals to control addictions. The nation has a huge problem with a dependence on simple sugars and the wrong kind of fats in their diet. Any combat against addictions is a monumental task. While conventional medicine has triumphed in some areas of the management of addictions, it has failed miserably in many areas. There are recent findings that there may be natural substances that can provide nutritional support for effects on the normal body functions of dependence. This is truly exciting news.

THE POWER OF KUDZU

The idea that herbs can reduce substance abuse is well described in traditional Chinese medicine. For centuries, people in Northern China have used herbal teas containing Kudzu as antidotes to drunkenness. These teas have been used extensively by Oriental individuals to relieve hangovers and restore sobriety. Studies at Shinn-Yang University in China, in the early 1990s, demonstrated that drunken rats consumed less alcohol and had reduced signs of intoxication as a consequence of the use of several Chinese herbs, including Kudzu.

Kudzu is an annoying weed for horticulturists. It was introduced from Japan into the United States in 1876, at the Centennial Exposition in Philadelphia. Kudzu became a popular plant because it was used in the early 20th century for soil-erosion control. These good intentions resulted in a massive spread of this vine in the southeastern United States. Kudzu grows like wildfire and it can take as long as ten years to kill with herbicides. The annoying Kudzu plant has been featured in recent research for its ability to help people reduce their alcohol consumption. Kudzu has been referred to as "the weed that whacks binge drinking" (WJ Cromie, Harvard News Office).

HARVARD UNIVERSITY STUDIES ON KUDZU

Ground-breaking studies by members of the department of psychiatry at McLean Hospital (an affiliate of Harvard Medical School) reported that Kudzu in extracted forms could reduce total alcohol intake, slow down the speed of drinking of alcohol and result in fewer hangovers, without any side effects. In this study, fourteen human volunteers were placed into an apartment and allowed to drink as much beer as they wanted, up to a maximum intake of six bottles of beer. This resulted in a baseline observation concerning how many bottles of beer each individual could drink under "normal" circumstances. Many young Americans may "think" that six beers represent modest alcohol intake. After this initial observation, half of the volunteers were given a capsule containing Kudzu and half were given an inactive capsule (dummy pill or placebo). The results of these experiments were startling.

Each individual that took Kudzu drank significantly less alcohol than those who took the placebo. Furthermore, the Kudzu-treated group was both slower in drinking alcohol and less likely to request a second or third bottle of beer. The individuals who took dummy pills (placebo) drank three or four bottles of beer, which was on average twice as much as the volunteers who took Kudzu.

The researchers noticed that the individuals who took Kudzu needed more gulps and swallows to finish a bottle of beer. This led to a suggestion that Kudzu may be acting directly on the brain by "telling" the body not to drink excessive amounts of alcohol. These researchers commented on an interesting observation that was made in a survey of Harvard University students where up to one half of all students admitted to binge drinking. These seem to be conservative estimates.

The research went further by the giving of low dosages of Kudzu over a period of one week. No side effects were noted. It was suggested that continuing use of Kudzu may cut down on the number and severity of hangovers, but no controlled studies have demonstrated that Kudzu will act in a way to eliminate established hangovers. The researchers criticized some commercially available forms of Kudzu and implied that they did not contain the putative active ingredient of Kudzu, which is called puerarin, a name taken from the family of plants called Pueriariae, of which Kudzu is a member.

HOW DOES KUDZU WORK?

There has been much speculation on how components within Kudzu may assist in helping people to reduce alcohol intake. Kudzu contains bioflavanoids, examples of which are isoflavones. Soy isoflavones have been shown to reduce alcohol intake in rats and the exact mechanism of this action of isoflavones remain unknown. Isoflavones could inhibit the enzyme in the stomach wall called gastric alcohol dehydrogenase (gastric A.D.H.). Inhibition of this stomach enzyme may act to increase blood alcohol levels following alcohol intake. It may be that isoflavones in Kudzu, or other Kudzu ingredients that have effects on alcohol metabolism, may have direct effects on the central nervous system.

The researchers at Harvard suggested that puerarin in Kudzu may cause increased blood flow to the brain and heart. The suggestion was that increased blood flow may deliver more alcohol to the brain and result in the individual being satisfied with smaller amounts of alcohol intake. I believe that these postulates are incomplete or naïve because the distribution of alcohol in the body is dependent on many factors other than blood flow.

There are five key studies on the value of Kudzu in the reduction of alcohol intake. These studies are listed in Table 34.

- Lukas SE et al. An Extract of the Chinese Herbal Root Kudzu Reduces Alcohol Drinking by Heavy Drinkers in a Naturalistic Setting. Alcohol Clin Exp Res., 2005 May; 29(5): 756-762.
- Benihabib E et al. Effects of Purified Puerarin on Voluntary Alcohol Intake and Alcohol Withdrawal Symptoms in P Rats Receiving Free Access to Water and Alcohol. J Med Food. 2004 Summer; 7(2): 180-6.
- Carai MA et al. Potential Use of Medicinal Plants in the Treatment of Alcoholism. Fitoterapia. 2000 Aug.; 71 Suppl 1:S38-42.
- Shebek J, Rindone JP. A Pilot Study Exploring the Effect of Kudzu Root on the Drinking Habits of Patients with Chronic Alcoholism. J Altern Complement Med. 2000 Feb.; 6(1): 45-8.
- Keung WM, Vallee BL. Kudzu Root: an Ancient Chinese Source of Modern Antidipsotropic Agents. Phytochemistry. 1998 Feb.; 47(4): 499-506.

Table 34 Five key studies on the value of Kudzu in the reduction of alcohol intake. The author has recorded anecdotal success with the use of Kudzu in obese individuals who "crave sugar."

ANTI-DEPENDENCE WITH SUPPLEMENTS?

One could argue strongly that addictions or circumstances of dependence are not necessarily diseases. Certainly, the use of a softer term "dependence" would not qualify as a disease. That said, alcoholism is a disease when chronic, excessive drinking occurs, but it is arguably a disease when it is in the form of binge drinking. The solution to any addiction, such as excessive alcohol intake, cigarette smoking or drug abuse, is intensive sociobehavioral interventions combined with positive lifestyle changes. However, natural substances that are safe and may assist in the nutritional support of anti-addictive behavior may be considered worthy of use. Furthermore, many standard or conventional treatments for addictions fail.

In supplements that may affect the body functions of dependence, high-quality extracts of kudzu can be combined with whole kudzu plant material, to which is added chamomile flowers for their "soothing" properties. Taking the "jitters away" from people with chamomile is useful approach for people who are trying to quit drinking or smoking. This is an important dimension of nutritional support for the "dependent personality."

NUTRITION AND LIFESTYLE FOR THE ADDICTED

Natural substances to control drug dependence cannot be expected to work without many other interventions that are required to correct addictions. The addicted person often has a substandard diet and people who drink alcohol excessively invariably have nutrient depletion. Many individuals who are dependent on substances of abuse will benefit from an optimal diet, together with multivitamins or mineral supplements or greens and berries.

Alcohol and cigarette smoke generate free radicals in the body and cause oxidative stress to tissues (Antioxidants, Chapter 4). This type of tissue damage results in many chronic diseases that are associated with substance abuse. Such diseases include, but are not limited to, heart disease, cancer, lung disease and premature aging. I believe that antioxidant intake is important nutritional support for many individuals who have addictions or dependence on substances, but disease prevention claims are not allowed for dietary supplements.

Withdrawing substances of abuse in many people may unmask the reasons for their habits. Many "addicts" require counseling and some require expert psychological assessments.

KEYNOTE SUMMARY: ANTI-DEPENDENCE

Humans have a distinct desire for dependence on relationships, food and chemical substances. If one has the privilege of speaking to a drug addict, they will describe cigarette smoking as one of the most powerful "urges" that they possess. Using small amounts of alcohol to encourage an alcohol abuser into controlled drinking has been shown to be a waste of time. The recent scientific discovery of natural substances that can assist in nutritional support of behavioral changes to combat dependence is very exciting. Medicine sometimes views dependence as a disease, but dependence may be best viewed as major deviations from acceptable lifestyles, especially in reference to alcohol intake.

A combination of botanical agents may provide nutritional support to alter the normal body function of a tendency to dependence on drugs or substances, especially alcohol. This suggestion draws upon recent scientific research that highlights the nutritional value of the plant Kudzu.

Dietary supplement products that claim to be a value in reducing the symptoms of a hangover should be rejected on grounds of common logic. In the place of "hangover remedies," one may substitute nutritional support that may have benefits in reducing the normal body function of the development of dependence. In fact, selling products to prevent or manage "hangovers" many encourage people to drink excessively. This practice has no role in holistic healthcare. It is completely contrary to the philosophy of natural medicine to produce a natural product that could encourage people to persist with their drunkenness or chemical dependence.

There has been much speculation on how Kudzu may work, but it contains compounds that have a structure similar to isoflavones which have wide-ranging potential health benefits. Chamomile, a popular "stress-busting" herb may help take the edge of the anxiety that individuals may experience during the withdrawal of alcohol or cigarettes. I emphasize that I cannot recommend supplements for the treatment of addictions, at law. I believe strongly that all addicted individuals should be assessed by a healthcare practitioner.

CHAPTER 29

MOOD

ALTERATION IN MOOD

COUNTLESS numbers of people experience negative moods, ranging from frank depression through to experiences of boredom, anxiety, isolation and restlessness. A conservative estimate of the need for psychiatric or psychological treatment involves an assumption that about 40% of the entire population may need such services at one or more times in their life.

There is no doubt that adverse lifestyle precipitates mood changes and it is known that people who smoke or drink excessively are prone to episodes of depression. Sleeplessness causes a depressed mood in many people. Therefore, before anyone discusses natural approaches to mood elevation, one must reinforce the importance of exercise, good diet, restoration of biorhythms and other lifestyle issues in the promotion of healthy and stable moods.

Temporary changes in mood are common and they are not always to be identified as mental problems requiring treatment. Modern society lives with a series of stressful life events which are best countered by planned resolutions and the use of relaxation responses. In this context, many forms of traditional medicine that teach ways to relax are valuable, e.g., Yoga, Tai Chi, martial arts, hypnosis, body work and meditation. Healthy sexual function and aerobic exercise elevate mood function to a substantial degree.

It is wrong for people to believe that they can self-medicate for significant emotional disturbances or psychiatric disease. In fact, such severe mental problems can impair an individual's judgment. Therefore, in cases of doubt, everyone should check with a socio-behavioral specialist. The manifestations of poor mental wellbeing are so varied that these disturbances are often overlooked as being the commonest cause of human suffering.

The body and mind are inextricably linked as the "body-mind" or "mind-body." The mind can tell the body to do almost anything and this is the basis of much common disease or disorder that is called functional disease e.g. irritable bowel syndrome (IBS). The gastrointestinal tract is a common site for functional disorders, where digestive symptoms occur in the absence of structural changes in the gut, such as inflammation or cancer (see Digestion, Chapter 9). Mood disturbance and gastrointestinal upset often go "hand in hand."

DYSTHYMIA OR DEPRESSION

Certain criteria are listed to help healthcare professionals diagnose negative mood changes. The most common and significant of all mental disorders is depression. It is accepted that anyone with five of the following eight symptoms is most likely a victim of clinical depression (Table 35):

1. Sleep disorder, insomnia or excessive sleeping.
2. Major appetite change with weight gain or weight loss.
3. Physical inactivity or too much activity.
4. Loss of pleasure or interest in day-to-day activities, e.g. sex.
5. Feelings of fatigue or energy loss.
6. Excessive guilt or sense of worthlessness.
7. Poor ability to remember, think or concentrate.
8. Thoughts about harming oneself or dying.

Table 35: Anyone with five of the eight symptoms listed above is probably depressed.

The word "dysthymia" has crept into classifications of negative mood. The symptoms of dysthymia are similar to those of clinical depression. Clinical depression is considered to be present when symptoms occur for at least 24 months in an adult, or 12 months in a child or teenager. I do not like these definitions because catching depression early with the correct interventions gives excellent outcome in most people. There is a specific mood disorder which is characterized by depression in the winter months. This depression may alternate with excessive mood elevation in the summer months. This disorder is believed to be related to changes in light exposure in many people. This form of depression is sometimes referred to as "seasonal affective disorder" and it can respond to special types of light therapy.

The disorder of mania must be considered a negative mood change, but the individual with mania often feels good. A person with mania may be elated, but they may also have inappropriate displays of anger or hostility. The manic person generally does not sleep, is hyperactive and pays little attention to well-being and health. Mania must never be self-managed because the manic person is often a danger to themselves and others, as may be the person who is seriously depressed. Alternating mania and depression is called manic-depression or bipolar disorder. These people suffer and make others suffer around them. This disorder must be managed by an expert. I have been impressed by the use of fish oil as a mood-stabilizer (Chapter 18).

THE SPECTRUM OF NEGATIVE MOODS

It is clear that depression can be mild, moderate or severe. There are at least 20 million Americans who suffer from frank depression each year and about 30 to 40 million Americans take antidepressant drugs or tranquilizers. There has been an increasing tendency to overuse antidepressant drugs. For example, many women in the transition of menopause are prescribed antidepressants, which does not seem a logical approach to this natural life event.

Anyone with a mood disorder must consider the correction of precipitating circumstances including: correction of adverse life events or poor diet, consideration of the depressing effect of some drugs, hormonal changes, allergic reactions and recovery from common diseases, such as flu. It is well-recognized that common infectious disease may precipitate negative mood changes which usually last only for a few weeks. The role of environmental toxins in causing mood change is an active area of research; and there is a link between some household chemicals, food additives, agricultural chemicals or heavy metals and mood changes or disorders of the central nervous system. The 9/11 rescue and recovery workers who were poisoned by toxic chemicals often complained of severe mood disturbance and detachment from their families.

The person with a negative mood must review smoking habits, levels of alcohol or caffeine intake and exercise. Negative lifestyle must be converted to positive lifestyle with the addition of optimal nutrition. Any person with a mood disorder is advised often to take a multivitamin and a multimineral on a regular basis. Fruit, vegetable, berry and greens powders are quite valuable (Chapter 4). The role of food allergies in the causation of mood disorders has been underestimated (Allergy, Chapter 30).

SUPPLEMENTS FOR NUTRITIONAL SUPPORT OF MOOD

There are many different nutrients, herbs or botanicals that might be proposed for the nutritional support of the normal body function of mood regulation. An overlooked way of nutritionally supporting mood is to use nutrients that have beneficial effects on brain structure or function. Such nutrients include lecithin for its phospholipid content, inositol, vitamin B6, folic acid, vitamin C and selenium (Memory, Chapter 23).

The popular herb Saint John's Wort has a long history of use for its mood elevating benefits and L-theanine, found in green tea has calming properties. An herb that has been underestimated in terms of its ability to mimic effects of chemical messages in the brain is Mucuna pruriens. These nutrients and botanicals form the basis of the formulations for the natural, nutritional support of "moods."

CONCLUSION

I stress that people with significant changes of mood or prolonged disturbances of mood should not self-medicate. Furthermore, people who are taking medications for mood disorders, e.g. antidepressant drugs are strongly advised not to mix dietary supplements with drugs, without adequate medical advice or supervision.

CHAPTER 30

ALLERGY

THE ALLERGIC RESPONSE

EVERYONE is aware of their potential to develop an allergic response. A true allergy involves immune reactions in the body which can occur as a result of exposure to a wide variety of substances, such as food, food additives, animal hair, etc. The substance that precipitates the allergic response is called an "allergen" (antigen); and even exposure to small amounts of allergens in the environment can result sometimes in quite serious symptoms of allergies. In simple terms, it is the allergen that triggers an immune response that involves cells and messenger molecules of the immune system. This activation of immune responses sets up an "inflammatory situation" that causes many different symptoms and signs. Allergies to antigens and allergens are very common.

The occurrence of allergies in the U.S. is difficult to estimate, but one in four people are allergic to one or more substances. Medications that are taken to control symptoms of allergies are among the most popular of all drugs. Many of these drugs belong to a group of compounds called anti-histamines. Anti-histamines have variable ability to treat allergic responses, but their use is often associated with side effects, especially drowsiness. This side effect has led to their questionable use as sleeping tablets and sedative inclusions in cough and cold products (Chapter 2).

Substances that trigger allergies can get into the body in many ways. They can be absorbed into the skin (e.g. artificial dyes in topical creams), or they can be eaten (e.g. food allergies), or they can be inhaled (e.g. pollen), or they can even be injected (e.g. bee or wasp stings). When the body is allergic to a particular substance, it often produces anti-bodies which combine with the allergen. This combining activity triggers a cascade of immune events that constitute the allergic reaction. Anti-bodies can signal cells of the immune system to release inflammatory compounds such as histamines etc.

Histamine and other inflammatory chemicals involved in the allergic reaction can travel through the body and cause many changes in body function. These allergy-induced changes include contraction of muscles in air passages (asthma), increase in mucus production in the nasal passages (rhinitis or sinusitis) and leaking of blood vessels with accumulation of fluid in body tissues (swelling or edema).

One may understand that these changes in body function manifest themselves in common medical disorders, such as hay fever, runny nose, swollen red eyes, cough, sneezing and even asthma. Some allergic reactions are more apparent by their effects on digestive function (food allergies), whereas others may be more obvious by their effects on the skin e.g. causing different types of skin rashes.

There are extreme cases of allergies that cause violent changes in body functions. These changes in severe allergic reactions include fainting, drop of blood pressure, shock, interruption of breathing, obstructive swelling in the mouth and throat, and even suffocation. There are cases of death reported on a regular basis from severe allergic reactions; and anyone with more severe forms of allergies must not self-medicate. If signs of severe allergies occur suddenly, individuals must present themselves at an emergency medical facility to receive intensive drug treatment or life support.

Fortunately, most people suffer with less severe forms of allergies, but allergic symptoms can make an individual quite miserable and provoke an ongoing state of inflammation in the body. Allergies are frequently misdiagnosed as infections, especially bacterial infections. It is known that allergies may even be part of the symptom complex of simple respiratory and ear infections. In other words, symptoms such as nasal congestion, cough, runny nose or sore eyes are symptoms that are present in both infections and allergic responses. There are many people who suffer from chronic ill health because they have undiagnosed allergies. It is sometimes forgotten that allergies may play a significant role in gastrointestinal upsets and even in chronic disorders such as arthritis.

Practitioners of holistic medicine view allergic responses as clear examples of imbalance in the immune system. Most drugs used for the management of allergies involve the blocking of the production of inflammatory substances, such as histamine or leukotrienes. However, there are simple, gentle and natural approaches to provide nutritional support for balancing immune functions that are involved in the allergic response. In fact, there are nutritional substances that have natural anti-inflammatory actions; and they may exert effects on body functions, similar to anti-histamine compounds that are used as drugs. However, drugs cannot be compared with supplements – at law.

NUTRITIONAL SUPPORT FOR BODY STRUCTURES AND FUNCTIONS INVOLVED IN ALLERGIES

Before anyone considers using nutrition or medication to manage allergies, they must do some "private investigation." The obvious way of managing allergies is to avoid the substances that cause the allergic reactions. This may be obvious to some people with allergies caused by common allergens such as pollen, shellfish, pet dander, peanuts, poison ivy or selected foods. However, in many circumstances the substance causing the allergy (allergens) cannot easily be identified. Identification of allergens can be an expensive and laborious process involving complicated skin or blood testing. Even with this kind of testing, the causative agent (allergens) may not be easily identified.

These days, we live with increasing environmental pollution, especially air pollution. Therefore, every day we may be exposed to multiple substances that can trigger an allergic response. We have little chance of avoiding this circumstance, especially if we live in urban areas where pollution is everywhere, or if we work in a closed building where air recycles and exposes an individual to all sorts of allergens.

Evidence exists that humankind is exposed to many different environmental toxins, which can act as potential allergens. The horrible experiences of rescue workers and recovery crews involved in the destruction of the World Trade Center on 9/11/2001 have taught us a great deal about the consequences of exposure to synthetic chemicals and other poisons found in building structures and our environment. Many individuals who were exposed to the toxic clouds produced after the 9/11 disaster suffered from allergic responses due to a variety of toxins that persisted in their body and caused tissue damage by oxidative stress and other mechanisms.

9/11 is a date that has gone down in infamy, but the medical consequences of this event for many thousands of people remain under-explored. Political arguments aside, the medical needs of rescue workers and adjacent citizens of New York and New Jersey have been supported by a process of gross inefficiency. While epidemiologists plot the adverse medical outcomes of 9/11, preventive medical strategies to intervene with detoxification have not received appropriate attention. Environmental toxin exposure during the 9/11 events involved asbestos, toxic heavy metals, other inorganic or organic disease-causing chemicals and perhaps other unidentified health-damaging agents. Evidence-based strategies exist to minimize toxin load following exposure to several toxic agents (detoxification, Chapter 32).

The New York Rescuc Workers Detoxification Program have applied classic detoxification methods to hundreds of exposed victims, using a vitamin supplement regimen, sauna, aerobic exercise and lifestyle advice, with clearly documented improvements in presenting symptoms that could be attributed to toxin exposure during the 9/11 events. These detoxifying interventions have shown objective evidence of reduction in toxic load of certain chemicals (e.g. PCBs), as measured by laboratory testing in a selected number of victims. With clarity, the victims reported consistently a reduction in allergies and the need for drug prescriptions, in circumstances where some rescue workers were receiving extreme, conventional polypharmacy (oral drug medication and inhalers).

Progression of disease from the toxic exposures of 9/11 is evolving and documented in the medical literature, including: deaths, reports of low birth weight, chronic respiratory disability and other disorders. The consequences of heavy metal exposure and excessive free radical load can be inferred or loosely forecast in the exposed populations, but a concerted effort at detoxification remains quite limited by resources and continuing arguments about the lack of efficacy or an evidence-base for detoxification methods. While meritorious outcome appears to be present in open-label observations of a simple initial detoxification program, further planning of continuity of more prolonged detoxification and lifestyle interventions require urgent attention for 9/11 victims.

The medical consequences of 9/11 are a "ticking time-bomb." The premature disability and death that could affect thousands of citizens in a significant radius of one of the highest population densities in the world is a major public health initiative that remains somewhat mismanaged. There is an urgent need for amalgamation of outcome data on detoxification practices, utilizing non-allopathic interventions. These circumstances of modern environmental pollution reinforce the importance of body cleansing or detoxification, which has great relevance to managing allergies, at least indirectly.

Any activity that helps reduce exposure to allergy causing substances is beneficial to many people. This activity may be as simple as regular household dusting or avoidance of foods containing artificial food additives, etc. There has been a major increase in asthma over the past few years, especially in children. In this disorder, the air passages in the lungs become narrowed and air flow is interrupted. It is known that allergic responses are often involved in the precipitation of asthma. Asthma should not be self-medicated because severe asthmatic responses can be life-threatening.

KEYNOTE SUMMARY: ALLERGY

A rational, simple and gentle approach to promoting comfort in individuals with allergies is to use several substances that have a long history of beneficial effects on the nutritional support of people with allergies. Many different natural substances have been proposed as useful in the reduction of allergic responses, but in some cases, the evidence for their benefit is not strong. Natural approaches to allergy reduction include the use of homeopathy, external techniques and an array of herbal remedies.

Based upon a review of literature in the natural health field, together with clinical experience, one may identify a combination of nutrients, herbs or botanicals, for which there is good scientific agreement to support the opinion that they can be used for nutritional support of normal body structures and functions that are involved in allergic responses.

In brief, these substances include bioflavonoids (especially quercetin), vitamin C, B vitamins, magnesium and several botanical substances or extracts. The herbs and botanicals that are valuable in the management of allergic responses include Picrorhiza kurroa, Astragalus, Devil's claw, Nettle, Thyme, Fennel, Milk thistle and Bitter orange.

There are some general principals that should be applied in the nutritional support of balanced immune functions involved in allergies. Individuals with allergies are advised to take a multivitamin because of the special role of vitamins A, B, C and E in supporting immune function (see Chapter 1). It is vitamin C that seems to star as "a kind of natural anti-histamine." Vitamin C is a powerful antioxidant that is able to stabilize white cells and inhibit release of inflammatory substances such as histamine. It is important to understand that the potential benefits of vitamin C, in this context, are usually seen at higher dosages of vitamin C, taken on a continuing basis.

Quercetin and other bioflavonoids exert "helper effects" with vitamin C and result in stabilizing effects on cells that release histamine (e.g. Mast cells). In fact, there is a prescription drug that is a synthetic flavonoid that is used in the treatment of asthma (cromolyn sodium). The absorption of quercetin from the gut is sometimes poor and this commonly occurring flavonoid is best taken with other mixed flavonoids.

A little known herb, with potential benefit in stabilizing body functions involving allergies, is Picrorhiza kurroa. This herb is well known in the ancient medical discipline called Ayurvedic medicine. In brief, components of Picrorhiza kurroa seem to interfere with histamine release and airway constriction in experimental animals. It appears that components of Picrorhiza kurroa can also prevent the release of inflammatory substances from mast cells. These nutritional effects of Picrorhiza have not been documented to the same degree as drugs that are used to treat airway constrictions. Individuals with asthma must not self-medicate for "asthmatic attacks," especially if they have serious allergies.

Astragalus (Astragalus membranaceus; huang ch'i) is an herb that has been used in traditional Chinese medicine. It is reported to balance immune function with specific effects on allergies. Astragalus is quite popular with traditional Chinese herbalists who use this herb in combination with many other botanicals; because it is believed that it may promote the function of other herbs that are taken for the same reason (synergy). Devil's Claw is mentioned in German literature as having specific value in the management of allergies and it appears to have anti-inflammatory actions.

The natural substances bromelain (an enzyme from pineapples), nettle leaves, milk thistle, thyme and fennel have all been proposed as useful in balancing immune functions by a variety of different mechanisms, including the provision of antioxidant or detoxifying effects. Other valuable natural antioxidants include grapeseed extract and Citrus aurantium.

A synergistic blend of natural substances with a variety of different effects on body structures and functions may provide nutritional support to balance immune functions that are involved in allergies. These supplements contain bioflavonoids, selected vitamins and specific botanicals with a precedent for their use, in the contexts of this discussion. A word of caution is required because plant substances may themselves cause allergic responses. In any cases of doubt, an individual must check the contents of any product, (food, dietary supplement or drug etc.) against known allergies and obtain the advice of a knowledgeable healthcare practitioner.

CHAPTER 31

SPECIFIC ANTI-AGING FACTORS FOR NATURAL CLINICIANS

CONCEPTS OF AGING

WHILE many seek the "fountain of youth," no one has found it. Aging is a complex process which can be modified only by multi-pronged interventions. Positive lifestyle is pivotal in the promotion of health and wellbeing. While one can extol the virtues and benefits of good lifestyle for health maintenance and longevity, the investment in "behavior change today for health tomorrow" is a difficult pathway of intervention. Mental and physical idleness result in loss of vitality. An important promoter of aging is lack of mind or body activity, resulting in the "disuse syndrome," with its hallmark of premature aging.

Many theories of aging have been proposed, but no single explanation suffices (Table 36). Despite uncertainty about aging theories, modern antiaging research has identified several key disorders or processes that promote tissue aging. These processes include: immune impairment, sleep deprivation, obesity, adverse lifestyle, genetic programming, poor nutrition, hormonal deficiencies or deregulation, inflammation, oxidative stress to tissues, deficient methylation and the formation of glycated proteins (Advanced Glycation End Products, or AGEs).

A wide range of natural substances have been identified that can provide favorable nutritional or chemical effects on several of these common disorders or processes that accelerate tissue aging. Modern research has identified many natural substances with antiaging properties, but simple interventions or single supplements (or drugs) cannot address the multifactorial aspects of tissue aging in an efficient or comprehensive manner. The intricate, biochemical cascades of events involved in aging require a synergistic approach to the formulation of antiaging substances, specifically anti-aging dietary supplements.

The objective of this chapter is to review and focus on antiaging interventions using dietary supplements, in order to induce youth preserving improvements in body functions and structures. This compilation of information will permit the natural clinician to adopt a synergistic approach to the correction or retardation of tissue aging using evidence-based, dietary supplement strategies.

HYPOTHESES OF AGING	COMMENTS
Free radical theories	Free radicals cause oxidative damage. Antioxidants of many types are valuable.
Cross-link theories	Cross linking of sugars or aldehydes and proteins cause major alterations in body structure and function. Concept of AGEs.
Immunologic theories	Autoimmunity increases with age. The thymus shrinks and white cell function or antibody production is often compromised.
Mutation and Error Theories	Mistakes in DNA replication or RNA function result in aging or age related disease e.g. cancer.
In-built Programs of Tissue Aging	A program exists in genetic material to control a number of cell functions.
Stress Theories	Stress is cumulative and lifestyle related, nutritional deficiencies enhance body stress. Adaptogenic herbs may be of benefit.
Repair budget Theories	Environmental and lifestyle issues alter the investment of an organism in tissue repair.
Miscellaneous	Obesity, metabolic syndrome X and diabetes mellitus are disorders of premature aging, sleep deprivation and restoration of biorhythms are important. Need for correction of hormonal deficiencies or deregulation. Alter biochemical malfunctions e.g. poor methylation. Combat chronic inflammation. Lifestyle change pivotal.

Table 36. Theories and hypotheses of aging with comments about age promoters and putative "age eradicators."

DIETARY SELECTIONS

The optimal "Antiaging Diet" should be reduced in simple sugars and saturated fat, while being supplemented with omega-3 essential fatty acids (EFA). The diet should contain modest amounts of protein of mixed origin (vegetable, meat, dairy and fish origin), high in fiber and dense in vital nutrients, such as vitamins, minerals and phytochemicals. Perhaps the most important dietary adjustments involve the reduction of useless, dietary calories (e.g. simple sugars, saturated fat or alcohol) and a restoration of the balance of omega-3 EFA to omega-6 EFA intake. The widespread, relative deficiency of omega-3 EFA and imbalance of omega-6: omega-3 dietary intake ratios have been implicated in proinflammatory states, increased risks of cancer or cardiovascular disease risk and the general promotion of chronic disease.

Omega-3 EFA supplementation is a pivotal step in antiaging, nutrient supplementation, but many fish oil supplements are obsolete. The amounts of active omega-3 EFA (EPA, eicosapentanoic acid and DHA, docosahexanoic acid) required to achieve disease prevention or therapeutic benefit are much higher than hitherto supposed; and such amounts cannot be administered efficiently in regular fish oil liquids or capsules. The optimum way to supplement omega-3 EFA is in well tolerated, absorption-enhanced, pure, concentrated forms of fish oil that are best presented in delayed release, targeted, enteric-coated, capsule delivery systems. While omega-3 EFA appear of great importance in supplements, the health benefits of omega-9 EFA is apparent in Mediterranean diets that are often enriched with olive oil. Macadamia oil has few advantages over olive oil and it is much more expensive.

There are many accounts of the role of mineral enrichment in the diet of certain ethnic groups that enjoy longevity. Enhanced mineral intake has been proposed as one explanation for the longevity of individuals in Okinawa, Japan and people who live in mountain regions of Pakistan (Hunzas). These observations form the basis of the putative benefit of holistic concoctions of minerals, trace mineral supplements, coral calcium and cell salt therapies. While good mineral intake may be important, other dietary or lifestyle factors combine to play a role in the promotion of an extended, healthy lifespan.

OXIDATIVE TISSUE DAMAGE

Tissue aging, due to free radical damage, is widely accepted as a tenable theory of aging. Reactive oxygen species are formed during normal body metabolism and especially during exercise. Many environmental toxins have pro-oxidant effects on tissues. The body has efficient ways of defending against the propensity to cause tissue damage. Endogenous antioxidants can "mop up" free radicals. These antioxidants include superoxide dismutase (SOD), glutathione, catalase, selenium and vitamins A, C and E… to name a few.

Multifunctional, natural antioxidants are ubiquitous in fruit, vegetables and berries (Chapter 4). To provide adequate antioxidant coverage, many physicians are using vitamin supplements (e.g. A, B complex, C, D and E) combined in complex mixtures of berries, greens and vegetable powders. These blended powders contain a vast array of antioxidant phytochemicals and micronutrients. This complex approach has started to replace the use of multivitamin supplements in the modern practice of Integrative Medicine. The key to antioxidant supplementation is to attempt to cover all body tissues with an antioxidant "blanket" of compounds that access many tissues (lipophilic and hydrophilic antioxidants). This approach should use antioxidants with different REDOX potentials, in order to maximize oxygen radical absorbance capacity (ORAC).

Cell membranes are particularly vulnerable to free radical damage. This circumstance demands the use of lipophilic antioxidants such as turmeric, vitamin E (tocopherols) or essential fatty acids of the omega 3 series (indirect antioxidants). Particularly valuable common antioxidants include pycnogenol, lutein, lycopene, ellagic acid, alpha lipoic acid, co-enzyme Q10, green tea or coffee polyphenols, bioflavanoids and isoflavones.

Co-enzyme Q10 (ubiquinone) is a powerful antioxidant with well documented benefits in the management of cardiovascular disease (angina, congestive cardiac failure, hypercholesterolemia etc). This antioxidant may play a role in the management or prevention of macular degeneration, prostate or breast cancer, cognitive decline, Parkinson's disease, skin aging or muscle weakness and it is valuable in chronic fatigue syndromes. Idebenone is a modified form of CoQ10 which may have a greater antioxidant action than CoQ10, but its cost-effectiveness remains unclear.

TISSUE GLYCATION

Glycation or glycosylation results from the undesirable combination of aldehydes, glucose or fructose with proteins. During cell membrane damage by free radicals, aldehydes, such as malondialdehyde (MDA), are released. These aldehydes can cross link sugars and proteins, causing protein aggregation with consequential loss of the functional and structural integrity of several tissue proteins. The linking of proteins with sugars or aldehydes involves a process of "carbonylation." This process of protein-linking and aggregation attracts further free radical damage, resulting in the formation of advanced glycation end-products (AGEs). These AGEs make cellular attachments which induce tissue destruction and the generation of disruptive end-products (e.g. nitric oxide or inflammatory mediators, including tumor necrosis factor (TNF) and undesirable interleukins (IL-6)).

The generation of AGEs can be interrupted by the use of carnosine that causes "carnosinylation." This chemical reaction is protective against the process of "carbonylation." Carnosine can combine with MDA, thereby inhibiting the process of glycation. Glycation results in severe compromise of tissue structure and function in many organs. The development of AGEs in metabolic syndrome X and diabetes mellitus explains, in part, the hallmark presence of premature aging in these disorders. Glycation is clearly related to the development of atherosclerosis, beta amyloid deposition in the brain (typical of Alzheimer's disease) and skin aging. Furthermore, glycation can involve cross-linking of sugars or aldehydes with both protein and DNA. This circumstance impairs the normal genetic functions of DNA. Carnosine and other anti-aging compounds fall into the category of "genomeceuticals" or "genome-nutraceuticals."

Carnosine and its variants (anserine, homocarnosine, N-acetyl carnosine and carcinine) contain alanine and histidine. Emerging evidence shows the benefit of carnosine in a variety of disorders or illnesses including: states of chronic inflammation, rheumatoid disease, hypertension, vascular thrombosis, peptic ulceration, delayed wound healing, skin aging, radiation-induced tissue damage, cancer and cataracts. Carnosine has well defined antiaging properties by extending the lifespan of laboratory mice; and it has been shown to expand the lifespan of human cell lines grown in tissue cultures (fibroblasts), in several lab experiments.

METHYL DONATION (METHYLATION)

The maintenance of the structural and functional integrity of several key chemical compounds in the body involves the donation of methyl groups. Examples of vital compounds that require methylation for optimal function include: high density lipoproteins (HDL), DNA, phospholipids, serotonin and adrenaline. Without a continuing ability of the body to methylate many of these pivotal body chemicals, normal tissue functions cannot proceed. A common result of impaired methylation is the damaging accumulation of homocysteine. Homocysteine accumulates as a result of its lack of conversion of homocysteine to methionine (a methyl donor).

Elevated levels of homocysteine are found in states of inflammation and are associated with several diseases, including: cardiovascular disease, dementia, osteoporosis, diabetes mellitus, systemic lupus erythematosis (SLE) and other autoimmune disorders. These circumstances benefit from the availability of methyl donors such as S-adenosyl methionine (SAMe) or tri-methyl-glycine (TMG), which are present in popular dietary supplements.

Deregulation of methylation tends to occur with age and exercise increases the need for methyl group donation. For these reasons aging or over-exercised tissues may suffer protein and DNA damage. A particular problem occurs with collagen destruction in individuals who over-exercise. In competitive athletes, tendon, periarticular and ligamentous disruptions result from compromised or sub-optimal methyl donation. Committed or elite athletes may benefit from methyl-donating supplements (TMG and SAMe), to engage in the preservation of youthful musculoskeletal function.

HORMONAL DEFICIENCY OR IMBALANCE

There is no evidence to support the naïve notion that hormone deficiencies provide a comprehensive explanation of the aging process. While specific hormonal deficiency or deregulation contributes to tissue aging in the mature individual, simple hormone replacements with growth hormone (HGH), DHEA, melatonin or sex hormones are not "stand-alone," antiaging interventions. That said, hormonal therapies show promising benefits for antiaging when used in the correct context. The relative deficiency of several hormones that occurs with advancing years is perceived by some physicians as a simple opportunity to reverse aging by hormone supplementation. Other physicians perceive reductions in certain hormones as a normal healthy adjustment made by the aging body. Of course, neither perspective is completely correct and these issues remain debatable among medical practitioners. All types of hormone replacement therapy remain "on trial" between conventional and alternative physicians.

The administration of human growth hormone (HGH) has become very popular in antiaging medicine, but its use remains controversial. While a number of studies have shown favorable physical and physiological outcomes with HGH administration, recent meta-analysis studies of HGH treatments fail to show real advantages or acceptable safety and efficacy. Proponents of growth hormone use in antiaging medicine report muscle mass increase, gastrointestinal benefits, improved visual acuity, enhanced exercise tolerance, blood pressure reductions, improved libido, promotion of immune function and enhanced cognitive activity.

Such benefits are undeniable in anecdotal reports, but the duration of some of the recorded benefits of HGH may be limited. The consequences of long term use of HGH in antiaging strategies remain uncertain.

The observed benefits of growth hormone supplementation must be balanced against known side effects which are most often experienced at high dosages of injected HGH. Adverse side effects of HGH include: soft tissue swelling, entrapment neuropathy, diabetogenic tendencies, gynecomastia, fluid retention, acromegalic features and hepatic enlargement. The risk of HGH as a promoter of cancer growth is a residual concern. Notable evidence exists that HGH treatments may enhance risks of colonic cancer. Insulin resistance is associated with dysregulation of IGF1 production which is the end-product of HGH injections. This change in IGF1 status has been proposed to explain the known link between Syndrome X and cancer. Claims that HGH can actually accelerate tissue aging remain challenged. On balance, it is clear that HGH treatments must be carefully planned and monitored by a knowledgeable physician. The formal prescribing guidelines for HGH use in anti-aging practice remain confusing, but many physicians believe that HGH administration is indicated when mature adults have documented low blood levels of HGH or IGF1.

Natural ways of boosting HGH release by applying hormonal or nutritional secretagogues are more portable than HGH injections in clinical practice. The classic way of enhancing the secretion of HGH involves the use of growth hormone releasing hormones (e.g. GHRP-6). It may be possible to take GHRP in sublingual or water formulations. Other hormonal secretagogues include GHRH analogues, Ghrelin, ProHGH, with or without GHRH cofactors. Some growth hormone-releasing products are administered by oral capsules or tablets, sublingual or oral sprays, with a variable evidence-base for safety and efficacy. Growth hormone releasing co-factors include glutamine, combinations of arginine, lysine and ornithine, L-dopa or plant derived mimetics (Mucuna pruriens), Carnosine, Homeopathic preparations, Gamma hydroxy butyrate (GABA), yeast extracts and mixed mineral supplements. The use of growth hormone secretagogues over extended periods of time may sometimes result in their ineffectiveness, as the pituitary or its effector mechanisms become tolerant to initial growth hormone releasing actions.

De-Hydro-Epi-Androsterone (DHEA) is a hormone that is readily converted to several sex hormones (estrogen, progesterone and testosterone). The decline in the endogenous availability of DHEA with age is associated with several disorders of aging including chronic inflammation, reduction in IGF1, immune impairments, neurodegenerative disorders (e.g. Alzheimer's disease) and risks of death in the elderly. The administration of DHEA in several of these disorders of aging has been reported to produce an overall benefit. Adverse effects of DHEA administration include severe depression and growth promoting effects of DHEA on the prostate (and perhaps other organs).

While the benefits of DHEA supplementation appear attractive, this supplement should be administered under medical supervision because of its relatively narrow benefit/risk profile. The combined use of melatonin with DHEA may have added antiaging benefits. Melatonin is a potent antioxidant hormone which may improve menopausal symptoms, partially restore age-related declines in thyroid function, exert anti-cancer effects and help restore the biorhythm of sleep. Recent research highlights the potential value of topical melatonin in reversing many changes found in aging skin, as a result of its powerful antioxidant effects.

ADAPTOGENIC HERBS AND BOTANICALS

The term adaptogen is often used in a loose manner in alternative medicine jargon. Adaptogens are most specifically defined as naturally occurring plant substances that assist in the adaptation of the body to continuing stress. However, this terminology is restrictive and many natural substances exist that can act as biological response modifiers (BRM) in a favorable way. The terms adaptogen and BRM may be used interchangeably to advantage. A large number of nutrients or botanical agents have adaptogenic qualities (Table 37). Clearly, a good, balanced nutritional intake of vitamins and phytochemicals is pivotal in a comprehensive adaptogenic body status (Chapter 4).

ADAPTOGEN	ACTIONS
Ginseng (Panax, Eleutherococcus)	Panax (Chinese/Korean), Eleutherococcus (Siberian), Panax quinqufolius (American) have variable antioxidant, brain supporting, cholesterol lowering and estrogenic actions.
Ashwagandha (Withania somnifera)	Ashwagandha contains alkaloids and antioxidants that may have anti-inflam-matory, cognitive-enhancing, anxiolytic and aphrodisiac qualities.

Dandelion (Taraxacum officinale)	Dandelion extract has a diuretic, liver supporting, anti-cancer, antioxidant, blood glucose-balancing and antithrombotic properties. It may inhibit IL6 and TNF alpha (anti-inflammatory)
Ganoderma (lucidum, Reishi)	Ling Zhi (Reishi) mushrooms have anti-cancer, antiangiogenic, DNA-protective, anti-inflammatory effects.
Schisandra (chinensis)	Schisandra has anti-stress, anti-inflammatory, energizing, immune stimulating and hormone balancing actions.
Rhodiola (rosea)	Rhodiola has anti-stress, memory boosting and antidepressant actions
Bacopia (monnieri)	Bacopia has anti-stress, brain supporting and rejuvenating properties.
Resveratrol (skin of red grapes)	Many benefits with adaptogenic effects on apoptosis.

Table 37. Botanical agents that have adaptogenic or biological response modifying effects. These natural substances can be combined in synergistic formulations to constitute a baseline, natural-antiaging approach.

CALORIE RESTRICTION OR CALORIE RESTRICTION "MIMICS"

Restriction of calorie intake, combined with the maintenance of nutrient density of food, has powerful antiaging benefits in rodents and probably humans. Experimental calorie restriction may improve protein metabolism with the elimination of cross-linked protein products by down regulation of "chaperone molecules," with resulting increases in hepatic protein elimination. Calorie restriction has been associated with reductions in blood cholesterol, blood markers of inflammation and improvements in glucose tolerance. Many of these benefits may be related to loss of adipose tissue, but the proposed actions of calorie restriction are legion (Table 38).

- Lowering of blood pressure
- Insulin sensitization
- Reduction of body temperature
- Apoptosis regulation
- Decreased oxidative stress
- Enhanced brain function

- Stimulation of growth factors
- Diminished death risk
- Improved tissue repair
- Lowering body weight
- Lowering of blood cholesterol
- Increased muscle mass
- Altered hormone profiles
- Increased energy
- Anti-stress actions
- Modulation of protein metabolism

Table 38. Proposed or documented effects of calorie restriction on body structures and functions.

Several natural compounds or drugs have been proposed as agents that can mimic variably the effects of calorie restrictions. These putative, calorie-restriction mimetics include resveratrol, hydroxycitrate, Gymnema alkaloids, alpha lipoic acid, cinnamon (methylhydroxychalones), indoacetate, metformin and thiazolidinediones. Much interest has focused on the antiaging benefits of resveratrol. These benefits are potent and versatile. They include: regulation of apoptosis, antioxidant actions, anticancer effects, cardiovascular benefits and specific gene-regulating actions. The aging gene in question is SIRT1. This gene modulates tissue aging by inhibiting apoptosis. Resveratrol exerts complex, poorly understood effects on apoptosis regulation, with an ability to upregulate or downregulate cell death.

TOXICITY AND PREMATURE AGING

The 20th century witnessed the increasing use of synthetic chemicals and the new millennium is a time to experience the adverse effects of these toxins (toxicants). Toxins are ubiquitous in our environment and the body tissues of animals and humankind. The association between toxicant exposures (derived from food, buildings, or consumer goods) and chronic disease is becoming increasingly obvious in contemporary medical research.

Attempts to avoid or ameliorate exposure to environmental toxins by lifestyle change, consumption of organic vegetables and body cleansing programs are valuable antiaging tactics (Chapter 30). Integrative medicine now stresses the use of non-toxic alternatives to many items that contain health-damaging toxins. Among the undesirable actions of organic chemicals (toxicants) are the promotion of weight gain, propagation of oxidative stress to tissues, direct mutagenic effects and the exertion of unwanted hormonal actions e.g. xenoestrogens.

While not prominent in antiaging advice, the avoidance of unnecessary pharmaceuticals and conventional hormone replacement therapy (HRT) for menopause appears to be prudent recommendations. Adverse side effects of medications and iatrogenic drug catastrophes are a major cause of death and premature disability in the US. There appears to be little doubt that the use of conventional sex hormone replacement therapy, with animal estrogens and synthetic progestins, appears to have more risks than benefits in the management of menopause. The proposed safety of bioidentical hormone treatments remains to be defined, despite the rhetoric.

IMMUNE FUNCTION

Immune senescence is characterized by both deficiencies and deregulation of immune function. Much interest in natural medicine has focused on the correction of Natural Killer cell function (NK cells), at the expense of considering needs to modulate other components of the aging immune system. While immune function involves a complex cascade of bio-physiological events, attempts to enhance or modulate immunity, using natural medicines, has often focused inappropriately on the use of single agents of botanical or nutritional origin, with the limited actions on the complex immune cascade of events.

My colleagues and I have tested the hypothesis that complex immune functions are best addressed by synergistic formulations of multiple herbs, botanicals and nutrients. In vitro and in vivo comparisons of dietary supplements with effects on immune function show that synergistic formulations of substances with known immune modulating effects provide more potent and versatile effects than single or limited compositions of immune stimulating supplements. This approach is summarized in Table 39 which identifies a combination of natural substances that are associated with specific research. This research shows profound stimulating effects on NK cell activity and cell mediated immunity with associated actions on immune, molecular cascades. It is noteworthy that complex immune modulating formulations can incorporate botanicals with antiviral properties (e.g. Andrographis paniculata), or extracts of Ecballium elaterium to further enhance immune protection. In brief, evidence has accumulated that improvement in immune function may promote longevity.

- Andrographis paniculata
- Acanthopanax Senticosa
- Green tea
- Turmeric

- Grape seed extract
- Zinc
- Vitamin C
- Ashwagandha
- Oregon grape
- Shitake mushroom
- Echinacea purpurea
- Goldenseal
- Golden thread
- Aloe Vera
- Garlic
- Astragalus
- Korean ginseng
- Coriolus versicolor
- Active Hexose Correlated Compound (AHCC)
- Beta glucan

Table 39. Nutritional and botanical agents with an evidence-base for use in combination to modulate and promote immune function. Courtesy of Holt MD Technologies. Treatment claims with natural substances that alter immunity have to be avoided.

SLEEPLESSNESS

Sleep deprivation has many adverse, social, psychological, psychiatric and physical consequences. Sleeplessness has been associated with alterations in appetite that promote weight gain, the induction of inflammation and chronic stress, together with linkage to several chronic diseases. Unobtrusive consequences of lack of sleep include mood change, depression, poor mental function and metabolic changes similar to syndrome X. An arguable association exists between abnormalities of sleep and premature death.

Standard prescription sleeping pills or over the counter hypnotic drugs are common causes of iatrogenic problems. Natural approaches to induce restful sleep are to be preferred over pharmaceutical approaches. Such interventions include lifestyle change, behavioral modifications and the use of synergistic combinations of herbs and nutrients that are part of "The Sleep Naturally Plan." Certain herbs with adaptogenic or antioxidant properties can be selected as natural ways of promoting healthy sleep. This approach is a viable alternative to using hypnotic drugs which may carry inherent risks of troublesome or dangerous side effects and perhaps premature death.

ANTI-AGING NUTRACEUTICAL STRATEGIES

In view of the many factors that contribute to aging, a holistic approach to antiaging is required, with due consideration for positive lifestyle change. The challenge in using remedies of natural origin as recuperative factors involves the creation of synergistic, natural formulations that can be administered in a convenient, cost-effective format that may result in reasonable patient compliance. Such formulations should include sufficient ranges and amounts of evidence-based, antiaging agents that can access the multiple aspects of the physiological and chemical cascades of aging. In summary, this combined approach requires a group of nutraceutical, antiaging factors that can be administered in a convenient, well-tolerated protocol (Table 40).

AGING FACTORS	ANTIAGING NUTRACEUTICALS
Poor nutrition	Preference for multivitamins combined with minerals in powder blends of fruit, berries, greens and functional herbs or nutrients.
Anti-aging factors to correct pivotal biochemical imbalance, incorporating methyl donation and antioxidants to interfere with tissue glycation and oxidative stress. Recommendations include putative secretagogues or HGH "helpers."*	Carnosine, Glutamine, S-Adenosyl Methionine (SAMe), Tri-Methyl-Glycine (TMG), Siberian Ginseng (Eleuthorococcus senticosa), Rhodiola rosea, Ashwagandha (Withania somnifera), Dandelion root (Taraxacum officinale), Schisandra chinensis, Ganoderma lucidum, Bacopa monnieri, Acetyl-L-Carnitine, N-Acetyl Cysteine, Citrus Bioflavonoids and Alpha Lipoic Acid with Folic acid, Vitamin B6 and B12 (Homocysteine relief).
Sleep deprivation	Initial lifestyle change with combination synergistic formulations of melatonin, 5 HTP, adaptogenic or sedative herbs.
Membrane lipid damage and prevention of chronic disease and inflammation.	Omega-3 essential fatty acids in enteric-coated fish oil capsules (at least 2g/day of 30:20 ratio of EPA/DHA). Cofactors required, e.g. minerals.
Immune impairment	Use of complex formulations that modulate immune cascades with antiviral activity.
Hormonal declines	Evidence-based GH secretagogues and DHEA

Combat diseases of premature aging	Cardiovascular health promotion, management of obesity, metabolic syndrome X and diabetes mellitus. Cancer prevention.

Table 40. The author's recommendations for the rational use of combination supplements in antiaging medical practice. A universal, baseline approach to body recuperation involves nutritional corrections and specific formulations of antiaging substances.*

CONCLUSION

A focus on a holistic approach to antiaging using positive lifestyle change and natural medicine is a key initiative in modern healthcare. Once relegated to the realms of quackery, remedies of natural origin play a major role in the promotion of longevity. The physician involved in antiaging medicine should consider "staged strategies" of intervention, starting with the most natural and simplistic approach of healthy lifestyle recommendations, followed by well designed and tailored nutritional approaches. Popular hormonal interventions can be exercised in these staged strategies, but physician supervision must be involved in interventions that alter endocrine profiles by hormone replacement.

CHAPTER 32

MISCELLANEOUS TOPICS

INTRODUCTION

D IETARY supplement technology changes rapidly. Certain product categories become of great consumer interest and many single-item products dwindle in their popularity. This section of the book serves two purposes. First, product categories of great interest, at the time of writing, are reviewed and second, a basic A to Z of commonly used botanicals is described. This chapter is intended to make this educational program more complete, but it is a mammoth undertaking for the reader. . . good luck!

HERBAL JARGON DEFINED

Abortifacents-Capable of bringing on a spontaneous abortion (To be feared and not recommended).

Alterative-An herb that works slowly to alter body chemistry. The effects are not immediately noticeable. Restores health and vital functions by cleansing the blood.

Analeptic-Having restorative or stimulating effects.

Analgesic-A pain reliever.

Anodyne-See analgesic.

Anthelminithic-Botanicals that rid the body of worms.

Antiarrhythmic-Preventing or relieving irregular heart rhythms.

Antiemetic-Controls vomiting.

Antihistamine-Counteracts histamine production in colds and allergies.

Antiphlogistic-Reduces inflammation.

Antipyretic-Lowers fevers.

Antiscorbutic-Botanicals that fight scurvy (these are high in vitamin C).
  Antiseptic-Prevents infection by inhibiting the growth of micro-organisms.

Antispasmodic-Controls muscle spasms.

Aperient-Gently stimulates bowel elimination.

Aphrodisiac-Arouses or intensifies sexual desire.

Aromatic-Substances that contain volatile oils. They stimulate digestion.

Astringent-These herbs help contain tissues; effective in stopping the flow of
  bodily fluids.

Bronchodilator-Widens air passages; relaxes the smooth muscles of the
  bronchi; eases breathing.

Cardiotonic-Enhances heart function.

Carminative-Induces the expulsion of gas, soothes digestion.

Cathartic-Rapidly brings bowel eliminations.

Cholagogue-Increases bile flow.

Choloretic-See cholagogue.

Demulcent-Soothing irritated tissues. Used for sore throats and upset
  stomachs.

Deobstruent-Clears obstructions from the body ducts.

Depurgative-Tends to bring about purification or cleansing.

Diaphoretic-Stimulates perspiration; aids in eliminating wastes.

Disinfectant-An agent that destroys or neutralizes the growth of disease-
  causing microorganisms.

Diuretic-Increases amount of urine passed.

Eliminative-Encourages elimination of bodily wastes through the colon,
  kidneys, lymph, and skin.

Emetic-Causes vomiting.

Emmenagogue- Promotes menstruation.

Emollient-Used to soothe the skin.

Expectorant-Promotes discharge of mucus and phlegm from respiratory passages.

Febrifuge-see antipyretic.

Galactagogue-Stimulates lactation.

Hemostatic-Stops bleeding.

Hepatic-Beneficial to the liver.

Hypotensive-Tends to lower the blood pressure.

Immunotonic-Strenghtens the immune system.

Laxative-Brings about bowel movements.

Nephritic-Used to treat kidney problems.

Nervine-Used to calm nervous conditions.

Ophthalmic-Used to treat the eyes.

Oxytoic-Intensifies labor and speeds childbirth.

Phytohormone-A hormone produced by a plant; plant hormones control such physiological functions as germination, growth, and metabolism.

Potentiator-An herb that increases the action of another herb.

Purgative-Brings about radical bowel evacuation.

Rubefacient-Substances that irritate the skin, producing redness.

Salivant-Stimulates secretion of saliva.

Secretagogue-Stimulates secretion of vital body fluids.

Sedative-Reduces anxiety, stress, or excitement.

Somnifacient-Sleep inducing.

Spasmolytic-Relieving or preventing spasms.

Stimulant-Temporarily arouses physiological activity.

Stomachic-Stimulates the production of digestive juices; relieves stomach disorders.

Styptic-Stops bleeding.

Sudorific-Induces or increases perspiration.

Sympathomimetic-Produces physiological effects that resemble those caused by the sympathetic nervous system (i.e., reduction of digestive secretions, contraction of blood vessels, increase in heart rate).

Tonic-Invigorates, refreshes, or restores the whole body.

Vasodilator-Expands blood vessels; promotes circulation.

Vermifuge-Expels worms from the intestines.

Vulnerary-A substance used to treat wounds.

The following list summarizes some common disorders that may be amenable to herbal interventions. The herbal substances in the table were selected because supporting data exists for their use. However, the evidence-base for certain botanicals to benefit certain diseases varies greatly. Remember that dietary supplements cannot carry treatment claims.

COMMON CONDITIONS AND THE HERBS USED TO TREAT THEM

Alzheimer's disease	St. John's wort, Ginkgo biloba
Arthritis	see Chapter 8, Joint Care
Asthma	Aniseed, celadine, licorice root, valerian
Blood pressure	Mistletoe, garlic, ginger
Boils	Chamomille, marjoram, marsh mallow, nasturtium. sanicle, compress of thyme
Bronchitis	Comfrey, camphor
Burns	Raw onions, potatoes, and aloe
Cholesterol (high)	Guggulipid, soybean extract (isoflavones, lecithin)
Colds	Andrographis, chamomile inhalations, cinnamon, Echinacea, ginger, marjoram infusions, peppermint, sunflower seed oil, thyme, yarrow etc.
Constipation	Elder blossom, hyssop, peppermint etc.
Depression	St. John's wort etc.
Diarrhea	Infusion of blackberry root, cinnamon, peppermint, peppers (teas)
Dyspepsia	Caraway, fennel, peppermint
Fatigue	Agrimony, marjoram, peppermint, rose hips, yeast tablets
Fevers	Andrographis, tinctures of aconite, feverfew
Flatulence	Caraway, tincture of cardamom, charcoal biscuits, fennel, garlic, turmeric, dill

Gout	Hyssop, juniper, capsicum
Headache	Chamomile, lavender (topically), mint, poppy, feverfew
Heart disease	Andrographis, foxglove, motherwort
Insomnia	Aniseed, bergamot, hops, valerian
Immune disorders	Andrographis, echinacea, garlic
Menstrual problems	Lady's mantle tea, rose hips
Piles	Lesser celandine, plantain (pulped leaves applied locally)
Rheumatism	Boswellia, chamomile, hyssop, mugwort, onion (rubbed on joints), rosemary (externally)
Sore throat	Stinging nettle (gargled), honey
Sprains and bruises	Arnica (externally), bromelain, homeopathic arnica
Stings and bites	Horseradish (externally), dock leaves (topically)
Stomach ulcers	Boswellia, garlic, licorice, peppermint
Toothache	Oil of cloves, elder, tansy
Urinary disorders	Birch chamomile, infusion of chickweed, cowberry, saw palmetto, Pygeum africanum, stinging nettles, cranberry
Varicose veins	Fresh coltsfoot leaves in a poultice, valerian
Vomiting	Chamomile, peppermint, spearmint, rhubarb

The examples of botanical healing given in the above list are often used by master herbalists who dispense rather than use fixed supplement formulations. These are examples of botanical applications and they are not necessarily recommendations of the author, even though the author is a skilled herbalist and medical doctor.

A TO Z GUIDE TO COMMONLY USED HERBS

Alfalfa (Medicago sativa)

Alfalfa has been used to lower cholesterol, promote good circulation, treat diabetes and provide general stimulating effects as a tonic and a promoter of appetite. However, the evidence for all these benefits is quite arguable. Alfalfa is quite nutritious, containing fiber, protein, unsaturated fatty acids, calcium, phosphorous, iron, other trace elements, organic acids, and vitamins K and C, together with chlorophyll pigment. Evidence for its documented benefit in the promotion of health is quite scant. Alfalfa should be taken in moderation because some evidence exists that it may cause blood abnormalities, such as a form of anemia and perhaps aggravate lupus (systemic lupus erythematosis, an autoimmune disease). In fact, alfalfa should probably be avoided by those who have autoimmune diseases.

Aloe (Aloe vera, barbadenis)

Aloe is used in the unapproved treatment of immune deficiency, diabetes mellitus, cancer, asthma and AIDS. It has a long history of use as a topical agent for a variety of dermatological problems. Aloe products have become the focus of intensive multi-level marketing activity and aloe products are ubiquitous in health food stores and grocery stores. Aloe is very beneficial in the topical treatment of abrasions, burns (especially sunburn), and dry skin. While the evidence for aloe as a therapeutic agent in a variety of skin disorders is quite convincing, the evidence for the oral use of aloe in several disease states remains debatable.

Contemporary research has focused on the presence of chemicals called acemannans. These are promoted as important active compounds in aloe preparations. There is some evidence that they may exert a beneficial effect on immune function. In order to obtain sufficient acemannan from many regular types of aloe, an individual may have to consume very large quantities of this botanical.

There is limited evidence that aloe has been useful as a complementary therapy in the treatment of AIDS, with some reports of synergistic effects with AZT. The postulated antiviral effects of acemannans require further clarification. Unfortunately, claims that aloe is a body cleanser, antiseptic, fever-reducing agent, nutrient, or anti-inflammatory agent are not supported conclusively by controlled studies or clinical information, but anecdotal benefit is apparent.

There are multiple sources of aloe, but the two main sources are Aloe vera gels, prepared from the leaf of the plant, and Aloe juice (or Aloe latex) which may be derived from dried plants or plants treated by a variety of chemical or mechanical processes. It has been observed that many aloe preparations may lose their "activity" if stored. Several dietary supplement manufacturers claim that their type of aloe extract contains active ingredients, without showing much evidence of health benefits.

You should also be aware that the word "aloe" can be applied to commercial products that contain minimal amounts of putative, active constituents. Many aloe products are reconstituted from extracts or concentrates of variably prepared aloe derivatives.

Angelica (Angelica archangelica)

Angelica, which is variably produced from the root, stem, leaves, or fruits of angelica plants, has been used in folklore medicine in the belief that it prevented gas and encouraged the passage of perspiration and urine. There is limited evidence to support that Angelica has these functions. Angelica has been used to induce abortion in a completely illegal manner, and if used in large doses in these circumstances, it is very dangerous. Extracts of Angelica contain compounds that may make the skin more susceptible to damage by sunlight. This susceptibility is called photosensitivity.

Apricot Pits (Laetrile)

Laetrile-commonly compounded of extracts from apricot kernels-was a very popular alternative cancer cure in the 1960's and 1970's. Several research studies subsequently brought into question the efficacy of laetrile and related compounds in cancer therapy.

The Food and Drug Administration took sanctions against the sale of laetrile in 1971, but it was not until the 1980's that multi-center clinical trials were performed with laetrile by the National Cancer Institute. These studies concluded that laetrile may be ineffective in cancer therapy, but many alternative medical practitioners questioned the NCI studies. Today, laetrile is not commonly used in the United States, but it is still used as a cancer cure by clinics in adjacent countries (e.g. Mexico). The alternative medicine community has continued to take issue with the conclusions of the clinical trials performed by the National Cancer Institute (NCI). At present, no solid evidence exists that amygdalin (the compound in apricot pits) or "laetrile" in any form has major benefits in the treatment of cancer, but many disagree with this statement, which has cost me friends.

Barberry (Berberis vulgaris)

Barberry is a Native American remedy that is said to be a general tonic. It contains alkaloids of uncertain pharmacological effects and probably has a limited role in contemporary herbal therapy, except in the management of intestinal parasitosis, or usage in small dosages as a COX-2 enzyme inhibitor.

Bayberry (Myria cerifera)

Bayberry root and bark contain compounds that may have steroid-like effects, but some concern exists about bayberry's ability to cause cancer in experimental animals. Bayberry may have some health benefits, but its safety is questionable in large dosages.

Betony (Stachys officinalis)

Betony was formerly used as a health panacea, but its only real value is as an astringent. Its astringency comes from its content of tannins. Tannins are used in the tanning of leather hides. Betony "mouthwash" has some use for gingivitis, and the herb has been reported to be effective in the management of some types of diarrhea, but I do not recommend it.

Bilberry (Vaccinium myrtillus)

Much interest exists in the use of bilberry extracts that contain chemicals (anthocyanosides or flavonoids) which are known to be antioxidants. Several studies have shown that anthocyanosides (anthocyanidins), in bilberries, can improve visual acuity at night; and enhance the ability of the eyes to adapt to the dark. The active components of bilberry work on retinal cells, and favorable results of the administration of bilberry extracts have been reported in a variety of ocular disorders, including diabetic retinopathy, macular degeneration, and several causes of night blindness. British Royal Air Force pilots who used bilberry reported improvement in their nocturnal eyesight during bombing raids on Germany in World War II.

Bilberry is a component of several dietary supplements that are sold to promote ocular health. Standardized bilberry extracts have much to offer in ocular health. They remain under-investigated and under-applied in clinical practice.

Black and Blue Cohosh (Cimicifuga racemosa and Caulophyllum thalictroides)

Black and blue cohosh have similar names, but their effects on the body are like "chalk and cheese". Black cohosh is very valuable in standardized form for the relief of menopausal symptoms and premenstrual syndrome. There is evidence in animals that black cohosh may contain compounds that bind to estrogen receptors, but the evidence for estrogenic effects in humans remains debatable. Blue cohosh has little if any role in modern herbal treatments and it may be toxic.

Borage (Borago officinalis)

Borage is a classic astringent containing tannins. It has a reputation for relieving symptoms of depression. In addition, much interest has focused on borage oil as a source of health giving polyunsaturated fatty acids (essential fatty acids). Some borage preparations contain certain alkaloids that may be carcinogenic or damage the liver. Only borage oil free of toxins should be used.

Boswellia (Boswellia serrata)

Boswellic acids are extracted from gum resins derived from the tree Boswellia serrata. The extract belongs to a class of compounds called gugguls, which have been described in ancient Ayurvedic medicine as possessing potent, antirheumatic properties. The active ingredients of boswellia extract are beta-boswellic acid and other acids.

Many studies have confirmed the benefit of standardized boswellia extract in the management of osteoarthritis and rheumatoid arthritis. Boswellic acids can protect against artificially induced arthritis in animals. This herb's anti-inflammatory actions have been well documented in soft tissue inflammation and it is a valuable agent for acne. Detailed laboratory experiments have shown that extracts of Boswellia serrata resin protect the main constituents of bone and cartilage (chondroitins), by reducing the activity of several enzymes that degrade important structural components of cartilage (glycosamino-glycans). Boswellia extracts inhibit leukotrienes (inflammatory chemical messengers).

Some scientists have referred to Boswellia as a nonsteroidal anti-inflammatory agent. This terminology is not to be confused with standard nonsteroidal anti-inflammatory drugs (NSAIDs), such as ibuprofen and naproxen, which often cause stomach upset and may produce stomach or duodenal ulcers. It is notable that Boswellia exhibits anti-ulcerogenic activity, in contrast to the ulcerogenic potential of NSAIDs.

Dietary supplements containing standardized extracts of Boswellia have been reported repeatedly to reduce joint swelling and morning stiffness, increase joint mobility, and produce an overall improvement in quality of life in individuals with arthritis. These effects have been seen in patients with a variety of rheumatological disorders such as: osteoarthritis, gouty arthritis, rheumatoid disease, nonspecific rheumatism, fibrositis, myositis, cervical spondylolysis, and backache due to vertebral disorders. Boswellia is finding an increasing role as a dietary supplement or a topical preparation in the treatment of arthritis in humans, but this role has not been accepted by the FDA. It has been used effectively by holistic veterinarians in dogs with hip dysplasia, and lame horses. The importance of the standardization of Boswellia products for their content of boswellic acids and pentacyclic triterpene acids should not be underestimated. I prefer it to be used in combination with other agents.

Bromelain

Bromelain is a mixture of certain protein-digesting enzymes (proteolytic) that are found in the stems of pineapples. Collaborative laboratory research studies show that most bromelain is contained in the stem of the pineapple, nearest to the fruit. High concentrations of bromelain are also found in the woody core of pineapples.

There are more than a couple hundred scientific studies supporting the use of bromelain as potential therapy for arthritis, sports injuries, and soft tissue trauma. In fact, bromelain has been used as a prescription medication for improving recovery from trauma and bruising. Bromelain has anti-inflammatory effects, including some demonstrated ability to block the production of compounds that mediate inflammation. Bromelain is sometimes a component of dietary supplements used to promote joint health, and the supporting evidence for this application is quite plausible. Bromelain has a new-found use as an important ingredient in products that accelerate wound healing and trauma recovery following medical aesthetic procedures. It can be used effectively in combination with homeopathic Arnica Montana for trauma recovery (vide infra).

Bran/Insoluble Fiber

Bran is a form of dietary fiber that has many potential health-giving properties. Dietary fiber resists digestion by the human gastrointestinal tract. Well-conducted epidemiologic, clinical, and experimental studies imply that bran supplementation can assist in the treatment or prevention of several diseases, including coronary heart disease, varicose veins, diverticular disease, hemorrhoids and colon cancer. Bran has been used as a way of promoting a feeling of fullness in the treatment of obesity, and good evidence exists that it can lower blood cholesterol. Many of the beneficial effects of bran are related to its ability to hold water, while it resides in the colon. Supplementation of the diet with approximately 25 gm of fiber per day is effective treatment for irritable bowel syndrome (IBS) in many sufferers of this condition. Bran affects many symptoms of IBS but it is not universally successful in managing abdominal pain due to spasm.

Butcher's-broom (Ruscus aculeatus)

Butcher's-broom, used in some herbal medicines, defies clear definition. This is because different plants have been used to produce several products that bear the name "butcher's-broom." Extracts of stems of certain types of butcher's-broom contain compounds that affect blood vessels by working on receptors in the adrenergic nervous system. These agents are believed by some to be beneficial in assisting in the restoration of vessel tone, especially in the lower limbs. These are probably naïve thoughts.

Butcher's-broom has been used to promote beneficial effects on the circulation. The overall effect on this herb is to cause constriction of blood vessels. Self-medication with butcher's-broom cannot be recommended because vasoconstriction can have serious consequences, if applied in the wrong context.

Caffeine-Containing Products

Caffeine is ubiquitous in the American diet and it is addictive. Herbals or beverages containing caffeine are best taken in moderation. The practice of combining ephedrine and caffeine in diet pills is dangerous and ill advised. I proposed this advice in 1995 in medical literature. One important issue must be raised among natural medical practitioners. The beneficial health effects of several herbs containing caffeine have been documented only with naturally caffeinated herbs, e.g. green tea. There is little evidence that decaffeinated herbs are effective, e.g. green tea or green coffee bean extract. The amount of caffeine found in extracts of green tea or green coffee beans is so small that it is not of clinical significance in most people.

There is no argument that caffeine has potent pharmacological effects, especially stimulatory effects. Individuals with healthy hearts as well as those with heart disease may suffer irregular heartbeats as a consequence of consuming excessive caffeine. Many people forget that excessive amounts of caffeine can cause nervousness, anxiety, insomnia, excess stomach acidity, high blood glucose, and high cholesterol levels. Furthermore, the lay public is not universally aware that caffeine can cause deformities in the fetuses of experimental animals.

Pregnant women should limit caffeine intake.

Calendula (Calendula officinalis)

Calendula is an ancient remedy that has unequivocal benefit when applied topically. Calendula assists in wound healing and the management of dry and chapped skin. Amazingly, relatively little research has been done with topical calendula, despite the continuous reporting of its beneficial effects.

Capsicum (Capsicum frutescens) or Cayenne

Capsicum (capsaicin) is found in several different types of pepper, and it is used both in topical and oral forms. The active ingredient of capsicum is capsaicin, which may have stimulatory effects on gastrointestinal function, anti-clotting effects, and cholesterol-lowering ability. It is believed that capsaicin depletes a particular substance (substance P) that facilitates the transmission of pain through peripheral nerves. Capsaicin is used in topical preparations to control the pain of skin eruptions, such as cold sores or herpes, but it burns when placed on the skin. It is a "reflex counterirritant" for pain control.

When taken orally, capsaicin has variable effects. It may even protect against peptic ulceration, although spices in the diet may exacerbate symptoms of peptic ulcer disease. Capsicum should not be used in high dosages.

Chaparral (Larrea tridentata)

Chaparral is mentioned because of its historical interest. This plant grows wild in many Southwestern states in the United States and it is an old Native American remedy (alleged) for just about every disease. Chaparral contains a substance (nordihydroguaiaretic acid) that some believe can cure cancer. Because this component of chaparral is very toxic, certain preparations of this herb should not be consumed by humans. Avoid chaparral.

Comfrey (Symphytyum officinale)

Comfrey has been used mainly in topical applications as a poultice for wound healing. It may be toxic when taken internally and preparations of comfrey may be contaminated with compounds derived from deadly nightshade. The most significant problem associated with comfrey ingestion is the possibility of liver toxicity, believed to be related to its content of certain alkaloids. Comfrey is unsafe for internal use.

Cranberry (Vaccinium macrocarpon)

Extracts of cranberry, whole cranberries, and cranberry juice are widely promoted for their benefit in the management of urinary tract infection and kidney stones. The beneficial effect of cranberry in urinary tract infection has been documented. Certain components of cranberries have antibacterial properties. These components seem to prevent bacteria from sticking to cells that line the urinary tract. Because cranberry juice is acidic (it contains hippuric acid), large amounts can cause acidification of the urine. This urinary acidification does not appear to be the main mechanism for the beneficial effect of cranberry in urinary tract infection.

Curcumin (Turmeric)

Curcumin is the yellow pigment of Curcuma longa, or turmeric, a spice used in the preparation of Indian curry. Curcuminoids are active constituents of turmeric and they deserve special mention because of their newfound, abilities to act as natural pain killers. Curcumin is known to be an effective antioxidant and anti-inflammatory substance. Animal experiments show that turmeric has anticancer effects, and several human studies are underway to assess the treatment potential of turmeric.

Mixtures of curcuminoids have wide ranging health benefits, which have led to their classification as "bioprotectors." The best known qualities of curcuminoids relate to their antioxidant qualities, but other biological effects of curcuminoids have been defined in laboratory and clinical studies in humans. Of great interest is the use of curcuminoid extracts as analgesics. The chemistry of curcuminoids appears to be complex and several claims have been made about the isolation of active principles. These active principles (curcuminoids) derived from turmeric, have been chemically complexed to improve absorption and rapidity of onset of action as a pain killer. It would appear that the effects of curcuminoids in pain control require dosages that are approximately equivalent to about 1200 mg of pure curcumin. In this form, curcuminoids have received approval by certain overseas regulatory agencies to be used in the direct treatment of symptoms or disabilities caused by different types of arthritis or musculoskeletal problems (Australian Regulatory Authorities).

The use of curcumin for pain control is a major advance in nutraceutical technology because of the potential or serious toxicity that has been encountered with over-the-counter or prescription pain killers e.g. aspirin or NSAID or acetaminophen. Controlled clinical observations show that curcuminoids may relieve arthritic pain in osteoarthritis or rheumatism or rheumatoid arthritis, with distinct abilities to relieve muscular aches or pains, joint stiffness, joint swelling and inflammation, to a variable degree. Data has been presented to regulatory agencies in Australia and these health claims have been endorsed by the government. Unfortunately, such endorsement has not been made by the U.S. Food and Drug Administration.

The toxicity of pain killers is well known. Acetaminophen (Tylenol® and many other brands) has been associated with liver toxicity and it carries a high risk of death from liver failure in circumstances of overdosage, such as those encountered with attempted suicide. The side effect profile of Aspirin and NSAID requires no amplification because these classes of drugs have common and onerous side effects, including in specific circumstances, the following: dyspepsia and stomach upset, peptic ulcer formation and complications, occasional life threatening bleeding from the upper and lower digestive tract, liver toxicity, renal toxicity and a yet to be completely defined overall risk of stroke or heart attack (most relevant to COX-2 types of NSAID).

Is it important to note that the focus of activity in turmeric chemistry is on curcumin content. Certain levels of curcumin have been shown in clinical trials to be useful for the effective management of pain and inflammation in arthritis. I stress that these findings are presented in peer-review medical literature, but they have not been endorsed by all regulatory agencies, especially those in the U.S. Providing curcumin in a specific form can enhance effectiveness and onset of action for pain relief. In brief, curcuminoids have well described antioxidant, anti-inflammatory, antiallergic, antispasmodic, antibacterial, antifungal and anticancer effects. These claims cannot be made in the U.S., except antioxidant claims.

In one important clinical trial, curcumin was given at a dosage of 1200 mg per day for up to six weeks in 18 patients with rheumatoid arthritic and significant improvement in symptoms of morning stiffness, restricted walking and joint swelling were observed (Deodhar SD, S.R., Srimal, RC. Indian J. Med. Res., 71:p. 632-634, 1980). Further studies in 182 patients with rheumatoid disease showed favorable clinical outcome after 16 weeks of administration of curcumin (1200 mg daily) (Chopra et al, J Rheumatol, 27(6): p. 1365-72, 2000). Direct comparisons have been made between curcumin and the powerful, potentially toxic NSAID, phenylbutazone, as a way of reducing post operative pain (Satoskar R, S. Shah and S. Shenoy, Int J Clin Pharmacol Ther Toxicol, 24(12): p. 651-4, 1986). In these studies, curcumin was found overall to be more effective than phyenylbutazone in reducing pain and tenderness at wound sites. A general review of several human clinical trials has shown that dosages of curcumin up to 2.5 g per day have potent anti inflammatory effects, with benefits for pain control (Chainani-

Wu, N, J Altern. Complement. Med., 9(1): p. 161-8, 2003). Curcumin has several actions including an ability to inhibit COX-2 enzymes.

Holt MD Technologies has recently proposed an amplification of the diverse effects of curcuminoids by the addition of a natural herbal blend that may inhibit COX-2 enzyme systems (Joint Care, Chapter 8). Scientific literature shows that curcumin blocks pro-inflammatory mediators (interleukin-IL-1, PGE_2). Curcumin also inhibits the incorporation of arachidonic acid into phospholipids in platelets; and it has other "blocking effects" on TNF-alpha, IL-1 beta and IL8. The antioxidant/anti-inflammatory effects of curcumin are well described in studies that show its ability to bind superoxide radicals, thereby inhibiting lipid membrane damage by lipid peroxidation. One can infer that curcumin has wide ranging potential application in many inflammatory disorders and these actions may explain observed benefits in Alzheimer's disease and obesity (obesitis)… to name a few conditions.

The addition of a COX-2 inhibitor herbal blend provides a greater spectrum of biological activity than curcumin alone and this permits the daily reduction of the total dosage requirement of curcumin. The proposed herbal blend added to curcumin includes: Phellodendron amurense, Barberry bark, Goldenthread root, Feverfew Herb, Ginger Root, Green Tea extract, Polyphenols, Tulsi leaves, Hops flower, Oregano leaves, Rosemary leaves, Chinese Skullcap Herb, Turmeric root, Nettle leaves and Devil's claw root. Boswellia serrata can be added for its leukotriene inhibitory effects. The biochemistry of the actions of these herbs is quite complex and wide reaching in its effects on chemical cascades that promote pain and inflammation. It should be noted that the optimum dosages of combined herbal preparations for pain control remain to be defined, but synergistic formulations appear to amplify overall effects on body structures and functions. The formulation of this kind of product gets into a very gray area in regulatory issues, but the expression of cyco-oxygenase-2 enzymes is readily defined as an expression of normal body function.

Dandelion (Taraxacum officinale)

Dandelion has enjoyed widespread use in the treatment of a host of conditions. Its use in folklore medicine is supported by much precedent. Dandelion appears safe, with some valuable anti-aging properties (see Chapter 31).

Devil's Claw (Harpagophytum procumbens)

Devil's claw may be useful as an appetite stimulant and carminative (flatulence-reducing substance). It is used widely in several European countries and is touted as a cure for many chronic degenerative diseases. Some practitioners of herbal medicine believe that this herb has antirheumatic and antiviral properties, but more supporting data are required.

Dong Quai

Dong quai is the classic female herbal supplement. It must not be used in pregnancy, but it has many anecdotal reports of its successful use in the treatment of painful menstruation, premenstrual syndrome, and menopausal symptoms. It is believed that Dong quai can have a modulating effect on the activity of estrogen. This herb may contain compounds that can make people sensitive to light. Dong quai is used widely in Asia and is a principal component of several traditional Chinese and Ayurvedic medicines, applied in women's health.

Echinacea

The North American Indians have used Echinacea for centuries. Today, Echinacea is a staple dietary supplement that is widely used in North America and Europe as an alternative treatment for cancer, as a treatment of yeast infections, and for enhancement of immunity and wound healing. Most of the research on Echinacea has been performed in Europe, even though the plants from which this herbal supplement is commonly derived are native to North America. There is good scientific agreement that the herb contains compounds which stimulate the immune system in a variety of ways. Data supporting the use of Echinacea to enhance the body's defenses is so strong that the German government has recommended the herb to be used as supportive therapy for a variety of recurrent infections. Echinacea is here to stay with evidence of benefit, even if some of the claims are overstated.

The reader should remember that all types of echinacea are not "born equal" in terms of their biological effects. Readers are advised to revise and recognize different species and extracts of Echinacea and their documented biological effects.

Ephedra (Ephedra sinica)

Ephedra is an ancient Chinese remedy that is often used in the treatment of respiratory illness and allergy. The active constituents of ephedra, known as ma huang in China, are ephedrine and related compounds. These compounds form the basis of commonly used, modern, over-the counter (OTC) cough and cold remedies (e.g., pseudoephedrine). In high doses, ephedra can excite the mind and stimulate the central nervous system. It can raise blood pressure, increase heart rate, and cause insomnia and mental agitation. Ma huang should not be used in conjunction with caffeine. Ephedra should not be used by individuals with significant heart disease or high blood pressure or Syndrome X.

Young people have very foolishly used ephedra to enhance athletic performance or as an illicit drug. Controls now exist on the use of ma huang in some states. There would appear to be little advantage for health in any of the components of Ephedra other than its content of ephedrine. Since ephedrine is freely available in a standardized format, a good argument existed to ban the use of ma huang completely. This happened. Unfortunately, the ban has not prevented some individuals from abusing over-the-counter sources of ephedrine, in their quest for a short-lived, but dangerous "buzz." Ephedra has been used as "herbal speed" and its use for this purpose has been encouraged by some unscrupulous people who have infiltrated the dietary supplement industry.

Evening Primrose (Oenothera biennis)

Medical literature supports the potential benefit of the fatty acid components of this oil in the management of premenstrual tension, menopausal symptoms, fibrocystic breast disease, diabetic kidney disease, and even attention deficit disorder (ADD). Each manufacturer of evening primrose oil claims that its product is better than others. The evidence for superiority is variable.

Evening primrose oil's health-giving constituent appears to be a precursor of hormone-like substances (prostaglandins) that mediate such physiological functions as metabolism, smooth muscle activity, and nerve transmission. While some nutritionists rave about evening primrose oil and its benefit, other oils of plant origin (e.g., soybean, safflower, pumpkin seed, and blackcurrant) also have potential benefits in terms of their contents of essential fatty acids.

In Western society, most people's diets are deficient in omega-3 fatty acids, which are found predominantly in fish oil. Although some plants contain precursors of these fatty acids, there is doubt that they can be efficiently utilized by the body to produce friendly types of hormone-like substances (prostaglandins). Evening primrose oil may have been overrated as a health-giving dietary supplement. Fish oil has more evidence for a health benefit than evening primrose oil.

Fennel (Foeniculum vulgare)

Fennel is a classic carminative (flatulence-reducer). It can be used with peppermint oil in a delayed release formula to manage irritable bowel syndrome (IBS) and lower digestive upset. Fennel relaxes smooth muscle in the gut and it may have value in blood sugar regulation. Sugar coated fennel seeds are commonly taken after a meal in India to stop halitosis and promote digestion.

Feverfew (Tanacetum parthenium)

Feverfew is used by some herbalists to treat nonspecific headache, abdominal pain, and fevers. As the name suggests, much anecdotal evidence supports feverfew's ability to reduce fevers. Several double-blind, controlled studies indicate that feverfew may be a useful treatment for headaches of diverse causes.

One of the most interesting applications of this herb in natural medicine is in both the prevention and treatment of migraine headaches. Its precise mechanisms of action in this context remain to be defined, but some evidence suggests that this herb may assist in normalizing blood vessel tone, by modulating the release of vasoactive compounds in the body. The active ingredient of feverfew is believed to be parthenolide.

Fo-Ti (Polygonum multiflorum)

Fo-ti, known as "ho shou wu" in China, may be useful in bringing about bowel evacuation, though its long list of potential beneficial health effects has defied plausible documentation, despite its longtime use in traditional Chinese medical practice. There is some evidence that fractions of fo-ti may be beneficial in treating circulatory disorders such as inadequate blood flow in veins. The herb has been used for nocturnal cramps in the lower limbs and in the management of "heavy leg syndrome" or "restless leg syndrome."

Garlic (Allium sativum)

Garlic is a very popular dietary supplement with beneficial effects on cardiovascular health. A voluminous amount of literature exists to support its use in several areas of health promotion.

Ginger (Zingiber officinale)

Ginger is a carminative (flatulence-reducer), and it has value in the treatment of motion sickness. It can be taken in several forms but seems to exert most benefit when taken as a capsule containing high quality ginger powder. The active constituents of ginger remain somewhat a mystery, but gingerosides are well-defined and well-studied compounds.

Ginkgo (Ginkgo biloba)

Ginkgo has a long history of use in traditional Chinese medicine. It is most commonly used in Western society for its potential benefits in promoting blood flow, the management of asthma, the promotion of sexual function, comfort in the menopause and the management of Alzheimer's disease and other types of dementia. Ginkgo is used very commonly by German physicians. Many scientific studies provide good evidence that Ginkgo can exert beneficial effects on blood circulation and memory. Of most significance are studies using Ginkgo that show improved cerebral circulation in the elderly. Ginkgo is rapidly finding a widespread role in the modern practice of Integrative Medicine.

Ginseng, American (Panax quinquefolium) and Ginseng, Asian (Panax ginseng)

Ginseng of various types is regarded as a panacea of health. Ginseng varieties are regarded as classic adaptogens and general tonics. It is believed that ginsengs can enhance the body's ability to ward-off disease. Unfortunately, finding standardized or authentic ginseng is often difficult.

The story of ginseng and health typifies one of the major problems in the dietary supplement industry. Several studies performed with one type of ginseng or an extract may show unequivocal benefit. These studies are then quoted as support for the sale of other types of ginseng. Favorable reports about one type of herb, grown in a specific location and manufactured in a certain way, do not constitute evidence supporting the benefit of all ginseng products as dietary supplements. This is the limitation of "borrowed science" in the dietary supplement industry.

Ginseng appears to be generally safe, although arguments prevail as to whether adverse effects occur following the use of large amounts of ginseng as a dietary supplement. Manufacturers of various ginseng products must focus their studies on demonstrating that their brand or preparation has biological activity and reasonable consistency.

Goldenseal (Hydrastis canadensis)

Goldenseal is a Native American remedy that has been used, in an unapproved manner, to treat infections, cancer, and liver disease. Goldenseal is combined with Echinacea in some dietary supplements. It has been proposed that Goldenseal has beneficial effects on mucous membrane linings in several body cavities. This herb may exert some benefit on infectious diarrhea, but well controlled studies are required. Some individuals think they can cheat drug-screening blood or urine tests by taking Goldenseal. They are mistaken.

Guggulupids or Guggulsterones

Guggulupids are extracts of a tree resin (see Boswellia) that has been widely used in Ayurvedic medicine to promote cardiovascular health and treat rheumatic disorders. A significant number of controlled clinical studies show that guggulupids can lower blood cholesterol. The active constituents of guggulupid are called guggulsterones. This Ayurvedic resin's effect on lowering blood cholesterol can be enhanced by adding vitamin C. Guggulupid appears quite safe. It is "related" to Boswellia. These resins are great acne treatments that are forgotten! The word Guggulipid® is a trademark of Sabinsa, NJ.

Hawthorne

Hawthorne is emerging as an herbal preparation for the management of cardiac and circulatory system disorders. Some studies imply that it may be useful in the management of angina; and it appears safe at recommended doses. Hawthorne may lower blood pressure by inhibiting certain enzymes, in a fashion similar to commonly used antihypertensive medications. Self-medication with Hawthorne in the presence of severe cardiac disease is not recommended. Abnormalities of heart rhythm have been alleged to occur with high dosages of Hawthorne.

Licorice (Glycyrhiza glabra)

Licorice has been used to treat peptic ulcer, menopausal symptoms, liver disease, inflammatory conditions, and even AIDS. Many studies of licorice imply that this herb can, in certain formats, heal peptic ulcer disease. There is little evidence for the benefit of licorice in the treatment of disease other than the peptic ulcer. Licorice is not valuable in reflux disease (GERD), despite erroneous recommendations. Unfortunately, licorice contains steroid-like molecules that cause fluid retention, swelling (edema), and high blood pressure.

Licorice is commonly found in candy. Large amounts of "quality," candy containing licorice may result in toxicity, especially in the elderly. A preparation called deglycyrrhizinated licorice was marketed as an approved drug for ulcer healing in Europe (Caved-S®).

Milk Thistle

Milk thistle is used by herbalists for liver disease, and some evidence exists that it may protect the liver against a variety of toxins. The active ingredient of milk thistle is silymarin, a flavonoid that has shown some benefit in limited human clinical trials in patients with hepatitis and cirrhosis. Milk thistle appears safe and very valuable.

Mistletoe (Viscum album)

Mistletoe is good for eliciting kisses, but it is quite toxic when taken orally. The toxicity of mistletoe varies by species or hybrid. It has unpredictable effects on the cardiovascular system and should be avoided. Mistletoe may be anti-angiogenic, but it should not be used in supplements.

Myrrh (Commiphora myrrha)

Myrrh finds its greatest use in perfumes and incense. It may be useful as an expensive astringent when applied topically. It has little use in health care.

Nettles (Urtica urens)

In general, nettles are very interesting plants. Stinging nettle is a significant and apparently effective component of natural remedies for prostate enlargement and urinary symptoms. Several clinical trials support the use of stinging nettles in the management of prostatic disease. Based on this evidence, several European countries have recommended that stinging nettle be used as a standard therapeutic agent for prostate disorders.

Papaya (Carica papaya)

Papaya is a delicious fruit that contains a mixed bag of enzymes which digest protein. The mixture of enzymes is referred to as papain. Because of its ability to digest protein, it is used in meat tenderizers. Papain deserves more study as an enzyme supplement to promote digestive health. Papaya has been promoted in encapsulated dietary supplements as a digestive aid. There are few studies in humans showing the effects of papaya, but clinical assessments show symptomatic benefit in individuals with a variety of digestive disturbances. Since the proposed benefit of papaya supplements is related to the enzymes it contains, only products that have demonstrated enzymatic activity should be used. Papaya enzymes can be applied topically to the gum margin to dissolve stickly plaque and help resolve gingivitis in a safe and effective manner (Oral Biocleanse®, Holt MD Technologies).

Parsley (Petroselinum sativum)

Parsley is an antiflatulent that also induces the expulsion of gas. It may have some diuretic (increasing the flow of urine) effects. Some components of the oils contained within parsley are toxic. Parsley oil should not be used in pregnancy because it may induce abortion. Parsley has been incorporated into some supplements that may freshen the breath. Extracts of parsley are safe in small doses, but possibly dangerous in large ones.

Pollen

Pollen has been used to treat almost every chronic disease known to man. Since 1920, it has been highly regarded as a cure for allergies. There is no question that pollen is a treasure chest of nutrients and bioactive compounds, and pollen of various types is available in several dietary supplements. Many types of pollen can cause allergic reactions, some of which can be very serious. Unfortunately, pollen defies standardization because the "active constituents" of pollen are not well defined. Many herbalists espouse its benefits, but controlled studies are few.

Propolis

Propolis is a substance that bees collect from the buds of certain trees and use as "cement" in their hives. It has demonstrable antibacterial and antifungal effects, which tend to be weaker than antibiotics. Propolis is often marketed in combination with pollen in the form of tablets or capsules. Evidence for a benefit for either of these substances in well controlled clinical studies is not readily available. Media evangelists in the U.S. have "hyped" the value of bee products.

Pycnogenol and Related Compounds

Called OPC (oligomeric-proanthocyanidins) by medical researchers, pycnogenol and related mixtures of flavonoids are a mixture of antioxidant molecules. These substances are botanical "vitamin C helpers" and they have become very popular as dietary supplements, because of their potent and versatile biological effects.

Used in antiaging approaches, these agents have been applied to the treatment of every chronic degenerative disease known to man. Their value as isolated therapeutic agents is doubted by practitioners of conventional medicine. While their application to many disease states has aroused healthy skepticism, good scientific agreement exists that they play a major role in the maintenance of general health, but more controlled clinical studies are required. OPCs are great for "sinusitis" of non-infectious origin.

Royal Jelly

Secreted by worker bees, royal jelly is the food of queen bees. Because queen bees live about twenty times longer than other bees in the hive, royal jelly is believed to have antiaging properties. Royal jelly has been proposed as an aphrodisiac and general tonic. It probably does not restore hair, but it has been known to cause allergic reactions. Royal jelly undoubtedly contains many interesting nutrients and compounds, which still require definition. There are many people who overstate the health benefits of royal jelly.

St. John's Wort

Given the existing evidence of the benefit of St. John's Wort in mild to moderate depressive illness, this herb is of great interest. It is documented to have antidepressant effects; and it has been proposed as an alternative to antidepressant medication (an unapproved use). It is applied in mild to moderate depression. It does not work in severe depression.

Unfortunately, many types of St. John's Wort are available for sale, but the content of active agents is not standardized. The herb appears quite safe at recommended doses, but the long-term safety of St. John's wort is not known. Cases of hypersensitivity and photosensitivity have been reported with its use and it may interfere with some anti-viral drugs (HIV treatments).

Saw Palmetto

Considerable evidence shows that extracts of saw palmetto may be useful in the treatment of prostatic disease. This herb is used in several countries as prescription medication for the treatment of benign enlargement of the prostate. Although several regulatory agencies outside the United States have accepted evidence of saw palmetto's benefit in the treatment of prostatic disease, the US Food and Drug Administration remains unwilling to accept its efficacy. There is some concern that only certain fractions of saw palmetto are active. Practitioners of complementary medicine remain convinced that several herbal extracts of saw palmetto or preparations of the whole herb are effective in the management of prostatic enlargement. It is best used in combination with other herbs and nutrients that support prostate structure and function (Prostate, Chapter 21).

Senna (Cassia senna)

Senna enjoys widespread, but sometimes reckless, use as a purgative (a substance that brings about forced and radical bowel evacuation). Although, the herb can be used safely on an infrequent basis, its chronic use can irreparably damage the colon by producing a disorder called "cathartic colon" or melanosis coli (pigmented colon).

Senna has appealed to some misguided people who think that their bowel must be emptied at least once or more in a twenty-four hour period. Such individuals fail to recognize that a reasonable range of normal bowel habit is from three bowel actions per day to one bowel action every three days. To force the colon to empty unnecessarily is not good practice. Irregularities of bowel habit in the absence of disease are best managed initially by lifestyle changes, such as increased exercise and more consumption of fluids, fruits, and vegetables. Gentle colon cleansing with synergistic herbs and magnesium is a safe (Colon Cleansing, Chapter 11). Change of bowel habit in an individual over the age of 40 should prompt colon-cancer screening (Chapters 8 and 11).

Skullcap (Scutellaria lateriflora)

Skullcap has been used for a variety of central nervous system diseases, but it is best known for its tranquilizing effects. There is some concern that extracts of skullcap may have toxic effects, especially liver damage. Unfortunately, there seems to be little general agreement about the best source of skullcap and even less agreement about its active constituents. Defined uses of Skullcap appear to be overall quite safe in modest dosages.

Soy Isoflavones

Isoflavones found in soybeans are an example of estrogen-balancing compounds derived from plants. They are not simple estrogens; they are more like an "adaptogen" or "biological response modifier." The principal soy isoflavones (genistein and daidzein) bear a structural resemblance to the female hormone estrogen and can modulate its effects. Soy isoflavones also have demonstrable anticancer effects and antioxidant effects in animals and humans. Isoflavone chemistry is often grossly misunderstood.

Spirulina (Blue-Green Algae)

Spirulina, a good source of a variety of nutrients, has been used, with alleged success, as a weight loss aid. It seems to have a high concentration of the amino acid phenylalanine, which has been "touted" as an appetite suppressant. Spirulina may be good food, but evidence that it has versatile "curative" benefits is lacking. It is an example of a greens "superfood" (Chapter 4).

Tea Tree Oil (Melaleuca alternifolia)

Incorporated into a variety of creams and lotions, tea tree oil has been used topically for wound healing and as an antiseptic. It appears to have widespread antimicrobial activity. Tea tree oil, however, may trigger allergic skin rashes. Overall, it is effective when applied topically to minor skin disorders, but other more potent and specific remedies are available.

Valerian (Valeriana officinalis)

Valerian root is an herbal sedative that has been used as a sleep aid for more than a century. This herb is used quite commonly in Germany as a treatment for insomnia, and it is regarded as a tranquilizer. It appears that valerian is quite safe and it has much to offer as a first-line option before an individual takes a drug tranquilizer. Tolerance develops to Valerian and it is best used in herbal combinations to support sleep (Chapter 2). Valerian has been called "Nature's Valium®" and herbalists have used it to withdraw individuals from Valium® and other benzodiazepine drugs (unapproved, effective, therapeutic interventions).

Yohimbe (Pausinystalia yohimbe)

Yohimbe is regarded as an aphrodisiac and it has been used by elderly males who wish to retain their sexual vitality. The herb, made from the bark of trees that grow in central Africa, does have stimulant and potential hallucinogenic activity. The active agent may have an effect on the transmission of certain nerve impulses, but it may cause excitation and induce agitation. Some physicians have expressed concern about yohimbe's potential to cause serious adverse effects. Still, this herb is sold widely in "raunchy" magazines, some herbal stores and sex shops. Yohimbine is a drug requiring a prescription, yohimbe is the herb.

Marine Nutraceuticals

The following dietary supplements of marine origin are included here because they have been combined with herbs or botanicals in some commonly used products.

Green Lipped Mussel

The New Zealand green-lipped mussel has been used alone or in combination with herbal products to treat arthritis. Several studies have examined the role of extracts of this mussel in arthritis treatment.

Seaweed

Seaweed has been used in the food chain from time immemorial; and there is a colorful history of its application for medicinal purposes. Seaweed belongs to a large group of plant life, called algae. There are two major categories of algae, including unicellular and macroalgae. Unicellular algae come in different colors such as green, brown and red. These primitive forms of life include spirulina, chlorella, and plankton. Unicellular algae have been widely applied in dietary supplements because of their content of vital nutrients. In contrast, macroalgae are much bigger organisms (macro=large). Macroalgae are commonly known as seaweed or kelp. These sea plants have some resemblance to plants on land; and they can range in size from centimeters to up to 200 meters in width or length. Seaweeds come in shades of yellow, brown, blue, green and red and there are more than 3,000 species of algae in the oceans worldwide.

Seaweed has been used for many medical purposes in several traditional medical systems. At the time of writing, much interest has been shown in the use of certain types of seaweed as weight loss supplements. The ability of many types of seaweed to be adjunctive to weight control has been known for many years. In recent times, interests lie with the ability of antioxidant compounds in seaweed, specifically fucoxanthin, to promote weight loss. While fucoxanthin has some support for its role as an enhancer of body metabolism (thermogenic effect), with direct effect on fat stores, there are other components of seaweed that may assist in promoting healthy weight control.

Many types of seaweed are excellent sources of dietary iodine which is an essential element for normal function of the thyroid gland. Deficiencies in the function of the thyroid gland may promote weight gain. Some seaweed contains a variety of trace minerals and vitamins which provide general nutritional support for individuals who may be engaged in calorie-restricted diets. The presence of certain poorly-absorbed polysaccharides (or types of fiber) present in seaweed may assist in providing bulk in the diet for enhancing a sensation of fullness in the stomach or regular bowel habits. Some of the complex sugars (fucoidans) in seaweed may stimulate immune function. Overall, there is a large amount of scientific literature on the use of seaweeds as health food, soil fertilizers and sources of medicinal compounds.

Many medical spas are using topical seaweed body therapies to promote skin beauty and health. This type of treatment is part of what is called thalassotherapy (ocean-derived treatments). Seaweed body treatments are believed to provide surface minerals that can diffuse into the skin; and they provide pleasurable and relaxing experiences when applied in the correct context. Cosmetic therapists believe that marine algae can enhance skin circulation, increase local metabolism in the skin and supporting structures, flush out toxins and assist in improving skin tone and smoothness, perhaps by inducing a mild dermabrasion. In addition, certain seaweed applications are believed to be moisturizing and toning for the skin. Specific applications of seaweed body treatments include attempts to detoxify the body, treat cellulite, enhance lymphatic drainage, clear limb swelling (edema) and even provide rejuvenating qualities. Seaweed scrubs are excellent for skin exfoliation. The evidence-base for these beneficial effects of the topical application of seaweed remains arguable in the medical literature.

In addition to the extensive topical use of seaweed, several types of macroalgae (kelp or seaweed) are treasured as dietary inclusions or dietary supplements. Several textbooks give extensive botanical profiles of different types of seaweed, with discussions of their nutritional or potential medicinal value. Examples of particularly valuable types of seaweed used in oral supplements include Irish Moss (Chondrus crispus), Fucose or Fucus vesiculosis (Bladderwrack), species of Laminaria, (especially Laminaria japonica), Sargassum muticum (Hondawara, Japan and Limu-Lala, Hawaii) and Undaria pinnatifida (Wakame).

Chondrus crispus or Irish Moss is an important source of mixed amino acids, magnesium and sulfur. There is some evidence that Irish Moss can reduce blood cholesterol levels and it may have antiviral properties. Other proposed properties of Irish Moss include neutralization of gastric acid secretion and it may exert a protective effect on the lining of the stomach and upper intestines. The sulfur containing mucopolysaccharides in Irish Moss form a gel when mixed with water and they are able to retain water up to 20 times their own weight. These gels may cause a sensation of stomach fullness, which is part of the simple, but valuable, "feel-full, weight-loss trick."

Fucus vesiculosis is a brownish green seaweed which is in common use in medicines. It is rich in minerals, trace elements, iodine and vitamin C. It has found application as a dietary source of iodine and a promoter of immune function. Fucoxanthins are abundant antioxidants found in Fucose or Fucus types of seaweed. Independent laboratory studies suggest that this antioxidant can exert significant thermogenic effects and assist directly in weight loss. These effects have been noted to be additive with exercise.

Several species of Laminaria are prized types of medicinal seaweed that have been used often in traditional Japanese medicine and by physicians in Europe. Laminaria seaweeds are a popular dietary inclusion in Japan and Korea. These species are rich in iodine, trace elements, polysaccharides (fucoidan) and antioxidants with the structure of fucoxanthins.

Sargassum muticum originates most often from Japan and it can grow to a length of several meters. This seaweed contains fucoidans and fucoxanthin-like antioxidants. It serves as an important source of alginates which have widespread use in the pharmaceutical industry. Sargassum species have been used as stimulants for plant growth in liquid plant foods and as a traditional Chinese remedy to deal with excessive mucus production in the body.

Undaria pinnatifida (Wakame) is a very large brown algae and it is related to the Laminaria types of seaweed. In common with other types of brown algae, it contains antioxidants and trace elements including the valuable antioxidant, fucoxanthin. Fucoxanthin has been described as having potential fat-burning actions. Undaria are rich sources of minerals and trace elements and they contain glucans which may stimulate immunity. This group of seaweeds is rich in calcium, niacin and vitamin C. Calcium may have special effects in weight control.

Japanese researchers have shown that the fucoxanthin components of Undaria (Wakame) may cause up to a 10% weight loss in experimental animals by direct effects on shrinking abdominal fat stores. The fucoxanthin component appears to stimulate a certain kind of protein that causes the oxidation of fat and its conversion to energy or heat (thermogenesis). This special body protein appears to be present in white adipose tissue (belly fat) and it is proposed that this mode of action of fucoxanthin may be quite valuable in reducing the size of a "pot belly." These animal experiments promoted researchers to recommend human clinical trials with fucoxanthin and studies, in Russia, seem to show notable thermogenic effects of seaweed antioxidants (fucoxanthin), found in Undaria and other seaweeds. In common with other similar types of seaweed, Undaria is believed to have beneficial nutritional effects in cancer and it may stimulate immune function.

Combining certain types of seaweed with other natural substances such as chromium or green tea polyphenols has formed the basis of dietary supplements that are used in the nutritional support of weight control (e.g. FucoseLean™).

Shark Cartilage

Considerable debate still exists over the potential benefit of shark cartilage in the treatment of cancer. Evidence to date does not support the notion that shark cartilage is a cancer cure, even though it may have some yet-to-be defined benefit in some patients with cancer. It appears that certain types of pure shark cartilage may exert an antiangiogenic effect and interfere with unwanted blood vessel growth, which is a major cause of several common, chronic diseases.

Some evidence has emerged that shark cartilage may be useful in the promotion of bone and joint health when administered orally as a dietary supplement. Evidence also exists that shark cartilage may exert benefit as a topical agent in the management of burns or wounds that are difficult to heal. There are many potent anti-angiogenic, natural compounds or botanicals, e.g. bovine cartilage, green tea catechins, soy isoflavones, mistletoe etc.

Nutritional Support for Hormone Replacement Therapy

Many women continue to take hormone replacement treatments, but little attention has been paid to the nutritional co-factors that are required for healthy sex hormone metabolism. In simple terms, supplying essential nutrients that assist in the control of the body chemistry of sex hormones is an important intervention for any woman with hormone imbalance or women who seek hormone replacement therapy (HRT). In my practice, I have seen the application of good balanced nutrition result in a reduced need for hormone supplements, variable restoration of hormone balance and better clinical results from hormone replacement treatments. The first line option in states of hormone imbalance is to make sure that baseline nutrition is covered. In this context, I have found multivitamins, mixed with berries and greens etc to be a very useful baseline nutritional insurance for beneficial effects on sex hormone imbalances. I believe that some physicians have been too quick with hormone prescriptions without addressing "baseline" issues.

While a general consensus in Integrative Medicine supports the use of bioidentical hormone replacement therapy (BHRT) versus synthetic conventional hormone replacement therapy (CHRT), balancing sex hormone administration remains often down to trial and error; and it is often variably or poorly monitored in clinical practice. Many physicians have embraced the benefits of hormone replacement with estrogen, progesterone or testosterone that more closely resemble the types of hormones produced in pre-menopausal years ("bio-identical" or preferably referred to as "bio-similar" hormones). Popular healthcare literature on HRT claims better symptomatic control of menopausal symptoms, improved health outcomes and fewer side effects with BRHT compared with CHRT, but evidence to support these notions is not yet conclusive in peer-reviewed scientific literature.

Given the current level of scientific knowledge, it has become quite difficult to define indications for sex hormone therapy in pre- or post-menopausal women. The alarming side effects of CHRT in the Women's Health Initiative studies in the U.S. and the One Million Women Studies in Europe have driven many mature females to seek viable alternatives to HRT. That said, there are a number of benefits of sex hormone administration in mature females, providing that the treatment is applied in a selective, supervised manner, with tailoring of management and close assessments of hormonal status. In addition, clinical and laboratory methods for administration and monitoring sex hormone status possess disadvantages and limitations. An ideal management approach would involve real-time assessment of hormonal status and its correction in a pulsatile or continuous manner. This approach would be ideal if it could be made synchronous with biorhythms, but medical technology has not advanced to a level that would permit this kind of approach.

Medical acceptance that there are limitations in the application of both BHRT and CHRT has been slow to dawn on practitioners of both Conventional and Integrative Medicine. There is increasing support for the utilization of services provided by compounding pharmacies that offer expertise in the mixing of sex hormones in efficient dispensation formats (e.g. University Compounding Pharmacy, California). Many modern pharmacists face two principle new challenges in healthcare-consumer preferences for menopausal management. On the one hand, the art of compounding is not taught in a widespread manner among pharmacists, whereas on the other the modern pharmacist may not have had complete training in natural therapeutics, e.g. pharmacognosy. Compounding pharmacies are very valuable for menopause and PMS management.

The objective of this section is to review the importance and application of nutritional or botanical support that can be utilized in the primary management of menopausal symptoms or health challenges. These matters are very important for the modulation or facilitation of exogenous sex hormone replacement. While the control of unpleasant symptoms in the peri-menopause or post-menopausal period is an important therapeutic target in many women, the major significance of the menopausal transition involves the onslaught of age-related diseases, such as cancer, osteoporosis, cardiovascular disease and cognitive decline.

I propose that management of the menopause with HRT alone has been "too often" considered, at the expense of recognizing the importance of nutritional, herbal or botanical supplementation. These natural approaches have a clear evidence base to provide first-line or complementary management to avoid or facilitate the application of HRT. In brief, there are two principle approaches to the use of dietary supplements for menopause management. First, their must be a clear recognition of the importance of the nutritional factors that are obligatory for the efficient action, metabolism or function of sex hormones. Second, the application of several botanical or herbal extracts may provide beneficial options as adaptogens that can act primarily through sex hormone receptor sites, especially estrogen receptors.

The Concept of HRT Nutritional "Companions" or "Helpers"

A large body of evidence supports the value of significant, positive, dietary change in the menopausal transition. Epidemiological information supports the value of phytonutrients with natural hormonal properties e.g. soy, fruit, vegetables, whole grains, nuts or plant lignans etc. Several isoflavonoids or lignans of vegetable origin are converted to phenolic compounds which can variably reduce vasomotor symptoms of the menopause, enhance vaginal secretion and assist in preventing certain cancers, notably breast and colon cancer. Some of these phytonutrients have been naively characterized in popular healthcare literature as simple "estrogens" or "phytoestrogens." While the effects of these phytochemicals on estrogen receptors have been identified, their effects are both pro-estrogenic and anti-estrogenic, depending on prevailing hormonal dominance in the body. These actions constitute "an adaptogenic effect" or "biological response modification."

Several individual or combined nutrient supplements have been demonstrated to be variably effective in suppressing unpleasant symptoms in the menopausal transition. Such supplements often and provide other general health benefits. Some of these studies, using single or combined nutrient supplementations, have led to the use of single or limited specific combinations of vitamins or minerals in dietary supplements that have been applied, with variable success, to manage PMS, the peri-menopause and menopause (Menopause and PMS, Chapter 3).

These studies on the nutritional support of menopause have often attempted to explain a specific role for a single nutrient in the management of menopause, without explaining the beneficial effect of the nutritional intervention in terms of the ability of several nutrients to promote effective actions of the nutrients on sex hormone chemistry and functions. The reported variability in the efficacy of single nutrient supplements for the management of menopause is readily understood. Single nutrient studies are fundamentally flawed in their construction, largely because single nutrients never work alone. All body structures and functions involve complex cascades of metabolic events and such events are quite clear in the complex metabolic pathways of estrogen and other sex steroids.

Dietary and nutrient deficiencies in menopausal women are often underestimated. The modern menopausal female is often challenged by weight gain which results in attempts to limit overall calorie intake in the diet. While the Standard American Diet (SAD) is rich in calories, it is often devoid of essential nutrients, such as minerals and vitamins. Therefore, limitation of calorie intake often results in selective nutrient deficiencies e.g. specific vitamins or minerals. Sex hormone metabolism requires many co-factors and therefore the facilitation of hormonal function may often depend upon adequate vitamin mineral intake. That said, there are certain nutrients that are quite critical in supporting sex hormone metabolism and function. These nutrients of specific importance include Vitamin B6, C and E, with magnesium, zinc and essential fatty acids (especially omega-3s).

The importance of Vitamin E in the management of hot flashes or vaginal disorders has been recognized for more than 60 years. Many of these observations of the benefits of Vitamin E on menopause are dated and they do not identify a specific benefit for one or other type of tocopherols. The biological function of Vitamin E has been most focused on its ability to act as an antioxidant that maintains the integrity of biological membranes. However, Vitamin E is known to regulate microsomal enzymes and membrane-associated enzyme systems, thereby acting as a key biological response modifier. In addition, it has a role in hormonal production, mitochondrial function and nucleic acid or protein metabolism.

The antioxidant functions of Vitamin E are believed to account for its benefit in cardiovascular disease, cancer prevention, cataract formation, maintenance of cognitive function and anti-aging properties. The functions of Vitamin E are dependent upon nutritional co-factors including Omega-3 fatty acids, selenium,

Vitamin C, beta-carotene and, to a lesser degree, iron and sulfur containing amino acids. Contemporary studies of Vitamin E supplementation in circumstances of dysmennorrhea, pre-menstrual syndrome and symptomatic menopause show benefits. In a prospective study of Vitamin E supplementation in breast cancer survivors, high dosage (800 IU per day) resulted in a significant reduction in hot flashes and other vasomotor symptoms, compared with placebo. High dosage vitamin E should be supervised.

Supplementation with Omega-3 fatty acids, in their active forms (enteric coated, fish oil with high concentrations of EPA and DHA) is advisable in most peri-menopausal and menopausal females because of protean health benefits. However, fish oil supplementation is best administered in enteric coated soft gels where the bioavailability of the active Omega-3 fatty acids may be enhanced up to 3 fold, resulting in superior therapeutic outcome, better patient tolerability and improved compliance. Regular fish oil capsules and liquids are becoming increasingly obsolete as scientific literature defines the need for relatively high dosages of active Omega-3 fatty acids to achieve treatment outcomes in a variety of disorders.

Several studies have highlighted the importance of B complex vitamins in the management of pre-menstrual syndrome, menopause and adverse effects of hormone administration in birth control pills. Most interest has focused on Vitamin B6 which has been shown to be variably successful in alleviating symptoms of women with pre-menstrual syndrome and menopause. However, Vitamin B6 does not work in isolation and it requires the presence of Vitamin B2 and magnesium to be maximally effective.

In summary, considering or starting hormone replacement therapy should always be accompanied by optimization of baseline nutrition. Viable alternatives to hormone replacement therapy are discussed in Chapter 3.

Toxin-Induced Lipogenesis (Environmental Toxins Causing Weight Gain)

The notion that toxic insults to the body may propagate obesity is a relatively new and novel concept. While the medical literature remains mired in discussions of "farmyard science" to explain the obesity epidemic, evidence accrues that environmental toxins may play a major role in our expanding waistlines. The repeated observations that excess calorie intake with idleness or adverse lifestyle have fueled the global epidemic of obesity, does not explain adequately the accelerating obesity epidemic. Indeed, these factors do not explain the rapid advent of weight gain in recent years (past 3 decades). I accept the importance of the classic explanations of obesity where genetic predisposition to "fatness" interacts with environmental influences, but the causation of obesity is obviously multi-factorial and not readily explainable by traditional epidemiological information. Something tipped the balance over the past three decades and this section probes the hypothesis that toxic exposures may have "tilted the scales" of the nation.

Toxin-Obesity Links

There is a positive correlation (strong relationship) between the increased use of synthetic chemicals and weight gain described in medical literature in recent years. While this link seems quite clear, it is not proof of a causal relationship. However, there are an increasing number of studies that link synthetic chemicals and weight gain. Most notable examples of chemicals causing weight gain are organophosphates, organochlorines, antibiotics, certain pharmaceuticals, several hormones and their analogues.

Although chemical pollution is the most obvious linkage between toxins and obesity, other "toxic insults" may play a role. The association of sleeplessness with obesity is well recognized in contemporary literature, but chronic insomnia may well be fuelled by "physical toxins" such as artificial illumination and other forms of electromagnetic radiation. Perhaps the least considered, but important, "toxic" causes of obesity may be viral infections or inflammatory states.

Several studies imply that environmental exposure to synthetic chemicals produce weight gain in humans and animals. The mechanisms of lipogenesis (fat storage) that is induced by chemical pollutants include, but may not be limited to: interference with fat metabolism and altered hormonal effects on the regulation of appetite. The list of chemicals that are associated with weight gain is growing in the medical literature. I reiterate that these compounds include several pharmaceuticals, herbicides, pesticides, certain heavy metals, household chemicals, industrial solvents and fire retardants … to name a few. The increasing evidence that environmental toxicity may promote obesity supports the routine use of body cleansing or detoxification as part of weight control programs.

Body Cleansing and Detoxification

Putrefying stool or feces with a prolonged residence time in the colon creates colorful biochemistry. Many volatile or soluble compounds including gases and organic acids are generated in the colon. These substances can have good or bad effects on the body and health or wellbeing. The colon is not merely a boring conduit or receptacle for stool. It is a dynamic organ that handles fluids and partially digested dietary intake in a regulated way. Contrary to some assertions, the large bowel has a very active lining and it is capable of absorbing many substances, including fluids, salts, drugs, some nutrients and toxins.

Varying degrees of colonic malfunction are almost universal on an intermittent basis. The healthy, functioning colon may not need to be washed out, cleansed or purged, but the unhealthy or unbalanced colon often requires this kind of attention. Many million Americans have engaged in "colon cleansing" by using laxatives, dietary supplements, enemas and elaborate colonic washouts, often with reported symptomatic benefits.

The Digesta (Contents of the Gut)

The notion that the contents of the gut play a major role in health or well-being has prevailed from time immemorial. Contents of the tubular digestive tract are best referred to as the "digesta." The digesta are formed as a consequence of inextricable linkage of the diet and gut function. The digesta is an ever-changing component of harmonious digestive function and it is the sum total of the contents of the gastrointestinal tract. The composition of colonic contents is particularly relevant to health in several contexts. These contents are created by ingested food or drink, modified by additions or deletions by the gut (digestive enzymes, mucus, gases, bile), all of which are modified by the gut microflora (bacteria, yeasts, molds, protozoa, parasites, etc.) The average colon contains many wanted and often some unwanted guests.

The gut contents form a very active biological soup (or slurry) that solidifies during its passage through the colon. This slurry is exposed to a large surface area of the gut, and, indirectly, a large surface area of the body. The chemical status of the body is usually defined in context of blood and tissue contents, without due consideration of the role that the digesta plays in determining this chemical status. The notion that the contents of the gut communicate with the body has strong scientific support, despite "conventional" rhetoric.

There are a large number of chemicals or metabolic products present or produced in the digesta, including: partially digested food, food additives, nutrients, organochemicals, end products of bacterial metabolism, oxidation products of food, ingested chemicals or altered bile and free radicals produced from bacterial metabolism…to name a few! In the presence of gut disease, different chemicals or bioactive end-products are produced. Such end-products include, but are not limited to, reactive nitrogen species and modified proteins that can act as potential allergens, toxins and biologically active molecules.

The oxidation status of the digesta may have a profound effect on body functions. The antioxidant status of the digesta is largely determined by food eaten, but it is modified by the complex ecology and inhabitants of the gut. Antioxidant status of the digesta may be quite important in the development of colon cancer or bowel inflammation. The digesta have been often ignored for their potential role in functional gut disorders, such as irritable bowel syndrome or common, structural, gut problems such as "leaky gut syndrome" (enhanced intestinal permeability). Leaky guts can let high molecular weight compounds into the body.

Many diffusible nutrients, phytochemicals or phytonutrients and their end products in the gut may be absorbed through the colon into the systemic circulation, or they may exert effects directly on the lining of the colon. Some of these proposals are contrary to popular belief among conventional medical practitioners, or they are dismissed as irrelevant in many contexts. However, the role of the colon in general health is a key consideration for practitioners of Integrative Medicine.

The Colon as a Source of Toxins

Allopathic medicine has discounted the role of the bowel and its inhabitants as a source of toxins for the body. For many centuries, physicians or healers believed in the phenomenon of "intestinal autointoxication." This belief was challenged in early part of the 20th Century, most likely by Dr. W.C. Alvarez (1924). This Physician published a classic paper entitled "Intestinal Autointoxification" in Physiological Reviews (4:352-393, 1924).

Dr. Alvarez stressed the notion that the mucous membrane of the colon is very efficient in preventing the passage of toxins into the general circulation. However, the defenses and functional nature of the colon is much more complex than was realized at the turn of the 20th century. While physicians and scientists have not denied the presence of many toxins in the gut, the conventional physician responds often to descriptions of the colon as an efficient, impenetrable barrier. Dr. Alvarez (1924) reinforced the continuing, but erroneous, beliefs that the colon is an effective barrier to "toxins."

Modern research has shown us to increasing evidence that the lining of the guts is variably permeable to unwanted agents. Several of these agents are present in the digesta, including infectious organisms, toxic chemicals, bacterial degradation products, etc. In fact, the colon may be a site where some agents are actually transformed and absorbed in the body, especially when transformation is by bacteria. Examples of this phenomenon include the cleavage of conjugated phytochemicals, such as conjugated soy isoflavones (glycones), by bacterial enzymatic activity in the colon.

The Importance of Residence Time of Colonic Contents

The residence time of stool in the colon is an important issue. Prolonged residence of the digesta is a measure of constipation or gut transit time. If stool stays around too long, fermentation or other biotransformations of chemicals or undigested food may occur. Increasing residence time of "toxic" chemicals in the digesta increases the time available for them to damage the colon or facilitate unwanted colonic absorption of these potentially noxious agents by the large bowel.

There is good reason to facilitate bowel emptying in many people who have constipation and this is ideally undertaken by correct lifestyle adjustments (e.g. adequate roughage, fiber in the diet, balanced nutrition, avoidance of toxic chemicals, exercise etc). On a selective or intermittent basis, purgation or the facilitated exodus of the colonic digesta by gentle means is often a refreshing or pleasurable experience with clear implications for good health (Colon Cleansing, Chapter 11). The idea of cleansing the body by the elimination of toxic reservoirs (e.g. stool or intestinal parasites) and the promotion of detoxification is neither novel nor new. Detoxification is a mainstay approach of the modern Naturopathic physician. Cleansing and detoxifying the body is deeply rooted in traditional medical practices, over a period of thousands of years, in Ayurvedic medicine, traditional Chinese medicine, and North American Indian medicine.

Lessons from Ayurveda

Ayurvedic medicine teaches prominently that the main cause of much illness is poor digestive function. For thousands of years this ancient discipline has proposed that food resides often for too long in the colon and becomes a source of toxins. This circumstance is likely to occur as a consequence of colonic fermentation, especially in the presence of unfriendly microorganisms, such as yeasts or miscreant bacteria. These concepts have led to special diets, or the use of specific botanical and herbal concoctions which are believed to cleanse the body via the colonic route of expulsion of toxins (Colon Cleansing, Chapter 11).

This ancient medical discipline with its focus on colon cleansing and body detoxification cannot be ignored, given its established precedent for health benefits. Prominent in Ayurvedic treatments are healthy lifestyle, Pancha

Karma (detoxification by cleansing) and the use of cleansing, detoxifying and rejuvenating herbs or botanicals (Chapter 11, Colon Cleansing).

Body Toxins and the Colon

Toxins are any agents that can damage cellular, tissue or organ function. Our "advanced" lifestyle, coupled with the modern industrial revolution has made environmental toxins ubiquitous. In modern times, humankind has produced greater levels of body toxicity. The modern, "intoxicating" environment has contributed greatly to the phenomenon of "autointoxification." Many books summarize common toxins that are present in our inner and external environment.

The colon may be a reservoir of inner toxins. It is accepted reasonably that many of these toxins (Chapter 11, Colon Cleansing) are the cause of acute, sub acute and chronic disease.

Many people can decrease their toxin load by altering day to day preferences. It is valuable to teach patients simple tips that may help them cut down on exposures to environmental toxins. While the advice in Chapter 11 of this book seems simple, it can make a profound contribution to health and well being.

An Expanded Understanding of Toxic Exposures

Many toxic substances do not remain in the environment in their original form or structure. These toxins are transformed by a variety of inorganic or biological processes. Chemical toxins (e.g. pharmaceuticals) are often degraded by the body and converted to molecules which become linked to other compounds or smaller molecules. In contrast, toxic metals are not broken down, but they are often converted into "available" or "non-available" chemical forms.

The speed with which organic toxins are broken down is very variable. For example, organophosphates may be metabolized in minutes or hours, whereas polychlorinated biphenyls (PCBs) are degraded only after many years. Understanding the chronological events of toxin activation or inactivation has major implications for attempts to cleanse the body. Organic toxins are most often ingested orally, making these latter concepts relevant to gut detoxification mechanisms and other factors such as colonic residence time.

Of particular relevance to the function of colon and its attempts to detoxify, are the modifications of toxic chemicals that can be made by microbial species. Bacteria can degrade toxins effectively in many contexts, but they can also elaborate toxins from otherwise non-toxic compounds. Organic toxins are most often degraded by microorganisms in the environment. Friendly bacteria in the colon (probiotics) are capable of degrading or detoxifying several organic toxins.

Industrial experiences, with attempts to undertake microbiological detoxification of the environment, have occurred by isolating and culturing bacteria that detoxify organic chemicals, after their successful seeding into a contaminated environment. We have a corollary in medicine where the same processes may occur with probiotic therapies which "clean" the colonic environment, while presenting added benefits, beyond the process of "detoxification."

Practitioners of alternative medicine are very familiar with the use of intravenous chelation for the removal of heavy metals within the body, but they may be less familiar with the ability of many herbal or botanical, natural compounds that can "detoxify" metals by the formation of complexes with organic compounds that share electrons through the process of chelation. Many phytonutrients can potentially chelate and produce unavailable metallic complexes which do not tend to cause body toxicity. In this form, metallo-complexes may be expelled more efficiently from the body. I do not propose oral chelation, in this manner, as a substitute for intravenous chelation, but the office practice of intravenous chelation can be made more efficient by the interval administration of oral chelators between intravenous chelation sessions.

An important example of these valuable concepts is the knowledge that elemental mercury has relatively low toxicity, but it is extremely damaging and hazardous in its methylated form. In brief, processes that complete detoxification depend on many different chemical reactions of an inorganic or organic nature. Against this background, I propose combined techniques for whole body detoxification in cases of significant toxin exposures. These recommendations include: direct cleansing procedures such as controlled fasting, well selected diets, herbal or botanical agents with "cleansing" ability, saunas, hydrotherapy and colonic irrigation…to name a few approaches.

Cleansing, Detoxification and Rejuvenation of the Gut

While this section attempted to focus on the colon for body cleansing, there are many body cleansing or detoxification procedures that can be used simultaneously to promote cleansing or detoxification. While I support the use of intravenous chelation of a very effective way of decreasing heavy metal contamination, I stress that it is only one of several pathways available for detoxification.

The liver is the key detoxifying organ with its ability to filter blood, engage complex chemical reactions and excrete bile. The skin excretes compounds in sweat and the kidneys are the main portal of excretion from the body. Less attention is placed to the lungs as a major organ of detoxification, but volatile chemicals are found in expired air in significant amounts in both states of health and disease. I assert the major importance of the colon in eliminating unwanted chemicals of all types and certain heavy metals can be excreted in the stool. It is important to remember that the tubular digestive tract has complex enzyme systems, unique physical environments and complex immune functions that can all contribute to detoxification.

While detoxification is important, the process of supporting or rejuvenating the harmony of the bowel is pivotal in sustained attempts to achieve body cleansing. My concepts are not complex. In general cleansing of the bowel and body are functions of good lifestyle habits including: optimum nutrition, avoidance of substance abuse, inappropriate or redundant drug treatments (e.g. NSAID) and toxins (Chapters 9 and 11).

Complex attempts at body detoxification are procedures that can be sometimes avoided by good patient advice. Such advice can result in less toxin exposure and overall disease prevention. Preventive efforts to avoid body toxicity may be the avoidance of potentially "toxic drugs" by the use of simple, gentle, natural first-line options to manage common ailments. For example, non-steroidal anti-inflammatory drugs (NSAID) are one of the commonest causes of gastrointestinal disorders, but they are the commonest drugs prescribed or used over the counter (OTC). These NSAID are frequent causes of dyspepsia, general gastrointestinal upset, liver dysfunction, impairment of renal function, upper and lower gastrointestinal bleeding and diffuse damage to gastrointestinal mucosal barriers. Aside from their selective propensity to cause heart attack or stroke, they have been overlooked as a common source of damage in the lower gastrointestinal tract where they break mucosal barriers and facilitate the entry of toxins or allergens. The use of NSAID is a highly relevant factor to consider in the promotion of body toxicity.

I believe strongly in the idea of cleansing the gastrointestinal tract with a high fiber, balanced diet combined with good fluid intake and exercise. An important adjunct to this cleansing activity is the use of osmotic laxatives that are combined with complex herbal formulas that have their roots in body cleansing in Ayurvedic or other forms of traditional medicine (Chapter 11). These botanical or nutrient approaches are often seen as complementary medical options that are often used by Naturopathic physicians (Chapter 11).

The reader should review Chapter 11 (Colon Cleansing), for an example of a colon cleansing formula that may be used on an intermittent, semi-continuous or continuing basis, depending on clinical circumstances. Detoxification is incomplete without supporting liver function (Milk Thistle) and using probiotic therapy. Good techniques for rejuvenation of gastrointestinal function which secondarily improves continuing detoxification include: the use of dietary supplements such as Omega-3 fatty acids, potent REDOX balanced antioxidants and probiotics, supported by prebiosis with fructooligosaccharides (FOS) or selected soluble fiber (especially hydrocolloid, soluble fractions of oat fiber, beta glucans).

Leaky Guts

The gut has to protect the body from unwanted intruders, but it also absorbs nutrients. Any circumstance that alters the permeability of the gut can have untoward consequences on health because a leaky gut can let in unwanted guests. Nutrients have several potential pathways or mechanisms of access across the walls of the gut. Much transport from the gut occurs in a relatively passive manner through spaces between cells that are normally kept closed by special (tight) junctions. Molecules can move through the lining cells of the gut, but many biomechanical factors restrict the cellular route of absorption for the active uptake of molecules, in general.

The tight junctions that exist between the lining cells of the intestines are fused together in a manner that closes the pathways between cells. These junctions very in structure and number (density) throughout the gut, and they go through a dynamic process of change to allow molecules of different size to pass. In simple terms, they act like a sieve with an adjustable pore size. Disruption of tight junctions can occur for a variety of reasons including inflammation, toxic damage to the lining of the gut (e.g. by drugs such as NSAIDs), as a consequence of disease of the bowel (gluten enteropathy or Crohn's disease) or as a result of general disease affecting the body (cancer, psoriasis, chronic viral infection, e.g. AIDS).

There is a host of diseases in which alterations of intestinal permeability have been described, but in some cases, "chicken-and-egg" argument rages, as to whether the enhanced permeability of the intestines or bowel is the cause or the result of the disease in question. Clinical observations have isolated several documented causes of increased mucosal permeability in the small intestine.

DISEASES LINKED WITH ENHANCED INTESTINAL PERMEABILITY:

Note that the association of several diseases with leaky guts does not necessarily mean that leaky guts caused the problem:

- **Autoimmune Diseases**: Ankylosing spondylitis, arthritis of diverse form (e.g. rheumatoid disease) and mixed connective tissue disease.
- **Gastrointestinal Disorders**: Gastroenteritis, Yersinia infection, ulcerative colitis, pancreatic disease, cystic fibrosis, Crohn's disease etc.
- **Trauma to Body**: Shock, endotoxemia from sepsis, burns.
- **Skin Disease**: Eczema, urticaria, psoriasis.
- **Miscellaneous**: AIDS, some cases of asthma, food allergy, some cases of schizophrenia, malnutrition following surgery, and yeast (Candida).

SOME CAUSES OF INCREASED INTESTINAL PERMEABILITY:

Drugs

NSAIDs are a common, dominant cause of leaky gut, but certain antibiotics, chemotherapy for cancer, gold compounds used in arthritis treatment, estrogen and drugs of abuse such as cocaine and amphetamine are potential culprits. Alcohol "rots" the guts and disrupts tight junctions.

Gut Infections

Bacterial and viral gastroenteritis can cause leaky gut, especially if food and water intake is limited. Some specific infections, like Yersinia, can lead to immune phenomena that result in arthritis and skin rashes, similar to Crohn's disease. Claims of "curing" Crohn's disease may just be examples of resolved infections (Yersinia). Claims of personal cures may be the "instruments of marketeers," sometimes.

Other Medical Interventions

Radiation therapy, surgical trauma (or burns and severe injury), and the institution of parenteral nutrition (TPN) can cause leaky guts.

Colloidal Silver

The use of heavy metals has been popular in several traditional medical systems, for at least one thousand years. There is much nonsense spoken about physico-chemical differences in medicinal silver preparations. Confusion prevails about the colloidal characteristics of silver, gold and copper in the promotion of the biological functions of these heavy metals. Several types of "chemical" statements are marketing propaganda, where some purveyors of silver containing supplements show pretty pictures of colloidal dispersions of silver. These pictures are attractive but quite meaningless. The effects of silver on the immune cascade of events are quite arguable and there is no real evidence that particle size is critical. The best measure of any silver colloid supplement is its ability to kill microbes, including yeasts, bacteria and viruses.

Some individuals who market colloidal silver preparations are attempting to mislead consumers and members of the dietary supplement industry when it comes to discussions of parts per million of silver in suspension. Naïve individuals believe that more parts per million are better. Higher concentrations of colloidal silver, above 45 parts per million, present safety concerns. Silver is a cumulative heavy metal and excessive silver deposition in body tissues must be avoided. Such deposition of silver has uncertain toxicity, including but not limited to possibilities of skin staining. In common with all heavy metals, silver is a tissue fixative and excessive amounts of heavy metals are best avoided (no continuous administration in higher dosages). To reiterate, the microbial kill of the product seems to be the most prudent way to assess biological activity. When it comes to amounts of silver in colloid supplements, "more is not necessarily better." The intravenous administration of silver colloids is reckless medical malpractice.

The activity of colloidal silver has been extensively studies by Holt MD Labs in collaboration with the research laboratories of Stuart Frank in Colorado. Extensive in-vitro research combined with clinical observation by credentialed medical practitioners shows that <u>augmented</u> silver colloid complexes are to be preferred. Laboratory results show that the addition of certain agents to augment the killing actions of silver colloid do not compromise biological activity of silver supplements.

These new types of silver colloid with "augmentation" perform better in microbial killing experiments than other silver colloid preparations including Silver Hydrosol™, Sovereign Silver™ and Argentyn™ (Trademarks of Natural-Immunogenics Corp). The use of augmented silver colloid preparations has been pioneered by Stuart Frank, Natures Benefit Inc and Natural Clinician LLC,

Little Falls, NJ. Augmented silver colloid is to be preferred in clinical practice. Remember it is not morphology or parts per million that matter, it is microbial kill.

Antiviral or Antimicrobial Botanicals and Herbs

Humankind remains challenged by many acute and chronic viral infections. When discussions of infections surface in natural medicine, there is a great risk of precipitating adverse regulatory action. No natural medicine or supplement can make a legal claim about viral treatment, but herbal compendia contain a large number of statements about the antiviral effects of certain plants or their extracts. The main solution proposed for many common viral infections in modern society is the use of vaccination. While certain vaccines appear effective at preventing viral disease (e.g. smallpox), others have been quite disappointing (e.g. HIV vaccines or Avian Flu vaccines). Antiviral drugs (pharmaceuticals) are notoriously ineffective in many circumstances. This situation has led to the use of natural substances that can promote immune function, with a view to improving overall general immunity to microbial infections. There are few drugs that are used to promote immunity, but there are many dietary supplements that have been shown to improve several different aspects of the immune cascade (Immune Function, Chapter 7).

Beyond the logical approach of enhancing immunity with safe and effective natural agents is the variable use of certain botanicals with known antiviral effects. Echinacea has become popular as a cough and cold preventive, but its effectiveness is sometimes arguable and it has little, if any, antiviral activity. Unfortunately, the beneficial effects of Echinacea are dependant upon the species and specific format or preparation of Echinacea that is used. Failure or inability to standardize natural medicine leads to easy criticism by individuals who will not accept the benefits of natural medicine. Against this background, all dietary supplement counselors must be very careful in avoiding treatment claims concerning viral infections. Therefore, I am limited to matter of fact and I shall not make claims. Recent scientific studies have shown great promise for the herbal management of certain viral infections, but approved treatment claims have not been assigned.

Recent, Egyptian studies of extracts of Ecballium elaterium (alone or in combination) in thousands of patients with Hepatitis C virus infection have revealed improvement in symptoms and reduction of viral load as measured by PCR (polymerase chain reaction). The herb Andrographis paniculata may interfere with cell cycling and HIV transmission. Administration of Lysine may be beneficial in some patients with genital Herpes. I provide these examples of modern research in herbal medicine to show the promise of this area of research. While certain drugs have been approved for the treatment of some of these chronic infections, problems exist with cost of treatment, portability of treatment, limited effectiveness and side effects. I encourage readers to carefully study some of these natural options which seem to be emerging with promise.

SPECIAL SECTION: DIETARY SUPPLEMENTS: CHILDREN AND TEENAGERS

Nutritional and Lifestyle Problems in Youngsters

Youngsters in industrialized societies are exposed often to the wrong kind of food. Excessive calorie intake from refined sugars in cereal, snacks and soda play a major role in promoting weight gain; and they contribute to insulin resistance. Resistance to the hormone insulin is the hallmark of Metabolic Syndrome X, where there is a variable combination of being overweight, having high blood pressure and abnormalities of blood cholesterol. While childhood obesity has obvious physical disadvantages, obesity related disease incubates in young people and it is a forerunner to type II diabetes. Recent surveys show an alarming increase in Syndrome X in teenagers, some children and many "young" adults. The occurrence of type II diabetes in children and teenagers has led to the strange medical label of maturity onset diabetes of the young (MODY). Type II or maturity onset diabetes is expected to occur most often in older adults, more than 50 years of age.

Many studies of the dietary intake of macronutrients (carbohydrates, fats and protein) in children show the consumption of too much simple sugar, not enough dietary fiber, the wrong type of fat and a preponderance of meat protein. In addition, many studies of micronutrient intake (vitamins and minerals) show inadequate dietary ranges and amounts of these essential nutritional factors.

Widespread media advertising pushes children to select processed food that is of low nutrient density while it is high in unwanted calories. Unfortunately, undernourished or malnourished youngsters become unhealthy adults; and obese children often become obese adults. These nutritional problems are made worse by the adoption of adverse lifestyle, notably lack of exercise. Attempts to correct adverse lifestyle or modify behavior towards health seeking activity can be quite difficult in children and adolescents. The fundamental nutritional approach for optimum health involves diets that are calorie controlled, reduced in saturated fats, enhanced in essential fatty acids of the omega 3 series, enhanced in fiber, reduced in simple sugar and salt, and adequate in protein intake from multiple sources (meat, fish and vegetable protein).

The emergence of risk factors for cardiovascular disease in childhood is very alarming. There are direct relationships between the body-weight of a child and the amount of time that a child may spend watching TV or playing video games. Children may be very receptive to education on healthy living, but they take their lead from adults. National Nutritional Survey data implies that more than 50% of all U.S. children may have at least one risk factor for heart disease. America has the most obese youngsters, per capita, in the world and weight control in children is often very difficult to manage. Some evidence-based weight control programs in children report positive clinical outcome as prevention of further weight gain, rather than sustained weight control or even significant weight loss!

There are other alarming problems affecting youngsters. In the 1990's the occurrence of autism may have increased by a factor of almost 200% and, in 2003, about 4.4 million U.S. children (age 4-17 years) were described as having attention deficit hyperactivity disorder (ADHD). It is alarming that more than 3 million American children are medicated with drugs for ADHD; and these drugs may cause dependence or serious side effects. Sleeplessness is an emerging issue in children and it is strongly associated in the medical literature with weight gain and stress which are key causes of ill health.

Assuring Good Nutrient Intake

Children who "pick" at their food or those who subsist on processed food will not achieve an optimum intake of vitamins, minerals or other nutrients. The main approach is to encourage children to eat in a balanced manner, but the palate of the modern child does not readily accept vegetables, fish or fiber. It is quite reasonable for any youngster on a standard American (SAD) diet to receive a children's strength multimineral/vitamin dietary supplement with omega 3 fatty acids. There are many valuable children's vitamin supplements available, in novel forms that make them attractive to kids. However, vitamin administration to infants or children below the age of toddlers is best supervised by a healthcare professional and adult dosages of dietary supplements should generally be avoided in youngsters, except teenagers over the age of 14 who are often "mini-adults."

Antioxidant intake is vital for health and these natural compounds are best found in fruits and vegetables. One way around a youngster's failure to take adequate amounts of fruit and vegetables in their diet is to use berries and/or greens formulae which can be given in metered dosages, depending on body size, reduced in amounts for children between the age of 4 and 14 years. Much concern has focused on lack of vitamin C intake in children which results in potential compromise of immunity or connective tissue growth. A common and underestimated deficiency in many children is essential fatty acids of the omega 3 series. Omega 3 fatty acids are required for the proper development of brain function and the nervous system. I stress that supplementation with omega 3 fatty acids, best found in fish oil, is the type of essential fatty acid most required. All children suspected or diagnosed with ADHD may benefit from fish oil sources.

Essential fatty acids cannot be manufactured by the human body and omega 3 fatty acids (DHA) is one of the most important and preponderant components of brain structure. Many people are confused about essential fatty acids and their supplementation. Western diets are often overloaded with essential fatty acids of the omega 6 series and restoration of the balance of omega 3 to omega 6 in the diet is often the most important objective. It is quite rare for any child to require omega 6 supplementation because of the widespread use of omega 6 vegetable oils in "standard food." I am convinced that fish oil supplements can contribute to good outcome in ADHD and autism.

SUMMARY: SUPPLEMENTS IN YOUNGSTERS

Age appropriate vitamin, mineral and omega 3 fatty acid supplements are often valuable in children. Adjusted dosages of berries and greens powders may be particularly ideal for children age 4-14. Children should be encouraged to increase their levels of aerobic exercise and control calorie intake in their diet by reducing amounts of simple sugars and unhealthy fats. The therapeutic use of natural medicine in children with herbs or homeopathic substances should be supervised by a healthcare giver. It should be noted that the safety of many herbs has not been well defined in children and parents should not be encouraged to medicate their children in the presence of significant illness.

NATURAL APPROACHES TO CLINICAL TRAUMA AND PROCEDURE RECOVERY

The use of herbs, botanicals, nutrients, topical natural agents or homeopathic remedies to support wound healing or trauma recovery has emerged as a very important medical intervention in Integrative Medicine. While acute trauma due to common accidents has most often been within the scope of practice of emergency room physicians, the massive expansion in the practice of plastic surgery, aesthetic surgery and topical laser therapy produces many cases of modest iatrogenic trauma. There is an emerging predilection from many patients and healthcare givers to manage minor to moderate degrees of trauma by simple, gentle and natural options.

The contemporary advent of many cases of skin trauma from aesthetic, medical intervention has created a large need for remedies of natural origin that may soothe post-medical procedure trauma by accelerating wound healing, and resolution of pain, bruising or swelling. On the one hand, many natural remedies have been applied to accelerate recovery from surgical trauma with a limited evidence base for their use. On the other hand, in recent studies, there has been clear documentation of good scientific agreement that certain natural remedies can accelerate recovery from trauma, as demonstrated in consistent open-label observations of physicians or controlled clinical trials.

NUTRITION AND TRAUMA

Many nutrients are reported to have specific activity in the healing of soft tissue wounds. Malnutrition has been known to result in major impairment in wound healing and associated tissue changes that result in swelling or bruising. While correction of nutritional deficiency in individuals with significant degrees of malnutrition is known to accelerate wound healing, the benefit of nutrient supplementation in the promotion of soft tissue healing, in otherwise healthy individuals, remains somewhat unclear.

The correction of overt malnutrition in any patient is mandatory and it constitutes standard medical practice before any elective surgical procedure. However, many cases of suboptimal nutrition cannot be readily detected on clinical grounds, even with somewhat complex laboratory testing. Many individuals who submit themselves to medical procedures for cosmetic reasons may be "conscientious dieters." Such individuals may have compromised often their intake of nutrient dense food to reduce body weight. Certainly, fad or extreme diets can produce selective nutrient deficiencies which may involve several nutrients that play a specific role in wound or soft tissue healing. Malnutrition in clinical practice must include consideration of the overweight or obese individual. The recognized association between obesity and poor dietary practices is well established. The overweight individual or individuals with Metabolic Syndrome X may be disproportionately represented in groups of patients who seek certain plastic surgery procedures, such as liposuction, facelifts or other "nips and tucks."

It is not cost effective to investigate the nutritional status of patients undergoing aesthetic procedures by using complex, laboratory investigations. It would seem logical and justifiable in the presence of any suspicion of suboptimal nutrition, to recommend a reasonably intensive and balanced nutritional supplement program prior to any form of elective surgery – at least in the short term. Dietary corrections combined with nutrient supplementation prior to elective surgery may assist in expediting the achievement of good nutritional status and good post-procedure outcomes.

Modern concepts in dietary supplement formulations have led to the development of products that have a good range of vitamins, minerals, phytochemicals, phytoantioxidants and other whole food nutrients that can provide a reasonable "umbrella" form of "nutritional insurance." Open-label observations with blends of powders that contain fruits, berries, greens and vegetable powders have resulted in testimonials of beneficial outcome due to rapid correction of minor degrees of suboptimal nutrition (Antioxidants, Chapter 4). Formal studies are required to define the benefit of this type of general nutritional approach. These types of supplement regimes can be included in protocols for the nutritional preparation of a patient for elective surgical or aesthetic procedures.

The application of general nutritional support in the individual with suspected malnutrition constitutes an evidence-based approach in clinical practice. Also, the use of remedies of natural origin to enhance wound or soft tissue healing should ideally have a demonstrated evidence-base in the practice of Integrative Medicine. Claims concerning the benefits of some nutritional supplements in improved wound and soft tissue healings are supported by controlled clinical observations, whereas others are not.

A number of specific nutrients have been defined to play a beneficial role in wound healing in both animal and human experimental studies. Specific nutrients with these properties include vitamins A, C and E, pantothenic acid, thiamine and minerals including: zinc, copper, manganese and others. Various combinations of specific nutrients have been utilized in studies of wound healing in animals or humans with variable outcome, but it is notable that a deficiency of essential fatty acids may retard wound healing.

The use of enteric coated fish oil supplements to provide extra nutritional support with essential omega 3 fatty acids prior to elective surgical procedures has become a focus of recent interest. There appears to be little need to supplement omega 6, essential fatty acids in most otherwise healthy people because of the ubiquitous occurrence of omega 6 fatty acids in the diets of most people (vegetable oil). The optimal ratio of omega 6 to omega 3 fatty acid intake has been recommended to be as low as 1:1, but the Standard American Diet (SAD) provides ratios of omega 6 to 3 fatty acids, up to 20:1. Evidence exists that this imbalance in the ratio of omega 6 to omega 3 fatty acids may be driving body metabolism towards disease states.

Nutritionally orientated physicians are increasingly using fish oil in enteric coated format, to prepare individuals for surgical intervention, because many such individuals may have Metabolic Syndrome X. Metabolic Syndrome X is most often associated with an overweight status and insulin resistance. Fish oil (EPA) contains the active omega 3 fatty acid, eicosapentanoic acid (EPA), which has desirable anti-inflammatory properties. A theoretical risk of the anti-coagulant potential of fish oil has resulted in some warnings about high dosage omega 3 fatty acid supplementation, but such warnings do not appear to be entirely justified at common daily dosages of fish oil (in the range of 2 grams of fish oil, enteric coated, with contents of key omega 3 fatty acids, Eicosapentaenoic Acid, 600 mg and Docosahexaenoic Acid, 400mg).

"NON-NUTRITIVE" DIETARY SUPPLEMENTS AND TRAUMA

The terms "non-nutritive dietary supplement" could be perceived as oxymoron. Regulations governing the use of dietary supplements only permit statements that refer to "nutritional support" for body structures and functions. Most herbs and botanicals contain nutrients to a variable degree, but extracts may not contain any significant concentrations of common nutrients, per se. Certainly, supplements such as enzymes, that have found a role in the management of wound healing, must be considered "non-nutritive;" but some may have indirect, nutrient-providing properties by assisting in the digestion of key nutrients.

Common herbs, botanicals or their derivatives with documented, but variable benefits on wound healing include Bromelain, Papain (Carica papaya), Centella asiatica (Gotu Kola), Aloe Vera (most often used topically), Chamomile (Matricaria chamomilla, most often used topically), mixed species of Echinacea and Procyanidolic Oligomers (OPCs or PCOs). The importance of the use of selected enzymes (bromelain) in wound healing is apparent in studies that show accelerated or enhanced healing functions following surgery or reduction in inflammatory responses to trauma or surgical interventions. It is believed that several enzymes, referred to for use in trauma, have beneficial systemic effects, not merely digestive-enhancing effects.

COMPLEX CASCADES WITH COMPLEX NUTRITIONAL APPROACHES

The complexity of the physiological cascade of events involved in soft tissue healing has led to the proposal that multiple substances can be formulated together to provide a more effective, synergistic way of achieving desired outcomes. The principles of synergistic formulation have been applied in several condition-specific formulations that are used in the nutritional support of key health challenges. Pivotal, well controlled studies of combined nutrients and dietary supplements that have shown benefit in several measured parameters of wound healing are documented in medical literature.

The variable combination of proteolytic enzymes, calcium and antioxidants has proven quite valuable in soft tissue healing in clinical trials. Preferred antioxidant incorporations in dietary supplements include vitamin C and vitamin C helpers such as Rutin and OPCs in grape seed or other fruit extracts. The ideal combination of these kinds of products remains to be accurately defined with dose-response studies. However, in one randomized, crossover, placebo-controlled trial, such combinations have proven valuable in accelerating soft tissue wound healing. In fact, recovery time with these kinds of supplement regimens, compared with placebo, may result in accelerated healing by a factor of approximately 17%, with full healing in about two weeks, compared with placebo.

BROMELAIN: A KEY APPROACH TO ACCELERATED HEALING

A natural mainstay for assisting in soft tissue healing, bruising and swelling is the use of proteolytic enzymes, such as bromelain and papain. In this context, the greatest evidence-base for benefit rests with the use of bromelain. Researchers described the introduction of bromelain as a valuable medicinal treatment of trauma in the mid 1950s. These researchers commented on the existence of more than 400 scientific papers that describe, variably, the overall benefits of the therapeutic use of this enzyme in reduction of inflammation, rehabilitation of sports injuries and prevention of soft tissue swelling and bruising following trauma or surgery. The aggregate scientific data on bromelain provide strong support for the use of bromelain in any dietary supplement or remedy of natural origin that may be used to provide nutritional support to enhance general healing.

Some of the most striking observations on the benefits of bromelain were made about 40 years ago, the time at which many Herbal Pharmacopeia were relegated in importance by the conventional medical profession, or even frankly discarded. Bromelain deserves considerable renaissance of interest in medical practice as a very safe and effective way of managing swelling, bruising and inflammation for traumatic or postoperative soft tissue damage. While high dosages of bromelain may inhibit clotting function, few documentations of this theoretical adverse effect exist; and high enzymatic activity is preferred to result in bioactivity in bromelain preparations, of the order of about 100mg of bromelain with around 2400 GDU (Gelatin Digestive Units). Pharmaceutical preparations of bromelain were made with special enteric coating many years ago, but these useful "drugs" have not remained very popular. If high enzymatic activity of bromelain is utilized, enteric coating of dietary supplements containing this enzyme may not be necessary.

SYNERGISTIC SUPPLEMENT APPROACHES

In summary, a dietary supplement protocol to provide nutritional support for the normal body functions of wound and soft tissue healing would contain at least Bromelain, vitamin C and vitamin C helpers such as OPCs and/or Rutin and/or Quercetin. This combination of natural substances has an evidence base for its application in the nutritional support of the normal body functions of cutaneous and soft tissue healing.

ARNICA MONTANA (LEOPARD'S BANE, MOUNTAIN SNUFF, MOUNTAIN TOBACCO, WOLF'S BANE, WOLFBANE)

Arnica montana is an endangered flowering herb found in elevated regions of Europe and Asia. In ethno-botanical literature, Arnica has been used most often in tinctures, pills and topical delivery systems to relieve traumatic injuries, pain, bruising, sore muscles and lacerations. Because of known toxicity, Arnica is not recommended to be taken as a dietary supplement in whole or extracted form.

The toxicity of Arnica montana used in whole or extract form in oral agents has included reports of heart damage, irritation of oral mucous membranes, upper gastrointestinal disorders and sudden increases in blood pressure. These adverse effects have <u>not</u> been found or described or observed with the use of <u>homeopathic</u> Arnica preparations. The irritation of mucous membranes induced by whole Arnica taken orally may be due to its contents of several sesquiterpeme lactones.

German Commission E recommendations for the use of Arnica include only topical application or only its use in homeopathic remedies. While few reported deaths have been related to the use of whole Arnica, one active component of whole or extracted forms of this plant (helenalin) can interact with many body enzyme systems, in a manner that creates risks that exceed possible benefits.

Topical Arnica montana preparations are advised to be used only when less than 15% of Arnica oil or less than 25% of Arnica tincture is present. It is reported that higher concentrations lead to skin irritation, especially when used for prolonged periods of time. Large amounts of Arnica taken by mouth in whole form may cause death and the use of Arnica on "raw skin" or open wounds may cause blistering and scarring, with or without the development of systemic toxicity and allergic dermatitis. There are no described drug interactions between Arnica montana in topical or oral forms. Homeopathic Arnica does not appear to alter various tests of blood coagulation in healthy volunteers (www.herbmed.org). There has been much confusion about the potential toxicity of Arnica Montana and I stress that homeopathic preparations of Arnica Montana are considered to be quite safe and variably effective when taken by mouth.

While ointments, gels and other topical forms of Arnica can be used with variable effectiveness for trauma and soft tissue healing, there may be problems with the use of high concentrations of Arnica in the presence of open wounds or damaged skin. Arnica Montana belongs to the Compositae family of plants, which are notorious for producing allergic skin reactions or eczematous lesions with chronic use. In one recent placebo-controlled trial evaluating the effects of topical Arnica on the resolution of laser-induced bruising after the treatment of telangiectasias, no real benefits were observed, but these results may not be generalized to other circumstances where beneficial effects of topical Arnica have been described in postoperative recovery. Some of the potential problems with topical Arnica have led to some degree of avoidance of its use in the postoperative patient with a surgical wound. Given these findings, there has been much recent interest in the study of homeopathic forms of Arnica that can be used in oral preparations for enhancing wound healing, treatment of bruises or contusions, dislocated bones, hematomas, phlebitis, post traumatic or post surgical edema and benign musculoskeletal disorders.

HOMEOPATHIC ARNICA MONTANA

There are several pivotal studies on the use of homeopathic Arnica for the treatment of postoperative or traumatic injury. The overall benefits of some of these reported studies have been argued in the medical literature. One review concluded that Arnica showed no overall benefit beyond a placebo effect. These conclusions may be questioned. The clinical trials that were evaluated in this aggregate review of the efficacy of homeopathic Arnica were not rigorous, as implied by the authors. The clinical trials that were analyzed were of variable scientific quality. In this reported synopsis of eight clinical trials with homeopathic Arnica, it was noted that the trials had serious methodological flaws, despite placebo control.

There is a great problem in attempting to draw conclusions from data aggregated from different clinical trials that have utilized different treatment regimens, with different homeopathic dosages of Arnica, in materially different clinical circumstances. These factors, and others, preclude a conclusion that homeopathic Arnica is ineffective in postoperative healing or recovery from trauma; and they do not take account of more recent clinical experiences with homeopathic Arnica montana that show benefit in these clinical circumstances. The preferred homeopathic strength of Arnica with evidence of good clinical outcome was 30X in studies of wound healing and sports injuries.

In the September 15, 2003 edition of The Journal of Plastic and Reconstructive Surgery, two randomized placebo-controlled clinical trials compared Arnica Montana in a homeopathic strength of 30X with placebo and reported overall benefits. There was less bruising and less swelling in the postoperative period following plastic surgery. In one study of homeopathic Arnica montana that examined the reduction of bruising after facelift surgery, the researchers reported 24% more bruising following facelift surgery in the placebo group which took 50% longer to recover than the group treated with the homeopathic Arnica. The results were defined from computer-imaging programs to analyze bruising and other parameters in the postoperative period of these patients. Overall, the results were found to be statistically significant with benefits for homeopathic Arnica noted on Day 1 and Day 7, in the postoperative period.

In studies that examined the reduction of bruising and swelling following liposuction, homeopathic Arnica montana was utilized in a randomized, prospective, double-blind, placebo-controlled trial. Michael Kulick, MD reported at the American Society of Aesthetic Plastic Surgery, (ASAPS, 2002) that homeopathic Arnica montana reduced bruising and swelling following liposuction surgery in female patients, in the age range of 18-45 years. The results of this study were derived from opinions of independent plastic surgeons who were asked to rank the sets of photos collected by Dr. Kulick following liposuction. In these studies, there was no substantial difference in the volume of fat removed from the 29 patients who were studied. The beneficial results of homeopathic Arnica in the reduction of bruising and swelling showed statistically significant improvement with the use of homeopathic Arnica when compared with placebo, under the conditions of this study

The Data Committee of the ASAPS has been reported to have reviewed the worldwide medical literature regarding the safety and efficacy of homeopathic Arnica. These committee members report the finding of studies with homeopathic Arnica that meet usual and customary standards of medical research. It is notable that the strength of Arnica that appeared to be optimal in the review of some studies by the data committee of the ASAPS was a homeopathic strength of 30X.

These conclusions taken with other information have led to the extensive marketing of homeopathic Arnica preparations with claims of safety and effectiveness. These claims may comply with Food and Drug Administration regulations for an over-the-counter claim of benefit of homeopathic Arnica in trauma induced bruising and swelling. In summary, scientific agreement exists that homeopathic Arnica may be variably effective in helping wound and soft tissue healing.

A LOGICAL INTEGRATIVE MEDICINE PROTOCOL FOR CLINICAL PROCEDURE AND TRAUMA RECOVERY

Practitioners of Integrative Medicine play a major role in the expanding areas of medical spa treatments and aesthetic surgical procedures. These interventions have been traditionally the focus of clinical practice among dermatologists and plastic surgeons. Women's health clinics have converted significant amount of clinical practice space and time to medical aesthetics, including popular procedures such as Botox injections, lip-puffing and eradication of facial lines by the injection of fillers or stimulants of dermal collagen production. In addition, there has been increasing practice of procedures such as liposuction and even limited skin surgical procedures by individuals without completion of a fellowship training program in plastic surgery or aesthetics. Several gynecologists have expanded the scope of their practice by performing aesthetic medical procedures for women. Overall, the use of modestly invasive surgical or medical practices for cosmetic reasons presents a newfound need, in many clinical contexts, for the natural management of postoperative trauma induced by such procedures.

In summary, the natural protocol proposed in order to provide nutritional support for wound and soft tissue healing for minor to moderate trauma involves:

Stage 1: general nutritional support to avoid the presence of isolated or general deficiency of nutrients that may inhibit healing.

Stage 2: the combination of homeopathic Arnica Montana with other dietary supplements that have an evidence base to support healthy healing. Of course, a healthy diet and good lifestyle change are strongly advised to promote any form of recovery.

BREAST HEALTH

I believe that many cases of breast cancer are either preventable or able to be delayed in their occurrence until later in life. Adverse lifestyle, genetic tendencies, conventional HRT and environmental toxicity appear to be major factors in the causation of breast cancer. Current breast cancer prevention strategies have major disadvantages and limitations. These strategies depend upon early diagnosis and intervention, but cancer may be quite advanced when it is detectable by manual breast exams or standard mammograms. Fortunately, there are new strategies that show promise of earlier and more accurate diagnosis or prediction, including breast thermography and emerging tumor antigen, antibody or genetic testing.

Many contemporary accounts about natural ways to prevent breast cancer have emerged in popular literature. In essence, the overall risk of breast cancer appears to be closely related to lifetime exposure to the sex hormone estrogen. Estrogen is made by the body (estradiol, estrone and estriol) and its metabolic pathways are complex. Certain types of estrogen appear to be more "friendly" for health, in comparison to others. Estradiol is the type of estrogen that is preponderant and linked to breast cancer risk. An ugly and dangerous form of "estrogenic stimulus" can occur as a consequence of exposure to synthetic chemicals found in plastics and other consumer goods (xenoestrogens). Conventional medical practices have contributed to the epidemic of breast cancer by the prescription of conventional HRT which has often combined estrogens from horse's urine (xenoestrogen) with synthetic progesterones (progestins).

There are many natural plant substances that have weak estrogenic activity e.g. soy isoflavones, certain lignans and red clover flavonoids. However, these natural substances are examples of biological response modifiers, not just simple estrogens. There is much misinformation about plant phytoestrogens, often perpetrated by the "antisoy brigade" who operates sometimes with questionable motivation. Every time soy foods go through a renaissance interest, the meat and dairy lobby "kicks" into focus on toxic components of soy. Many of the "soy knockers" present absurd or ignorant allegations about soy toxicity while they suffer from great amnesia about the negative health consequences that result from excessive meat and dairy intake.

Soy isoflavones (genistein, daidzein and glyceitin) can downregulate the effects of naturally occurring estrogenic hormones or xenoestrogens, especially in states of estrogen excess; and they can upregulate estrogenic stimuli in states of lack of estrogen. Therefore, they are best perceived as "a balancing act," rather than simple estrogens with potentially "nasty" effects. In fact, soy isoflavones have many health benefits that are unrelated to any affects on estrogenic stimuli. The health benefits of soy isoflavones include: potent antioxidant activity, antiangiogenic effects, platelet inhibitory effects and anticancer effects, by interfering with key enzymes that cause cancer expression. A comprehensive review of medical literature shows that soy foods are associated with breast cancer prevention. Therefore, I recommend soy foods for individuals with a history of breast cancer and I do not believe that soy is a risk for breast cancer. The breast cancer protective effect of soy foods is apparent when they are taken in childhood. These matters are discussed in detail in two of my books ("The Soy Revolution," Dell Publishing, NY, 2000 and "Soya for Health," Mary Ann Liebert Publishing Inc, NY, 1996).

A useful baseline support for breast health is to use multivitamins that are combined in powders that contain fruit, vegetables, berries and greens. The phytochemical content of this baseline nutrition provides potential cancer protection by antioxidant actions, inactivation of carcinogenic chemicals and inhibition of enzymes that cause cancer to grow. Phytochemicals with anticancer effects most notably include: Carotenoids, Flavonoids, Indole-3-Carbinol, Sulforaphane and D-Glucaric Acid (Chapters 3 and 4).

Attempts to detoxify the body intermittently are very important, especially in individuals who live in geographic locations that have a high occurrence of breast cancer that is most likely related to environmental contamination, e.g. Long Island or Staten Island, New York. The increasing industrialization of third world countries is occurring with questionable control of environmental toxins e.g. many Pacific Rim countries and China. The selection of fats in the diet plays a major role in breast cancer propagation. Omega-3 fatty acids and omega-9 fatty acids appear to be protective against breast cancer (Fish Oil, Chapter 18). Flax seed contains precursors of valuable essential fatty acids, but its benefit is most related to its fiber or lignan content. Flax oil is not a reliable source of active omega-3 fatty acids which are best taken in enteric-coated fish oil capsules.

Specific nutrients of phytochemicals best known for their antioxidant actions are ideal for use in synergistic formulations to promote breast health. These combination formulations may contain beneficial additions to alter eicosanoid metabolism or other biochemical actions. My recommendations for evidence based synergistic supplement approaches include: ellagic acid, Wakame seaweed, lycopene, bioflavanoids, garlic, green coffee been or green tea polyphenols, resveratrol, sulforaphane, evening primrose oil, Panax ginseng, calcium D-glucarate, flax seed, indole 3 carbinol, Maitake mushroom and turmeric. I am most impressed with the ability of ellagic acid to exert favorable effects in both breast cancer prevention and potential adjunctive management of established breast cancer.

THYROID SUPPORT

Thyroid hormones are important regulators of body metabolism. These hormones affect every organ system and most body functions. There are several causes of thyroid insufficiency (hypothyroidism), but the cause of hyperthyroidism is often unclear. A large number of cases of poor function of the thyroid may pass undetected with standard laboratory testing. Some estimates place the occurrence of hypothyroidism at about one in four of the elderly population.

Thyroid hormones are manufactured by the thyroid gland using tyrosine and iodine. Reports of widespread deficiency of iodine in the diet of industrialized communities have to be challenged. In fact, average iodine intakes in the US are about four times higher (600mcg/day) than the RDA for iodine at 150mcg/day. Arguments prevail about the availability of iodine in various elemental forms, but the body can often efficiently prepare iodine and tyrosine for chemical combination. Certain foods may trap iodine, directly or indirectly or result in relative iodine deficiency e.g. mustard greens, radishes, turnips and cabbage, all of which are otherwise healthy foods. Anyone with hypothyroidism should be cautious about excess intake of these foods, which may act as "goitrogens." Several vitamins or minerals play a pivotal role as cofactors for the synthesis of thyroid hormones.

In brief, valuable thyroid-supporting, natural substances include: vitamins A (best supplemented as beta carotene), B complex, C and E, amplified by the addition of bioflavanoids, zinc and copper. Parsley and Sarsaparilla are herbs with anecdotal benefit in the support of thyroid function. These nutritionals can be combined with L-tyrosine and L-tryptophan, plus iodine from natural sources, such as seaweed or kelp. Synergistic combinations of these natural substances permit the nutritional support of thyroid function, but they may not be adequate when used alone to treat established thyroid deficiency. Replacement of thyroid hormones is possible with drugs or natural sources of thyroid hormone (RLC Labs, Scottsdale, AZ). Thyroid function should be monitored carefully in any person with diagnosed hypothyroidism. The thyroid support group of nutrients or botanicals may be used with thyroid hormone replacement; and they have no described toxicity when used in individuals with hyperactive thyroid glands, but iodine replacement is not indicated in hyperactive states of thyroid function.

ADRENAL SUPPORT

Alterations of the hormonal secretions of the adrenal cortex or medulla are associated with chronic stress. Adrenal suppression may respond to "adaptogens." Chronic anxiety or stress may cause the adrenal medulla to secrete excess adrenaline and related catecholamines. This excess hormonal activity may respond to several adaptogenic or calming herbs. Of great importance in many people is the suppression of the hormone secretions from the cortex of the adrenal gland which relates to the availability of corticosteroids, aldosterone and dehydroepiandrosterone (DHEA). These "suppressors" act to exhaust functions of the adrenal gland. Many nutrients and herbs have been proposed to support adrenal cortical function which is most often suppressed by lifestyle or disease or drug stresses. An important cause of suppression of the adrenal cortex is the administration of steroid hormones, commonly used in the treatment of inflammatory disease or asthma etc. The adrenal cortex can be suppressed by cortisone administered by any route, including oral, topical and inhaled corticosteroids.

In brief, the nutritional or herbal factors that carry the best evidence base to provide nutritional support for adrenal cortical function include : Licorice, (Glycyrrhica glabra), Panax ginseng, Eleutherococcus senticosus, (Siberian Ginseng), Astragalus, Pantothenic Acid, Bupleuri falcatum (Chinese thoroughwax root), Curcuma longa (turmeric) and Vitamin C, B6, Magnesium and Zinc. Dietary supplement formulations for adrenal support are often incomplete and true synergistic activity results from comprehensive, simultaneous administration of the above natural substances.

CHAPTER 33

PETS

BACKGROUND

THE origins of human and veterinary medicine are closely linked. At the start of the 20th century, the disciplines of human and animal medical practice split. However, there are new attempts to bridge the gap between veterinary medicine and human health. Humankind has sought simple, gentle and more natural approaches to disease prevention and wellness promotion in recent times. This new era in medicine involves holistic healthcare that is portable to our pets. For more information on pet foods or supplements, readers are referred to the book entitled "Natures Benefit for Pets", Holt S., Bader D.R., Wellness Publishing, 2001. (www.wellnesspublishing.com)

In common with human medicine, veterinary medicine has experienced a shift in treatment paradigms towards "natural healthcare." Knowledge from human dietary supplement advances has been applied with benefit to companion animals. This aspect of care is at the basis of the powerful movement in holistic veterinary practice. Always, I encourage people to "love their pet and visit their vet."

As our elderly population is challenged by our thin bones and creaky joints, one may forget that our companion animals experience the same problems, but our pets may suffer in silence. It may surprise many individuals to learn that several of the most important nutritional technologies used in dietary supplements have been developed by veterinary scientists, but these advances have enjoyed their greatest application in human medicine, rather than veterinary practice.

It is striking that many common problems in companion animals (dogs, cats and horses) are similar to those experienced by humans of equivalent age. For example; about 50 million Americans have arthritis in one form or another and, up to 60 percent of all dogs over the age of five years may have some form of arthritis, such as hip dysplasia or osteoarthritis.

BONE AND JOINT HEALTH

There is no need to accept the concept of the "old lame dog, cat or horse." Advances in nutrition show good outcome with a variety of natural substances that can provide nutritional support and benefit common forms of joint problems in dogs, cats and horses. Controlled clinical trials with several natural products in domestic pets demonstrate the effective improvement in the symptoms and signs of arthritis and stress injuries. The serious and life-threatening side effects of anti-arthritic medication in humans have been recognized in dogs, cats and horses. Deaths and severe disability from non-steroidal anti-inflammatory drugs (NSAIDs) may occur in companion animals.

Useful dietary supplements that can be combined in the nutritional support of bone and joint health include: shark cartilage, glucosamine, hydrolyzed collagen, methylsulfonylmethane (MSM), Boswellia serrata, bromelain, vitamin C, saccharomyces and New Zealand green lipped mussel. Pet owners are encouraged to talk to vets about food supplements and there is always a preference to have an expert involved in pet care. The science of synergy in pet supplements is quite new.

SKIN AND COAT HEALTH

Pets share our pride when their skin and coat are healthy and vibrant. They feel "proud." Skin and coat health is a reflection of total body health in our companion animals. Several nutrients can support a vibrant, glowing coat in our pets including: powdered omega 3 fatty acids, collagen, flaxseed powder, wheat germ powder, beta carotene, vitamin C, vitamin E, horsetail, selenium, digestive enzymes, Lactobacillus acidophilus and saccharomyces. Pet owners should realize that some of the nutrients, used sometimes by holistic vets, are not generally recognized animal feeds (or AAFCO approved).

DIGESTIVE HEALTH

Digestive health in pets is an absolute requirement for good general health. Probiotics (friendly bacteria, such as Lactobacillus acidophilus, etc.) digestive enzymes and detoxifying herbs may be useful in balancing digestive function.

Good digestive function results in the optimal assimilation of nutrients from the diet of our pets. Recent studies in companion animals show that problems such as arthritis, allergies and frequent infections can all be related to poor digestive function. Useful supplements that can be used for digestive health include: enzymes such as protease, amylase, lipase, cellulose, lactase, bromelain, pepsin, papain, probiotics, L. acidophilus and selected botanicals, such as cranberry, garlic, spinach and fructooligosaccharides (prebiotics). Probiotics have been shown to improve exercise performance in horses.

EAR HEALTH

Dogs and cats with floppy ears invariably develop external ear infections or irritations. All natural ear drops containing natural antimicrobials such as garlic oil, Oregon grape, Mullein, Acetic acid, etc., can provide natural alternatives for external ear hygiene. These natural antimicrobials kill yeasts, bacteria, mites and they may repel several types of insects. These topical agents have been used by veterinary staff to get rid of ringworm. This is external hygiene the natural way.

IMMUNE FUNCTION

The whole area of immune deficiency in dogs and cats is a big problem. Important supplements for immune support in dogs and cats include adequate supplies of omega-3 fatty acids together with probiotics that balance digestive function and result in immune support. Many cats are at great risk of immune deficiency.

ORAL BIOCLEANSE®

Applying gel with papain, green tea and vitamin C is present in Oral Biocleanse® for gum hygiene. Dissolving sticky plaque this way may avoid needs for teeth-brushings and decrease the need for tooth scaling under anesthesia.

CONCLUSION

The administration of food supplements to animals is not governed by the Dietary Health and Education Act of 1994. The food supplements that I have described are reviewed in several text books of natural veterinary medicine, but supplements used in holistic veterinary practice may not be approved as "animal food." There are rules and regulations that govern pet foods and readers are referred to AAFCO standards.

In cases of doubt, pet owners are advised to seek advice from their veterinarian. Supplements of natural origin clearly demonstrate the benefits of nature for our beloved companion animals. Always check with your vet. "Love your pet and visit your vet."©

CHAPTER 34

WELLNESS EDUCATION

INDIVIDUALS who are willing to self-diagnose and self-medicate with nutri-ents, dietary supplements or drugs must make informed decisions about what they consume or advise others to take. The key to preventive medicine is the promotion of positive lifestyle with a special emphasis on food and nutrient intake. Wellness Publishing Inc. was formed to specialize in the publication of Wellness Guides© which cover a variety of conditions that represent key public health concerns in our modern society.

The notion of "wellness" goes beyond the idea of "health." The most significant improvements in public health will occur only by the application of preventive medicine where "knowledge is power." If there was one single way of improving the health of any nation, it would be to improve levels of education on health matters (edutherapies). This is a powerful approach to the promotion of well-being; and it is likely to achieve more than any new drug, supplement or surgical procedure.

Classic textbooks of conventional medicine describe disease treatments under the headings of general management, drug approaches and surgical management. Far too little emphasis is placed on general management principles of disease where first-line options for health promotion, such as nutrition, are found.

There is a powerful revolution of thought in modern medicine. These thoughts have been precipitated by public opinion and a "grass roots" consumer lobby. This revolution involves the use of simple, gentle and natural approaches to health and well-being. Many medical disorders are not an acute emergency and the application of remedies of natural origin may be followed by conventional medical treatments, if the natural approach does not work. This is the modern change in treatment paradigms towards Integrative Medicine.

Natural medicine may complement conventional medicine. However, individuals must be aware of potential, problematic interactions among medications and dietary supplements. In some cases, nutritional approaches with or without dietary supplements, could perhaps spare the need for higher dosages of a medication that may be required to treat a disease. There are many examples of the benefits of the "blending" of conventional and alternative medicine into new forms of Integrative or Pluralistic medicine. Again, I caution people to obtain expert advice if they wish to mix dietary supplements with standard medications.

Conventional medicine has triumphed in many areas, especially those that relate to needs for urgent treatment, e.g., heart attack, strokes and accidents. Alternative medicine has little to offer the acute medical crisis, but it has a great deal to offer disease prevention and the promotion of well-being. I must reinforce the enigma of modern medicine as a form of disclaimer. Dietary supplements are not to be used to treat or prevent disease at law. That said, many physicians and healthcare consumers use dietary supplements for these purposes!

Perhaps politicians should learn that they cannot legislate against the self-reliance that people have to improve their well-being with natural pathways to health. That said, the dietary supplement, food, pharmaceutical and medical device industries have a major responsibility to provide understandable information that will permit an individual to make an informed decision about their healthcare choices. Health education is a powerful form of treatment that I have termed "edutherapy" or "edutherapies."

At the time of writing, freedom of choice in healthcare is threatened by proposed legislation to limit a consumer's choice on how their well-being may be managed. This book has not been an attempt to interfere with any doctor/client relationship. Perhaps it is more appropriate to talk about healer/client relationships in the new age of pluralistic medicine, where many different types of medical disciplines, old and new, may be used to promote well-being.

Wellness Publishing titles (www.wellnesspublishing.com) include:

- Holt S and Bader D, Natures Benefit for Pets, Wellness Publishing, Little Falls, NJ, 2001
- Holt S, The Antiporosis Plan, Wellness Publishing, Little Falls, NJ 2002
- Holt s, Combat Syndrome X, Y, and Z, Wellness Publishing, Little Falls, NJ 2002

- Holt S, Digestion, Wellness Publishing, Little Falls, NJ, 2008 (in press)
- Holt S, Wright J, Syndrome X Nutritional Factors, Wellness Publishing, Little Falls, NJ, 2003
- Holt S, Menopause and PMS Naturally, The MenoPlan, Wellness Publishing, Little Falls, NJ, 2008 (in press)
- Holt S, Enhancing Low Carb Diets, Wellness Publishing, Little Falls, NJ, 2004
- Holt S, Sleep Naturally, Wellness Publishing, Little Falls, NJ, 2003
- Holt S, Supreme Properties of Hoodia, Wellness Publishing, Little Falls, NJ 2005

VERY IMPORTANT AND SPECIAL WARNINGS TO READERS

DIETARY SUPPLEMENTS ARE NOT FOOD AND THEY ARE NOT DRUGS. DIETARY SUPPLEMENTS CANNOT BE USED TO DIAGNOSE, PREVENT OR TREAT ANY DISEASE. DIETARY SUPPLEMENTS ARE SOLD WITH STATEMENTS THAT HAVE NOT BEEN EVALUATED BY THE FOOD AND DRUG ADMINISTRATION. DIETARY SUPPLEMENTS MAY CARRY LIMITED HEALTH CLAIMS FOR THE NUTRITIONAL SUPPORT OF BODY STRUCTURES AND FUNCTIONS.

THIS BOOK DOES NOT ATTEMPT TO PROMOTE THE USE OF SUPPLEMENTS AS MEDICINE. HOWEVER, THE RIGHT FOOD CAN BE GOOD MEDICINE! FEW DIRECT COMPARISONS EXIST BETWEEN THE CLINICAL OUTCOME OF THE USE OF DIETARY SUPPLEMENTS AND THE CLINICAL OUTCOME OF THE USE OF DRUGS. THIS BOOK IS NOT A DIETARY SUPPLEMENT LABEL AND IT SHOULD BE DISPLAYED IN A GEOGRAPHIC LOCATION SEPARATE FROM SUPPLEMENT PRODUCTS IN A RETAIL SETTING.

THE AUTHOR ACCEPTS NO RESPONSIBILITY FOR ANY INDIVIDUAL WHO ENGAGES IN SELF DIAGNOSIS OR SELF MEDICATION. INDIVIDUALS ARE STRONGLY ADVISED NOT TO SELF MEDICATE IN ANY CASES OF DOUBT AND ALWAYS ACCEPT ADVICE OF A SKILLED HEALTHCARE PRACTITIONER. DRUGS, FOODS, AND DIETARY SUPPLEMENTS MAY INTERACT WITH EACH OTHER IN COMPLEX WAYS. ANYONE WHO IS RECEIVING A DRUG PRESCRIPTION SHOULD INFORM THEIR DOCTOR ABOUT THE

SUPPLEMENTS THEY ARE USING.

INDIVIDUALS ARE STRONGLY ENCOURAGED TO SHARE ALL INFORMATION WITH THEIR HEALTHCARE PRACTITIONER. READERS ARE CAUTIONED THAT THE DESCRIPTION OF AN INTERVENTION AS "NATURAL" DOES NOT NECESSARILY MEAN THAT IT IS DEVOID OF ADVERSE EFFECTS. PLEASE SHARE THE CONTENTS OF THIS BOOK WITH YOUR HEALTHCARE PROVIDER. DIETARY SUPPLEMENTS CAN BE USED WITHOUT A PRESCRIPTION. PLEASE SECOND GUESS MARKETING PROPAGANDA ABOUT DIETARY SUPPLEMENTS.

This book has several unique characteristics. First, it must be understood clearly by all readers that there is no attempt to make any treatment claims whatsoever for dietary supplements. On occasion the word "treatment" may be used with information on herbs but this refers to "traditional" or folklore medicine. The discussions in this book try to focus on discussions of body structures and functions. However, these matters cannot be discussed in a manner that provides an understanding on the use of functional or dietary supplements, without some discussion of how body structures and functions may change in common diseases. I refer all readers to an article that I wrote more than ten years ago that describes the far-reaching consequences of the Dietary Supplement and Health Education Act of 1994 (DSHEA 1994) (Alternative and Complementary Therapies, 1995).

Dietary supplements can be sold with "limited health claims". Such claims involve the use of clumsy language such as *"product X or Y…. provides nutritional support for …. a body structure or function"*. Claims such as *"product X or Y… treats or prevents a disease"* cannot be applied to dietary supplements. When consumers are asked why they take dietary supplements, they respond often in a manner that leads to a conclusion that they are taking supplements for health reasons. In other words, many users of dietary supplements believe that they are taking supplements to prevent, manage or treat disease. This circumstance is part of a paradigm change in treatments in medicine, where modern healthcare consumers are increasingly willing to make a self-diagnosis and to engage in self-treatment. However, the law takes a different approach and it must be obeyed.

The author makes the following strong statements. Dr. Stephen Holt MD advises that self-diagnosis and self-management can be risky in some circumstances and he encourages all individuals who take dietary supplements to discuss their use with their healthcare-giver of choice, during clinic visits. These warnings and other warnings should be contained ideally within package inserts that are used in the sale dietary supplements. In this context of safe supplement usage, the retailer of dietary supplements must be knowledgeable.

Under no circumstances whatsoever can this book be considered to be a product label, at law. Within the DSHEA (1994) are advisory statements that third party literature can be used to inform healthcare consumers about dietary supplements, but the literature must have certain specific uses and characteristics. In particular, the information given must be truthful, must not make direct treatment claims, and it must be the subject of good scientific agreement. The author believes that the writings in this book represent "good scientific agreement".

At the end of this book, a reference section provides further reading and in the further reading are secondary references that support many statements made in this book. Of course, the content of this book represents the author's interpretation of scientific, folklore or traditional use of nutrients, herbs or botanicals; and the author is prepared to justify his conclusions which may not be shared by all scientists or healthcare givers.

Against this background the following disclaimer statement is used and applied to all material in this book. *"Dietary supplements cannot be used to diagnose, prevent, treat or cure any disease"*… at law. However, there is another enigma in modern medicine where many medical practitioners have started to use dietary supplements in disease management and treatment. It must be understood that some people do not think that this use of dietary supplements conforms to "usual and customary standards of medical practice". Because this book mentions supplements and ingredients, it is important that this book be separated from the point of sale of dietary supplement products. This is an important legal consideration because the contents of this book cannot be confused with product labeling.

The author believes that many dietary supplements are used inappropriately because the healthcare consumer is provided with inadequate or misinformation, and sometimes zealous marketing information, (knowingly or unknowingly). There has not been a significant attempt on the part of any agency or association to take responsibility for the education of retailers and consumers on the use of dietary supplements. There are many reasons why natural medicine is still considered "taboo"; but these reasons are disappearing, as more healthcare consumers attempt to seek simple, gentle and natural approaches to promote health and wellbeing. The author emphasizes that because something is "natural", it does not necessarily mean that it is safe. The author does not recommend the use of dietary supplements in pregnancy or childhood or in the presence of poly-pharmacy, without skilled medical guidance.

The readers of this book may question the need for these kinds of disclaimer statements. The author is not attempting in any way whatsoever to interfere with established doctor – patient or healthcare giver – client relationships. In fact the author encourages readers of this book to share information with healthcare givers in all settings, with the knowledge that there may be differences of opinion on the benefit of certain dietary supplements.

The book is for information purposes only and the author or publisher of this book cannot accept responsibility for the consumption of anything mentioned in this book. That said, dietary supplement manufacturers must be willing to demonstrate the fidelity of the products that they sell. The world of medicine is an imperfect world where there are modern trends for overmedication with drugs and, in some circumstances, dietary supplements. Dr. Stephen Holt is committed to trying to "keep the nation well" by using education as therapy. This is the concept of edutherapies (www.edutherapies.com).

ABOUT THE AUTHOR

STEPHEN HOLT MD, LLD (HON), CHB, PhD, ND, FRCP(C), MRCP (UK), FACP, FACG, FACN, FACAM, OSJ

D R. Stephen Holt is a best-selling author and medical practitioner in New York. He has been described as a visionary, a pioneer of Integrative Medicine and is world-renowned for his work on nutrition and dietary supplements. He is a frequent guest lecturer at medical and scientific conferences.

For many years, Dr. Holt has developed management pathways for several public health initiatives, with an emphasis on lifestyle changes and nutritional interventions. He believes that healthcare should be portable, widely available and free for children and the elderly. Dr. Holt has been described as the "doctor's doctor" because many of his patients are medical practitioners. Because of the major pressure on Dr. Holt's time as an international lecturer etc., he restricts his patient care to referrals only from other doctors.

Dr. Holt's principle training has been in allopathic medicine, but he has charted new treatment paradigms using natural medicines. He believes in the concept of "medical pluralism;" where many different medical disciplines come together to provide holistic healthcare. Dr. Holt supports the practice of most forms of medicine including: chiropractic medicine, naturopathic medicine, podiatric medicine, homeopathic medicine, as well as traditional medical disciplines that offer many alternative strategies for health maintenance.

He is an author of more than 20 books in the popular healthcare field and he has also contributed many chapters and articles for medical textbooks and journals. As well as publishing hundreds of scientific articles in leading medical journals, Dr. Holt has been cited thousands of times in the medical and lay press.

An honors graduate in medicine from Liverpool University Medical School, in England, UK, Dr. Holt holds sub-specialty qualifications in gastroenterology and internal medicine. He has practiced clinical medicine for 36 years. Dr. Holt has held the rank of full professor of medicine and bioengineering (adjunct) for many years and he has received awards for medical teaching and research, in the United States, China, Indonesia, Great Britain, Malaysia, Thailand, Taiwan, South Korea and other countries.

Dr. Holt was the recipient of an honorary appointment as a Professor of medicine at San Yat-sen University of Medical Sciences in China, an honor bestowed on only a small number of Western physicians. In 2005, Dr. Holt was honored with the degree of Doctor of Humane Letters for his contributions to education in medicine. He has been Knighted by the Holy Order of St. John and now holds the highest academic rank as a Distinguished Professor of Medicine, in his capacity as the Chairman of the New York Department of Integrative Medicine.

METABOLIC SYNDROME, SYNDROME X: SYNDROME X, Y, Z...?

INTRODUCTION

METABOLIC syndrome, or "Syndrome X," as it is often called, is the variable combination of obesity, hypercholesterolemia and hypertension linked by an underlying resistance to insulin. This condition is often associated with excess insulin secretion. The syndrome was first described by Gerald Reaven in 1998, but its principal component of obesity was not initially emphasized. Retrospective data from the National Health Nutritional Survey for the period 1988 to 1994 implied that 47-million Americans had metabolic syndrome. The current prevalence of the syndrome may now be approximately one in every four adults in the United States population, or about 70-million individuals. So common and so pernicious are the negative health outcomes of metabolic syndrome X that it qualifies as the number-one public health problem facing several Western societies.

Although the metabolic syndrome X is identified as a major cause of cardiovascular disease, it is less apparent that it increases deaths and disabilities from all causes, and underlies female reproductive disorders, polycystic ovary syndrome (PCOS), non-alcoholic fatty-liver disease, non-alcoholic steatohepatitis, gestational diabetes mellitus, significant changes in body eicosanoid status, inflammatory disease, poor cognitive function, Alzheimer's Disease and certain cancers…to name a few diseases.

RETHINKING THE MANAGEMENT OF METABOLIC SYNDROME

Excessive dietary intake of refined sugar, lack of exercise, poorly defined genetic tendencies, environmental toxins and adverse lifestyles contribute variably to the pathogenesis of the metabolic syndrome. Current pharmaceutical and surgical approaches to management of the syndrome have many obvious disadvantages and limitations. It has been suggested by Federal Government researchers that focused treatments of the individual components of the syndrome (hypercholesterolemia, obesity and hypertension) are unlikely to provide a better outcome than are "integrated" management strategies. This suggestion is consistent with dietary attempts to restrict refined, carbohydrate intake, and it helps to explain the short-term success of some low carbohydrate diets for weight control. The notion of "integrative" management strategies as first line options for Syndrome X opens the door for "alternative" management with dietary supplements.

FIRST-LINE MANAGEMENT OPTIONS FOR METABOLIC SYNDROME

Metabolic syndrome has variable clinical manifestations, which I have attempted to incorporate in a new, unifying concept of disease. This concept extends far beyond the existing definition of Syndrome X as obesity, hypertension and hypercholesterolemia, linked by underlying insulin resistance. In order to take account of this unifying concept, I have coined the term Syndrome X, Y and Z…to incorporate many other diseases linked to insulin resistance (Figure 1).

SYNDROME X IS THE NUMBER ONE PUBLIC HEALTH INITIATIVE IN INDUSTRIALIZED COMMUNITIES.

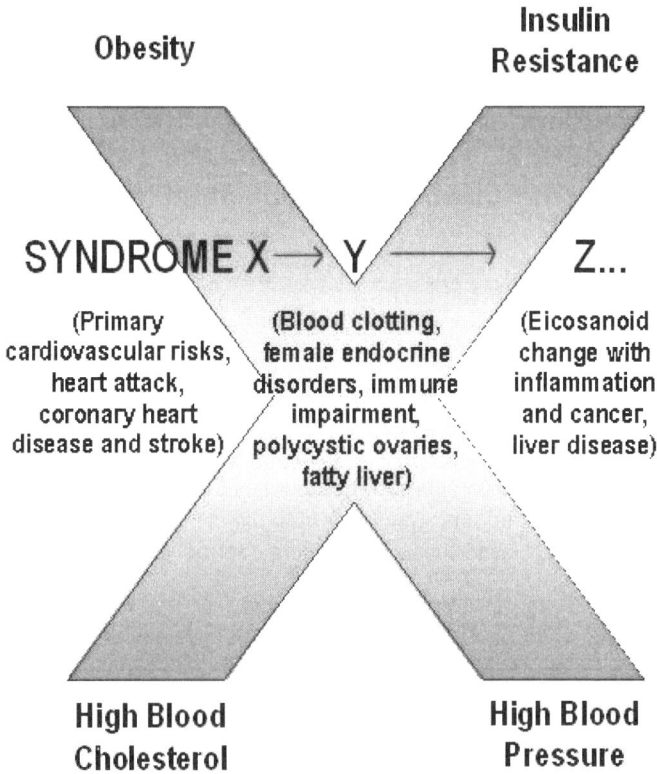

Figure 1: The concept of Syndrome X, Y and Z..., which includes the constellation of the four hallmark components of Syndrome X (metabolic syndrome) (large X in the figure), to which are added other diseases, accounting for the Y and Z...component. The terms Syndrome X, Y and Z... are designed to emphasize the wide range of disabilities associated with the metabolic syndrome.

Effective prevention and treatment of metabolic syndrome involves a multifaceted approach directed at all of its cardinal components. Current allopathic treatments (drugs) for syndrome X have been too specifically focused on the individual components of metabolic syndrome (e.g. anti-hypertensive therapy, cholesterol lowering drugs etc.) While pharmaceutical interventions should be applied where necessary, they most often form a "back-up plan" for its management. In contrast, the natural techniques of lifestyle modification, and nutritional or nutraceutical interventions or both, may provide versatile and potent first-line options for the management of syndrome X.

In many cases, treating obesity must involve the management of Syndrome X, but Syndrome X may occur infrequently in an individual of normal body weight and not all overweight people have syndrome X. (Table 1.) Failing to diagnose or manage Syndrome X in the obese individual is negligent, medical practice (Table 1.). There is no doubt that syndrome X is both under-diagnosed and under-treated in both conventional and alternative medical practices.

NUTRITIONAL FACTORS FOR SYNDROME X

FACTOR THERAPEUTIC EFFECTS

Factor	Therapeutic Effects
Soluble fiber e.g. oat beta glucan	Soluble fiber reduces post-prandial blood glucose, reduces blood cholesterol, improves glucose tolerance, regulates bowel function, primes the immune system, probably by a prebiotic effect. In addition, soluble fiber promotes satiety and it has other intrinsic metabolic effects. Plays a pivotal role in nutritional management of syndrome X and weight control, especially in children.
Soy Protein (25 g/day)	Soy protein reduces blood cholesterol and its isoflavone content may reduce platelet "stickiness" and exert valuable antioxidant functions. Value of vegetable protein rotation in diets. Soy has many other health benefits and it is an ideal dietary substrate for use in diabetes mellitus and syndrome X. Soy is not toxic.
Omega 3 fatty acids (EPA)	Omega 3 fatty acids are best taken in fish oil concentrates, high in EPA, presented in enteric coated capsules for greater compliance and bioavailability. Plant precursors of omega 3 fatty acids (e.g. flaxseed oils, walnut oils, macadamia etc. are not reliable sources of active fatty acids). Fish oil sensitizes insulin by acting on PPAR receptors and it has multiple health benefits including: cardiovascular benefits, anti-inflammatory actions etc.
Chromium	Several studies imply that chromium in various forms may assist in blood cholesterol reduction, weight control and they may sensitize the actions of insulin.
Alpha lipoic acid	A powerful anti-oxidant which plays a specific role in combat against advanced glycation end-products (AGES), with possible reduction in tissue complications in states of dysglycemia. Has a specific insulin sensitizing role, but should not be given by parenteral administration.
Vanadium	An insulin sensitizer of variable value.

Antioxidants	Including but not limited to anthocyanadins, ellagic acid, turmeric, bioflavonoids, direct or indirect anti-oxidant vitamins or minerals e.g. Vitamin E, C, A, selenium, zinc etc. Anti-oxidants are often misused and mis-formulated. Anti-oxidants should be given with REDOX balance to access all body tissues, hydrophilic and lipophillic properties. Single high dose antioxidants are best avoided, especially by unopposed intravenous administration.
Starch blockers and fat blockers	White kidney bean extract, soluble fiber, chitin of variable value.
Cinnamon	An insulin mimetic.
Maitake	Weak insulin sensitizing effect with both whole mushroom powder and fractions. Not a stand-alone weight control or syndrome X nutritional factor.
Green coffee bean extract	Polyphenols e.g. chlorogenic acid assists in correction of dysglycemia, with specific effects on hepatic glucose synthesis.
Green tea	Very potent antioxidant with widespread health benefits, including effects on glucose metabolism. Distinguished content of catechins, especially EGCG.
Hoodia gordonii	Proposed as a non-stimulant appetite suppressant due to its content of steroidal glycosides.

Table 1. Syndrome X nutritional factors are composed of nutrients, botanicals, herbs and extracts that are of potential value in the nutritional management of Metabolic Syndrome X, associated with obesity. Some listed substances may provide nutritional support for diets used in the management of diabetes mellitus. (Adapted from Holt S, Wright JV, Taylor TV, Holt F, "Syndrome X Nutritional Factors", Wellness Publishing, Little Falls, NJ, 2003)

CLEAR BENEFITS OF DIETARY FIBER IN SYNDROME X

Many types of soluble fiber may benefit individuals with metabolic syndrome, through their effects on appetite or satiety regulation, body weight, and blood cholesterol levels. Evolution of research into soluble components of dietary fiber has led to the discovery of fractions of oat soluble fiber (beta-glucans) that have been shown to effectively lower blood cholesterol, reduce postprandial blood glucose, induce satiety, and suppress appetite. Although the glucocolloids that contain these beta-glucan fractions of oat fiber have physicochemical properties that modulate upper gastrointestinal motility by delaying gastric emptying, or by retarding or impeding the absorption of specific (macronutrients such as glucose and fats), they also have intrinsic metabolic effects (IMEF).

These IMEF occur, in part, as a consequence of the prebiotic actions of fiber and fermentation of soluble fiber in the colon to yield short-chain fatty acids, including propionic, acetoacetic, and butyric acids. Of these, propionic acid can enter the portal circulation of the liver, and may interfere with cholesterol synthesis by blocking the activity of hydroxymethyl-glutaryl coenzyme A (HMG CoA) reductase, a key enzyme in the synthetic pathway of cholesterol. Other types of soluble fiber are of value in blunting postprandial blood glucose responses, e.g. soy fiber, pectin and guar gum.

The "Glycemic Index" and the glycemic load of food are relevant to the dietary guidelines or nutritional support that may counteract exaggerated glycemic responses in the metabolic syndrome. In simple terms, the Glycemic Index is a way of describing the ability of different foods to cause a post-prandial rise in blood sugar. Foods laden with simple sugars can be expected to cause a rapid rise in blood glucose to high levels which, in turn, triggers insulin secretion from the pancreas. Such foods have a "High Glycemic Index."

A major component of the glycemic index is related to altered rates of sugar absorption, at least after acute sugar intake. Upward swings in blood glucose are determined to a significant degree by rapid rates of transfer of glucose to its site of maximal absorption in the small bowel, which is a function of the rate of gastric emptying. Speedy absorption of sugar pushes blood glucose levels to high ranges (a high glycemic response). In simple terms, repeated, rapid, roller-coaster swings in post-prandial blood glucose tend to "flog the pancreatic islet cell mass to death." The concept of glycemic index or load becomes more complex with mixed diets.

ESSENTIAL FATTY ACIDS AND METABOLIC SYNDROME

The influence of eicosanoids on glucose and insulin homeostasis has been defined partially, but the effects of insulin resistance (or lack) on eicosanoid pathways are less clear. Many individuals with Syndrome X have a dietary status where eicosanoid pathways are driven towards the production of prothrombotic and pro-inflammatory prostaglandins. This may occur, in part, as a consequence of common dietary deficiencies of certain essential fatty acids (omega 3 fatty acids) or alteration in the ratio of omega 6 and omega 3 essential fatty acid dietary intake. This shift towards "deviant" prostaglandins is aggravated by insulin resistance, ketoacidosis and the diabetic diathesis.

There is evidence that eicosanoid production can be altered by insulin lack or excess and hyperglycemia. Animal studies show increases in a circulating metabolites of PGE2 production after the experimental induction of diabetes with streptozotocin. This rise in PGE2 metabolites is also found in diabetic humans. Thus, both the circumstances that contribute to the development of Syndrome X and insulin resistance within the metabolic Syndrome X can be expected to contribute to changes in the body eicosanoid status in a detrimental manner for health.

This metabolic change in eicosanoid status is manifested mainly a quantitative difference in the types of eicosanoid (prostaglandins) produced. "Active" Omega-3 fatty acids (EPA and DHA), found in fish oil supplements, can assist in correcting "deviant" pathways of eicosanoid production. The dosage of fish oil required to induce a therapeutic effect in this context is higher than dosages that are most often used in clinical practice (greater than 2g/day of 30:20, EPA:DHA).

Enteric coated fish oil capsules are to be preferred for clinical use because they can provide up to three times the bioavailability of active Omega-3 fatty acids (EPA and DHA) compared with regular fish oil capsules or liquids. Powerful arguments can be made to reject the use of "regular" fish oil capsules because compliance becomes poor with high dosages, which may be required for a "therapeutic effect."

Fish oil liquids are obsolete for use in professional practice because of their variable absorption, poor compliance and tendency to spontaneously decompose and form damaging lipid peroxides. Furthermore, it is known that among eicosanoid precursors, eicosapentanoic acid (EPA) can enhance insulin sensitivity, presumably through effects on PPAR-receptors, which regulate the actions of insulin. Natural clinicians must finally appreciate that Omega-3 fatty acid precursors, found in vegetable oils (e.g. flax, walnut, macadamia etc.) are not reliable ways of achieving the desired influence of active Omega-3 fatty acids. Omega 3 precursor conversion rates to EPA may be often as little as 2% conversion of the total precursor dose in a 24 hour period.

Diets intended to combat syndrome should have more liberal contents of omega-3 and where appropriate, omega-6 fatty acids, in the correct balance with one another, together with a strictly controlled intake of refined carbohydrates, a restricted salt intake, an increased intake of fiber intake, and an increased proportion of vegetable sources of protein. Refined carbohydrate-controlled diets require facilitation to make them more effective in the long term (by attempts to overcome insulin resistance). This usually equates to the effective management of the constellation of problems found within Syndrome X (cholesterol, blood pressure and insulin resistance). Table 1 presents a number of dietary components and supplements that can help in preventing and managing metabolic syndrome, accepting that dietary supplements are not to be used to diagnose, prevent or treat any disease… at law.

"OBESITIS": MORE THAN A NOVEL CONCEPT!

Obesity and excess body fat can be classified as inflammatory conditions and inflammation is a key factor in the pathophysiology of Metabolic Syndrome X. Not only does obesity raise the level of pro-inflammatory messenger molecules in the body, it precipitates or contributes to several disorders of inflammation, including cardiovascular disease, cancer, arthritis, Alzheimer's disease, liver disease and asthma. This inflammatory disease "link" with obesity further explains the undesirable effects of insulin resistance, introducing the novel term "**obesitis**".

The hallmarks of Metabolic Syndrome X and many cases of pre-Type II, or early Type II diabetes mellitus often involve the presence of insulin resistance. Insulin acts by specific receptor binding which precipitates many intra-cellular events. Current evidence suggests that insulin resistance is determined partially by chemical mediators that are released from immune competent cells or fat cells. For example, elevated levels of the inflammatory cytokine, tumor necrosis factor-alpha (TNF-alpha) are associated with overnutrition and reduction of TNF-alpha activity is associated with weight loss and improvements in insulin resistance. Many factors that link inflammation and tissue damage have come from recent studies of non-alcoholic, fatty liver disease which is a common component of Metabolic Syndrome X. I believe that Metabolic Syndrome X is a major cause of "cryptogenic" cirrhosis.

While the underlying biochemical basis of the relationships between obesity or Metabolic Syndrome X and inflammatory disease remains underexplored, these circumstances permit me to coin the term "**obesitis**" and propose that "anti-inflammatory" approaches should not be overlooked as an important part of obesity management.

Up to one third of blood levels of the inflammatory cytokine, IL-6, may emanate from adipose tissue and weight loss is often associated with reduction in blood markers of inflammation e.g. C-reactive protein (CRP), IL-18. Popular healthcare authors have attempted to link inflammation with many common diseases, but their interpretation of this important association is limited or "naïve" because only changes in eicosanoid status are emphasized (e.g. The Zone). While correcting eicosanoid precursor pathways with Omega 3 fatty acids is an important anti-inflammatory and insulin sensitizing maneuver, it is not the whole story.

Recent studies have confirmed the anti-inflammatory actions of certain substances that are found in fat tissue. These substances have been referred to as adipocytokines which include leptin, adiponectin, and visfatin. Adiponectin is manufactured by fat cells and blood levels of this protein are reduced in states of obesity, insulin resistance, type II diabetes mellitus and atheroma. Adiponectin exhibits potent anti-inflammatory effects by suppressing TNF-alpha synthesis and promoting the availability of anti-inflammatory cytokines, e.g. interleukin-10 or interleukin-1- receptor antagonist. The "plot" thickens in "**obesitis**" where imbalances of pro-inflammatory and anti-inflammatory cytokines exist. These issues are closely linked to immune dysfunction hat is common in obesity, syndrome X and Type II diabetes mellitus. The natural clinician can reverse these circumstances, at least partially, with holistic natural interventions.

The final common pathway of tissue damage in obesity or syndrome X often involves oxidative damage due to the generation of free radicals, perhaps exacerbated by a reduction in antioxidant defenses in the body. Of course, the progression of the complications of obesity and diabetes mellitus is related to oxidative tissue stress, with the development of advanced glycation end products (AGES). Therefore, the treatment of obesity related disease seems quite incomplete without supporting antioxidant body functions in the clinical management of the obese or overweight person, (Table 1 and 2), especially in the presence of co-existing syndrome X.

Insulin resistance-Chromium polynicotinate, vanadium, maitake, green tea polyphenols, mixed berry antioxidants and alpha lipoic may assist insulin function. Beta-glucan fractions of oat soluble fiber may lower blood glucose levels after sugar intake. Green coffee bean extracts alter hepatic glucose metabolism. Cinnamon is an insulin mimetic.
Abnormal blood lipids-Antioxidants and chromium with biotin may exert favorable effects on blood cholesterol. Ota beta-glucan may reduce blood levels of low-density lipoprotein (LDL) cholesterol, and triglycerides, and may variably increase high-density lipoprotein (HDL) cholesterol.
Obesity-Starch-blockers may inhibit sugar absorption. Oat beta-glucan may produce a sensation of satiety when taken before meals, and thereby assist in controlling calorie intake. Delayed appetite suppressant effects of fiber occur and smoothing out blood glucose responses may help to stop "sugar craving."

Hypertension-Variable but small reductions in blood pressure result from weight control and lifestyle changes, e.g. exercise, avoidance of substance abuse (alcohol, caffeine and smoking). Soluble fiber may have modest independent blood pressure-lowering effects.
Oxidative stress and advanced glycation end products. This may be reduced by bioflavonoids, ellagic acid, anthocyanidins, alpha lipoic acid and other antioxidants.
Homocysteine—Vitamins B6, B12, and folic acid may reduce blood homocysteine levels. Homocysteine and hyperuricemia must not be overlooked in the metabolic syndrome X. Beware of hyperuricemia.

Table 2. Elements of Syndrome X (Metabolic Syndrome) and Nutritional Factors that may counteract them

CIRCADIAN BIORHYTHMS, SLEEP, OBESITY AND METABOLIC SYNDROME X

Sleep deprivation, overweight status and Metabolic Syndrome X appear to be inextricably linked in many people. The mechanisms of this association are not fully understood. Reduction in sleep duration in healthy young men is associated with major changes in hormonal levels of substances (ghrelin and leptin) that increase hunger and appetite, thereby promoting weight gain. An established association between short sleep duration and obesity has led to the proposition that more sleep is necessary to prevent obesity. Sometimes, restoring sleep patterns alone can promote weight loss.

Chronic lack of sleep increases an individual's susceptibility to the Metabolic Syndrome X and it is known that "forced" sleep deprivation in healthy young adults appears to be "diabetogenic", as evidenced by detectible alterations of glucose metabolism. The diabetogenic effects of sleep deprivation may be hormonally mediated. Sleeplessness has been associated with decreases in the normal nocturnal surge of thyrotropin or growth hormone and increases in corticosteroid secretion. These hormonal changes are often present in the elderly, reinforcing the notion of a potential causal relationship among sleeplessness and/or obesity and premature aging.

The relationship between obesity and insomnia may be linked to the excitability of brain cells, most notably the stress-responsive hypocretin/orexin cells in the hypothalamus. Daily stresses may act on the hypothalamus, resulting in sustained stimulation of hypocretin/orexin cells which could precipitate insomnia and overeating. One may now postulate the link between obesity and other conditions such as fasting, periodic hypoglycemia and peri-menopause which are "stressors" that could all serve to excite hypothalamic neurons.

The restoration of sleep patterns of optimum quality and duration can be expected to improve the management of obesity, but stress management appears to be a very important additional factor in obesity management, because of its beneficial effect on sleep patterns or body metabolism that favors weight control. It has been suggested that common weight gain around the menopause is due to hormonal changes. I reject this hypothesis and propose that this peri-menopausal weight gain is more likely to be due to sleep deprivation which often accompanies the transition of menopause. Failure to restore sleep biorhythms in the menopausal female thwarts all attempts to control unpleasant transitional symptomatology.

Inducing sleep by the use of certain hypnotic drugs has to be seriously questioned in the management of the overweight individual and it may be quite undesirable in certain circumstances. For reasons that remain unclear, drugs such as Ambien® (Sanofi-Aventis) may cause weight gain, binge eating and bizarre behavior. Clearly, natural ways to healthy sleep are preferred over pharmaceutical interventions. Comprehensive plans to engage in positive lifestyle change, together with the use of synergistic dietary supplements are attractive first-line management options for common sleep disorders. Sleeping naturally has been described in programs that involve lifestyle change and the use of nutritional support for sleep with dietary supplements. Sleep is a major area for intervention with natural healthcare.

IMPLICATIONS FOR EFFECTIVE MANAGEMENT OF OBESITY (A SUMMARY)

Integrative medicine can offer the optimal pathway to the management of an overweight status and/or Syndrome X, if the modern science of allopathic medicine is complemented or/replaced by holistic care (Table 3). Many people can shed a few pounds of bodyweight in the short tem, but sustained weight control involves many management principles, other than diet, drugs or supplements alone.

A HOLISTIC WEIGHT MANAGEMENT PROGRAM
FOR NATURAL CLINICIANS

FACTORS TO ADDRESS	ACTION
Mutual acceptance of weight status, required commitments and targets for weight and health management	Weight assessment BMI measurement Fat distribution Definition of realistic weight loss targets with health focus. Avoid unrealistic weight loss expectations.
Identify and exclude specific secondary causes of obesity	Congenital disorder, thyroid disease, Cushings Syndrome, psychiatric disease, drugs, surgery, metabolism and insulin resistance syndrome, Metabolic Syndrome X, etc.
Is Metabolic Syndrome X present?	The overweight person with syndrome X has increased risk of many diseases (Syndrome X, Y, Z…) Failure to address insulin resistance syndrome in the presence of obesity is incomplete medical management.
Diet	Tailored to specific weight control targets and objectives. Short-term accelerated weight loss with low carbohydrate approach, Long term maintenance with balanced diets includes: restricted simple sugar, trans-fatty acids and saturated fats, moderate protein intake (1g/Kg) with vegetable protein inclusion, moderate salt intake. Planning required for special circumstances of liver disease, diabetes mellitus, hypertension and, again, beware of Syndrome X.
"Obesitis" Obesity is an inflammatory disorder	All factors that may suppress inflammation are worthy interventions. The common pathway of inflammation often involves oxidative stress. Various nutraceuticals may suppress inflammation and/or independently or simultaneously sensitize the actions of insulin, e.g. alpha-lipoic acid, hydrophilic and lipophilic antioxidants and the versatility and power of eicosapentanoic acid (EPA), given in enteric coated capsules for compliance and bioavailability.
Correct Biorhythm	Reductions in sleep duration and quality promote weight gain, abnormal glucose metabolism and insulin resistance. Without healthy sleep weight loss cannot be sustained and eating disorders emerge, especially nocturnal "fridge-raiding"

Behavior Modification	Many approaches, but altered attitudes to food and removal of positive reinforcements to overeating. Frequent social gluttony
Exercise	Movement is an absolute prerequisite for weight control. Energy into the body must be balance by energy expenditure. Aerobic exercise must be matched to physical fitness levels. Panacea benefits from exercise are apparent.
Adjunctive Approach	Dietary supplements for weight control are often associated with illegal treatment claims for obesity and many have a poor scientific basis for their use. Stimulant weight loss supplements should be avoided in the mature, obese person. Reductions in net calorie intake are the goal, but modern nutraceutical technology has combined appetite suppression with attempts to alter metabolic changes associated with obesity e.g. dysglycemia and insulin resistance syndrome, the hallmark of Metabolic Syndrome X. Drugs used in weight control have onerous side effects. Hoodia gordonii shows promise for non-stimulant appetite suppression and it can be combined with natural substances that alter dysglycemia e.g. green tea and chlorogenic acid (found in green coffee bean) etc
Surgical Intervention?	A variety of approaches with contemporary interests in non-invasive surgery e.g. gastric banding. Surgery for obesity results in a circumstance of forced malnutrition. The clinical course and natural history of the post-obesity surgery patient has not been evaluated in the long-term. The nutritional status of the post-surgical obese individual is often mismanaged. A big question mark exists with obesity surgery in children and teenagers. Careful selection required for surgery, but holistic care of these patients must occur to decrease post-surgical morbidity and mortality. Surgery is "the last ditch".

Table 3. A holistic management plan for obesity, with relevance to the concepts of "obesitis" and syndrome X, Y and Z..., proposed by Stephen Holt, MD

The last thing that is required in the new millennium is another diet promise for weight loss. That said, carbohydrate restriction in the short term can result in apparently safe and effective, accelerated weight loss. However, long term restriction of carbohydrate intake is probably neither safe nor effective and compliance is a problem. Low carbohydrate diets result often in rebound weight gain, largely because of lack of compliance and the documented failure of carbohydrate restriction alone to overcome insulin resistance (Syndrome X).

Without positive lifestyle change there cannot be a health benefit from any weight control program. I have great reservations about the increasing use of surgery for weight control, even though recent studies imply that laparoscopic, gastric-banding techniques are reported to be more effective than diet and lifestyle interventions for weight control. Furthermore, improvements in some components of syndrome X and obesity are to be expected as a consequence of certain surgical procedures; and short-term quality of life measures may improve.

Some recent comparative studies of obesity surgery have involved patients who would not normally receive surgery for obesity. However, obesity surgery comes with complications and its outcome is often related to the existing health of the patient and the skill of the surgeon. There may be at tendency to overestimate the value and safety of bariatric surgery and its use in teenagers poses worrisome issues because of lack of long-term follow up studies. It is not known exactly when the risk-benefit ratio of surgery is most favorable and non-invasive management obesity must always be perceived as the first-line option. Surgery has been proposed as able to reverse several components of Syndrome X, but the presence of Syndrome X, per se, cannot be considered an indication for surgery.

Drugs for weight control are often undesirable interventions because of side effect profiles. Nutritional approaches are often safe and they are assumed to be cost effective when used in an appropriate manner. Unfortunately, dietary supplements used for weight control are purveyed often with weak evidence of efficacy. Natural substances that reduce appetite by stimulant mechanisms may compound cardiovascular risks in the obese individual who may already have hypertension and cardiovascular risk factors (Metabolic Syndrome X). The removal of Ephedra (Mahuang) as a dietary supplement for weight control was appropriate because of the misuse of this otherwise useful dietary supplement.

The U.S. Federal Trade Commission has taken a strong position that dietary supplements cannot carry a weight loss claim which is regarded as a "drug claim"... at law. Recent studies with putative, non-stimulant appetite suppressants such as Hoodia gordonii and Caralluma fimbriata extract or wall are very promising because controlled intake of calories is the key initiative in weight control.

SUMMARY

Changes in lifestyle, and nutritional interventions with condition-specific dietary supplements, may have more to offer for the prevention and treatment of metabolic syndrome or obesity than do existing allopathic management strategies (Table 3.). Combating the specific components of syndrome X has become one of the most important public health initiatives in Western Society. This initiative continues to be often ignored. In particular, the increasingly global initiative for achievement of a healthy body weight must be comprehensive in its tactics and weight control diets require modification and facilitation with revised dietary guidelines and the help of lifestyle changes used with key dietary supplements or functional foods.

REFERENCES TO APPENDIX C

Reaven GM, Banting Lecture, 1988: Role of insulin resistance in human diabetes. Diabetes 37:1595,1998.

Ford ES, Giles WH, Dietz W. The prevalence of metabolic syndrome in the US population. JAMA 297(3):356-359, 2002.

Holt, S. Combat Syndrome X, Y and Z... Newark, NJ: Wellness Publishing, 2002.

Braaten JT, Wood PJ, Scott FW, et al. Oat beta-glucan reduces blood cholesterol concentration in hypercholesterolemic subjects. Eur J Clin Nutr 48:465-474.1994.

Inglett GE. Nutrient patent for beta glucan from cereals. U.S. Patent No. 6,060,519, 2000.

Glore SR, Van Treeck D, Knehans AW. Guild M: Soluble fiber and serum lipids. A literature review. J Am Diet Assoc 94:425-436, 1994.

Hallfrisch J, Schofield DJ, Behall KM. Diets containing soluble oat extracts improve glucose and insulin responses of moderately hypercholesterolemic men and women. Am J Clin Nutr 61:379-82, 1995.

Holt S, Heading CR, Carter D, et al. Effect of gel fiber on gastric emptying and absorption of glucose and paracetamol in humans. Lancet 1:636-639, 1979.

Holt S. The Soy Revolution. New York: Dell Publishing, Inc., 1999.

Holt S, Wright JV, Taylor TV. Syndrome X Nutritional Factors. Newark, NJ: Wellness Publishing, 2003 (in press)

Robertson RP. Eicosanoids as pluripotential modulators of pancreatic islet function. Diabetes 1988; 37:367

Axelrod L, Levine T. Plasma prostaglandin levels in rats with diabetes mellitus and diabetic ketoacidosis. Diabetes 1982; 31:994

McRae JR, Day RP, Metz SA, et al. Prostaglandin E2 metabolite levels during diabetic ketoacidosis. Diabetes 1985; 34:761

Handelsman Y. Guest Editorial. Metabolic Syndrome and Related Disorders. Mary Ann Liebert Inc. 2005: Volume 3, Number 4; 281-283.

Matsuzawa Y, Funahashi T, Nakamura T. Molecular mechanism of Metabolic Syndrome X: contribution of adipocytokines adipocyte-derived bioactive substances. Ann NY Acad Sci. 1999;892:146-154.

Bloomgarden ZT. Concepts of insulin resistance. Metabolic Syndrome and Related Disorders. Mary Ann Liebert Inc. 2005; Volume 3, Number 4; 284-293

Pirola L, Johnston AM, Van Obberghen E. Modulation of insulin action. Diabetologia. 2004;47:170-184.

Wellen KE, Hotamisligil GS. Inflammation, stress, and diabetes. J Clin Invest. 2005;115:1111-1119.

Bloomgarden ZT. Non-alcoholic fatty liver disease and malignancy as complications of insulin resistance. Metabolic Syndrome and Related Disorders. Mary Ann Liebert Inc. 2005; Volume 3, Number 4; 316-327

Grimble RF. Inflammatory status and insulin resistance. Curr Opin Clin Nutr Metab Care. 2002;5:551-559.

Sears B. The Anti-Inflammation Zone. Regan Books; 2005.

Bloomgarden ZT. Cardiovascular complications of insulin resistance. Metabolic Syndrome and Related Disorders. Mary Ann Liebert Inc. 2005; Volume 3, Number 4; 305-315

Fonseca VA., Bratcher C., Thethi T. Pharmacological treatment of the insulin resistance syndrome in people without diabetes. Metabolic Syndrome X and Related Disorders. Mary Ann Liebert Inc. 2005; Volume 3, Number 4; 332-338

Angulo P. Nonalcoholic fatty liver disease. N Engl J Med. 2002;346:1221-1231.

Spiegel K, Tasali E, Penev P, Van Cauter E. Sleep curtailment in healthy young men is associated with decreased leptin levels, elevated ghrelin levels, and increased hunger and appetite. Ann Intern Med. 2004;141:846-850.

Taheri S. The link between short sleep duration and obesity: we should recommend more sleep to prevent obesity? Arch Dis Child. 2006;91:881-884.

Kohatsu ND, Tsai R, Young T, VanGilder LF, Burmeister, Stromquist AM, Merchant JA. Sleep Duration and Body Mass Index in a Rural Population. Archives of Internal Medicine. 2006;166:1701-1705.

Holt S. Sleep Naturally. Little Falls, NJ: Wellness Publishing Inc.; 2003.

Horvath TL, Bing Gao, X. Input organization and plasticity of hypocretin neurons: Possible clues to obesity's association with insomnia. Cell Metabolism, Vol. 1, 279-286, April 2005

Barrett J., Underwood, A., Perchance to…Eat? Newsweek. March 27, 2006;54

Holt S. Enhancing Low Carb Diets. Wellness Publishing; 2004

O'Brien PE, Dixon JB, Laurie C, et al. Treatment of mild to moderate obesity with laparoscopic adjustable gastric banding or an intensive medical program: a randomized trial. Ann Intern Med. 2006;144:625-633.

Holt S. Supreme Properties of Hoodia Gordonii. Wellness Publishing; 2005.

Rajendran, R, Rajendran, K, Pregnane Glycoside compositions and caralluma extracts products uses and thereof. US Patent and Trademark Office. September 2005; 1

OTHER BOOKS BY THE AUTHOR (www.wellnesspublishing.com):

Skinner HA, Holt S, The Alcohol Clinical Index, Addiction Research Foundation, Toronto, 1993

Holt S, Soya for Health, Mary Ann Liebert Publishers, Larchmont, NY 1996

Holt S, and Comac L, Miracle Herbs, Carol Publishing, Secaucus, NJ 1997

Holt S and Barilla J, The Power of Cartilage, Kensington Publishers, NY, NY 1998

Holt S, The Sexual Revolution, ProMotion Publishing, San Diego, California 1999

Holt S, The Natural Way to a Healthy Heart, M. Evans Inc., 1999 (second printing 2002)

Holt S, The Soy Revolution, Dell Publishing, Random House, NY, NY, 1999 (third printing 2002)

Holt S, Natural Ways to Digestive Health, M. Evans Inc., 2000 (second printing 2002)

Holt S and Bader D, Natures Benefit for Pets, Wellness Publishing, Newark NJ, 2001

Holt S, Natures Benefit From Coral Calcium: Sorting Science from Speculation, Wellness Publishing, Newark, NJ 2002, First edition; Second edition, 2003

Holt S, Keeping the Nation Well, Wellness Publishing, Newark, NJ 2003

Holt S, The Antiporosis Plan, Wellness Publishing, Newark, NJ 2002

Holt S, Combat Syndrome X, Y, and Z, Wellness Publishing, Newark, NJ 2002

Holt S, Digestion Naturally, Wellness Publishing, Little Falls, NJ, 2008 (in press)

Holt S, Wright J, Syndrome X Nutritional Factors, Wellness Publishing, Newark NJ, 2003

Holt S, Menopause and PMS Naturally: The MenoPlan, Wellness Publishing, Little Falls, NJ, 2008 (in press)

Holt S, Enhancing Low Carb Diets, Wellness Publishing, Newark NJ, 2004

Holt S, Sleep Naturally, Wellness Publishing, Newark NJ, 2003

Holt S, Supreme Properties of Hoodia, Wellness Publishing, Newark, NJ 2005

Holt S, Sex Naturally, Wellness Publishing, Little Falls, NJ, 2008 (in press)

Dr. Holt's books are available in major bookstores, fine health food stores, and on the internet at www.wellnesspublishing.com.

REFERENCES

The references below are selected to be representative of information to support concepts of "good scientific agreement", concerning the use of nutrients, herbs and botanicals that can be applied in the nutritional support of body structures and functions. The author has reviewed thousands of medical references and the reference sections of this book must be considered incomplete. That said, most references that are listed have secondary references, within their content. This means, that the listed references are considered a good starting point for more complete knowledge on the subjects discussed.

The author has purposely chosen references that give conflicting opinions, in some cases, to permit an individual to get a more balanced view of supplement usage. Please note, this approach is not used commonly in popular healthcare literature that discusses dietary supplements. Readers must be aware of differing opinions and, in cases of doubt, the author recommends consultation with a knowledgeable healthcare giver.

Chapter 1: Multivitamins

Ascherio, A., Rimm, E.B., Giovannucci, E.L., et al. A Prospective Study of Nutritional Factors and Hypertension Among US Men. Circulation 86 (1992): 1475-1484.

Block, G. Vitamin C and Cancer Prevention: The Epidemiologic Evidence. American Journal of Clinical Nutrition 53 (1991): 270S-282S.

Blot, W.J., Li, J.Y., Taylor, P.R., et al. Nutrition Intervention Trials in Linxian, China: Supplementation With Specific Vitamin/Mineral Combinations, Cancer Incidence, and Disease-Specific Mortality in the General Population. Journal of the National Cancer Institute 85 (1993):1483-1492.

Chapuy, M.C., Arlot, M.E., Duboeuf, F., et al. Vitamin D3 and Calcium to Prevent hip Fractures in Elderly Women. NEJM 327 (1992): 1637- 1642.

Dietary Reference Intakes for Calcium, Phosphorus, Magnesium, Vitamin D, and Fluoride, Washington, D.C.: National Academy Press, 1997.

Duchateau, J., Delepresse, G., Vrijens, R., et al. Beneficial Effects of Oral Zinc Supplementation on the Immune Response of Old People. American Journal of Medicine 70 (1981): 1001-1004.

Enstrom, J.E., Kanim, L.E., Klein, M.A.. Vitamin C Intake and Mortality Among a Sample of the US Population. Epidemiology 3 (1992): 194-202.

Harlan, W.R., Hull, A.L., Schmouder, R.L., et al. Blood Pressure and Nutrition in

Adults: The National Health and Nutrition Examination Survey. American Journal of Epidemiology 120 (1984):17-28.

MRC Vitamin Study Research Group. Prevention of Neural Tube Defects: Results of the Medical Research Council Vitamin Study. Lancet 338 (1991): 131-137.

Rimm, E.B., Stampfer, M.J., Ascherio, A., et al. Vitamin E Consumption and the Risk of Coronary Heart Disease in Men. NEJM 328 (1993): 1450-1456.

Stampfer, M.J., Hennekens, C.H., Manson, J.E., et al. Vitamin E Consumption and the Risk of Coronary Heart Disease in Women. NEJM 328 (1993): 1444-1449.

Ubbink, J.B., Vermaak, W.J., van der Merwe, A., et al. Vitamin B_{12}, Vitamin B_6, and Folate Nutritional Status in Men with Hyperhomocysteinemia. American Journal of Clinical Nutrition 57 (1993):47-53.

Willett, W.C., Polk, B.F., Morris, J.S., et al. Prediagnostic Serum Selenium and Risk of Cancer. Lancet 2 (1983): 130-134.

Chapter 2: Sleep

British Herbal Pharmacopoeia, British Herbal medicine Association, UK, 1996

Blumenthal M et al, Herbal Medicine, Integrative Medicine Communications, 2000

Fugh-Berman A, Alternative Medicine: What Works, Odonian Press, Arizona, 1996

Holt S, Sleep Naturally, Wellness Publishing, Newark, NJ, 2003.

Mayell M, Off-the-Shelf Natural Health: How to Use Herbs and Nutrients to Stay Well, Bantam, New York, 1995

Murray MT, The Healing Power of Herbs, Prima Publishing, California, 1992

Reavley N, Vitamins etc, Bookman Press, Melbourne, 1998

The Complete Book of Natural and Medicinal Cures, The Editors of Prevention Magazine Health Books, Berkley Books, New York, 1996

Tyler VE, Herbs of Choice, Pharmaceutical Products Press, New York, 1994

Tyler VE, The Honest Herbal, Pharmaceutical Products Press, New York, 1993

Tyler VE, Herbs of Choice, Pharmaceutical Products Press, New York, 1994

Tyler VE. The Honest Herbal, Pharmaceutical Products Press, New York, 1993

Chapter 3: Menopause And PMS

Amato P, Christophe S, Mellon PL. Estrogenic activity of herbs commonly used as remedies for menopausal symptoms. Menopause. 2002; 9:145-50

Bardwick JM, Psychology of Women. Harper and Row, N.Y., 1971

Berg S (ed.). Women's Health Today. Rodale Press, Pa. 1999

Blumenthal M, Gruenwald J, Hall T, Rister RS (eds.): The Complete German Commission E Monographs: Therapeutic Guide to Herbal Medicine. Boston: Integrative Medicine Communications, 1998

Dalton K, Once a Month. Hunter House, Ca., 1994

Foley D, Nechas E. Women's Encyclopedia of Health and Emotional Healing. Rodale Press, Pa. 1993

Griggs B, Green Pharmacy. Healing Arts Press, Vt. 1991

Holt S, Phytoestrogens for Healthier Menopause. Journal of Alternative and

Complementary Therapies. June 1997.

Kronenberg F and Fugh-Berman A, Complementary and Alternative Medicine for Menopausal Symptoms: A Review of Randomized, Controlled Trials, Annals of Internal Medicine, Vol 137 No 10, 2002

Low Dog, T. Alternative Therapies and Menopause: A Review of the Evidence, Natural Pharmacy, Vol 7, 3, p.p.1, 8-9,14, 2003

Marshel JB, Konner L. Trouble-Free Menopause. Avon Books, N.Y., 1995

Murray MT. Natural Alternatives to Over-the-Counter and Prescription Drugs. William Morrow And Co., N.Y., 1994

U.S. Preventive Services Task Force. Postmenopausal Hormone Replacement Therapy for Primary Prevention of Chronic Conditions: Recommendations and Rationale. Ann Intern Med 137 (10):834-839, 2002

Whitaker J, Dr. Whitaker's Guide to Natural Healing, Prima Publishing, California, 1995

Chapter 4: Antioxidants

Bland, J., The 20 Day Rejuvenation Diet Program, Keats Publishing, 1997, pp 81- 97.

Decker, E.A., The Role of Phenolics, Conjugated Linoleic Acid, Carnosine, and Pyrroloquinoline Quinone as Nonessential Dietary Antioxidants, Nutrition Reviews, 53, No. 3 (1995):49-58.

Dragsted, L.O., Strube, M., and Larsen, J.C., Cancer-Protective Factors in Fruits and Vegetables: Biochemical and Biological Background", Pharmacology and Toxicology, 72S (1993): 116-34.

Messina M., and Messina, V.K. Vegetables: Rating the Healthiest. In Encyclopedia Britannica: Medical and Health Annual, pp. 289-94. Chicago: Encyclopaedia Britannica, Inc., 1996.

Parke, D.V., Nutritional antioxidants and disease prevention: Mechanisms of action. In Basu TK, Temple NJ, Garg M (eds): Antioxidants in Human Health and Disease. CABI Publishing, 1999, p 1.

Shils, M.E., Olson, J.A., and Shike, M., eds. Modern Nutrition in Health and Disease. Philadelphia: Lea & Febiger, 1994

Tyler VE, Herbs of Choice: The Therapeutic Use of Phytomedicinals. New York: Pharmaceutical Products Press, 1994.

Chapter 5: Antiaging

Caine KW, A Men's Health Book, Men's Health Today 2000, The World's Best New Advice on Living Longer, Stronger, Healthier, Better, Rodale Inc., Emmaus, Pennsylvania, 2000.

Chen LH, Nutritional Aspects of Aging, CRC Press, Boca Raton, FL, 1986.

Ebersole P, Hess P., Toward Healthy Aging, Human needs and nursing response, C.V.Mosby Company, St. Louis, Missouri, 1981.

Editors of Prevention Magazine, LifeSpan-Plus, 900 Natural Techniques To Live Longer, Rodale Press, Emmaus, Pennsylvania, 1990.

Eliopoulos C., Gerontological Nursing, J.B. Lippincott Company, Philadelphia, Pennsylvania, 1987.

Finch C.E. and Johnson, T.E., Molecular Biology of Aging, Wiley, New York, 1990.

Kanungo M.S., Biochemistry of Aging, Academic Press, London, United Kingdom, 1980.

Smith D.W., Human Longevity, Oxford Press, New York, NY, 1993.

Walford, R.L., The 120 Year Diet, How to double your vital years, Simon and Schuster Inc, New York, NY, 1986.

Walford R., Maximum Life Span, Norton & Co., New York, NY, 1983.

Walford R.L., and Walford L., The Anti-Aging Plan, Strategies and Recipes for Extending Your Healthy Years, Four Walls Eight Windows, New York, NY, 1994.

Winick M. (ed.), Nutrition and Aging, John Wiley & Sons, New York, NY, 1976.

Yu B.P., Free Radicals in Aging, CRC Press, Boca Raton, FL, 1993.

Chapter 6: Osteoporosis: Thin Bones

Bales C.W., Drezner M.K., Hoben K.P., Eating Well, Living Well with Osteoporosis: Duke University Medical Centre. Viking, Penguin Books Inc. NY, NY, 1996.

Brown, S.E., Better Bones, Better Body. Keats Publishing Inc., New Canaan, CT.1996.

Heaney, R.P. Nutrition and risk for osteoporosis. In: Marcus R., Feldman, D., Kelsey, J., (eds) Osteoporosis. Academic Press, San Diego, Ca, 483-505, 1994.

Heaney, R.P., Nutritional factors in osteoporosis. Annu Rev Nutr 13:287- 316, 1993.

Holt S, Irshad M, Howlen CW, Maneiro m. Nonsteroidal anti-inflammatory drugs and lower gastrointestinal bleeding. Dig Dis Sci 38:1619-1623, 1993.

Holt S, Saleeby G. Gastric mucosal injury induced by anti-inflammatory drugs (NSAIDs). Southern medical Journal 84, 3:355-360, 1991.

Holt S, The Antiporosis Plan, Wellness Publishing, Newark, NJ, 2002

National Osteoporosis Foundation, National Objectives for Disease Prevention and Health Promotion for the year 2000. National Osteoporosis Foundation, Washington D.C., 1988.

Nevitt, M.C. Epidemiology of Osteoporosis. Rheumatic Disease Clinics of North America 20.3 535:559, 1994.

NIH, Optimal Calcium Intake. National Institutes of Health 12.4. 1-24, 1994.

Strause, L., Saltman, P., Smith K., Andon, M., The role of trace elements in bone metabolism. In: Burckhardt, P., Heaney, R.P., (eds), Nutritional Aspects of Osteoporosis, Raven Press, New York, pp 223-233, 1991.

Chapter 7: Immune Function

Barilla J., Andrographis paniculata, Can herbs fight common ailments, cancer, and chronic viral infections? A Keats Good Health Guide, published by Keats, a division of NTC/Contemporary Publishing Group, Lincolnwood (Chicago), Illinois, 1999.

Beisel W., Edelman R., Nauss K, Suskind R., Single-nutrient effects of immunologic functions, JAMA 1981, 245:53-58.

Chandra R., Newberne R. Nutrition, Immunity, and Infection. New York: Pleneum Press, 1977.

Chang HM., But PPH eds. Pharmacology and applications of Chinese Materia Medica, Singapore: World Scientific, 1987: p 1041-1046.

Chu DT., Wong WL., Mavlight GM, Immunotherapy with Chinese medicinal herbs, J Clin Lab Immunol 1988, 25:119-129.

Dowd P., Heatley R. The influence of undernutrition on immunity, Clin Sci 1984, 66:241-248.

Havsteen B., Flavonoids, a class of natural products of high pharmacological potency. Biochem Pharmacol 1983, 32:1141-1148.

Hemila H. and Herman ZS, Vitamin C and the common cold, A retrospective analysis of Chalmers' review, J Am Coll Nutr 1995, 14:116-123.

Kusaka Y., Kondou H., Morimoto K., Healthy lifestyles are associated with higher natural killer cell activity. Prev Med 1992; 21:602-615

Palmblad J., Hallberg D. Rossner S., Obesity, plasma lipids and polymorphonuclear (PMN) granulocyte functions. Scand J Heamatol 1977; 19: 293-303.

Sanchez A, Reeser J, Lau H et al. Role of sugars in human neutrophilic phagocytosis. Am J Clin Nutr 1973, 26: 1180-1184.

Chapter 8: Joint Care

Bland J.H., Cooper S.M., Osteoarthritis: a review of the cell biology involved and evidence for reversibility. Management rationally related to known genesis and pathophysiology, Sem Arthr Rheum 1984, 14:106-133.

Brooks P.M., Potter S.R., Buchanan W.W., NSAID and osteoarthritis – help or hindrance, J Rheumatol 1982, 9: 3-5.

Felson D.T., Naimark A., Anderson J., The Prevalence of Knee Osteoarthritis, The Framingham Study, Ann Intern Med 1988, 109:18.

Holt S., Barilla J.R., The Power of Cartilage, Kensington Publishers, NY, NY (in press), 1998.

Holt S., Irshad M., Howlen C.W., Maneiro M., Nonsteroidal anti-inflammatory drugs and lower gastrointestinal bleeding, Dig Dis Sci 38: 1619-1623, 1993.

Holt S., Saleeby G., Gastric mucosal injury induced by anti-inflammatory drugs (NSAIDS), Southern Medical Journal 84, 3: 335-360, 1991.

Holt S., The Antiporosis Plan, A Wellness Guide, Wellness Publishing, Newark, NJ, 2002.

McAlindon T.E., Jacques P., Zhang Y et al, Do antioxidant micronutrients protect against the development and progression of knee osteoarthritis? Arthritis Rheumatism 1996, 39:648-656.

Pujalte J.M., Llavore E.P., Ylescupidez F.R., et al. Double-blind clinical evaluation of oral glucosamine sulphate in the basic treatment of oesteoarthrosis, Curr Med Res Opin 1980, 7: 110-114.

Reddy C.K., Chandrakasan G., Dhar S.C., Studies on the metabolism of glycosaminoglycans under the influence of new herbal anti-inflammatory agents, Biochemical Pharmacol 1989, 20: 3527-3534.

Staines N.A., Suppression of collagen induced arthritis by oral administration of type II collagen: Changes in immune and arthritic responses mediated by active peripheral suppression. Autoimmunity, 16:189-199, 1993.

Wrigth V., Treatment of osteo-arthritis of the knees, Ann Rheum Dis, 1964, 23: 389-391.

Chapter 9: Digestion

Fugh-Berman, A. Alternative Medicine: What Works. Tucson, Ariz.: Odonian Press,1996.

Gershon, M.D. The Second Brain. N.Y.: HarperCollins, 1998.

Griggs, B. Green Pharmacy. Rochester, N.Y.: Healing Arts Press, 1991.

Herbal Drugs and Phytopharmaceuticals. N.G. Bisset, editor. Boca Raton, Fla.: CRC Press, 1989.

Holt, S. The Soy Revolution. N.Y.: Dell, 2000.

Holt, S. The Natural Way to a Healthy Heart, M. Evans and Company, Inc., New York, NY, 1999.

Holt S., Natural Ways to Digestive Health, M. Evans and Company, Inc., New York, NY, 2000.

Holt, S. and Comac, L. Miracle Herbs. N.Y.: CRC Press, 1995.

Nutrition and Health. F. Bonner, editor. N.Y.: CRC Press, 1995.

Pert, C.B. Molecules of Emotion. N.Y.: Scribner, 1997.

Present Knowledge in Nutrition, 7th ed. E.E. Ziegler and L.J. Filer, editors. Washington, D.C.: Textbook of Natural Medicine, 2nd ed. J.E. Pizzorno and M.T. Murray, editors. N.Y.: Churchill Livingstone, 1999.

Stanway, A. Alternative Medicine: A Guide to Natural Therapies. London: Chancellor Press, 1979.

Taylor, T.V., Surgical Gastroenterology. Oxford, U.K.: Blackwell Scientific Publications, 1985.

Upper Digestive Surgery: Oesophagus, Stomach and Small Intestine. T.V. Taylor et al, editors. London: W.B. Saunders, 1999.

Chapter 10: Heartburn

Baik SC et al, Increased oxidative DND damage in Helicobacter pylori-infected human gastric mucosa. Cancer Res, 56: 1279-1282, 1996.

Beil W, Birkholz C, Sewing K.F., Effects of flavonoids on parietal cell acid secretion, gastric mucosal prostaglandin production and Helicobacter pylori growth, Arzneim Forsch, 45:697-700, 1995.

Holt S., Management of gastroesophagealreflux disease – Part I, Internal Medicine for the Specialist 11, 11:100-106, 1990.

Holt S., Management of gastroesophagealreflux disease – Part II, Internal Medicine for the Specialist 11, 12:57-63, 1990.

Murakami S., Isobe Y., Kijima H., Nagai H., Muramatu M., and Otomo S., Inhibition of gastric H+, K+ATPase, and Acid Secretion by Ellagic Acid, Planta Med. 57 (1991)

Chapter 11: Colon Cleansing

Gotschall E., Breaking the vicious cycle, Kirkton, Ontario: Kirkton Press, 1994.

Hentges DJ, ed. Human intestinal microflora, In: Health and disease, New York, NY: Academic Press, 1983.

Holt S., Natural Ways to Digestive Health, M. Evans and Company, Inc., New York, NY, 2000.

Sonnenberg A, Koch T.R., Epidemiology of constipation in the United States, Dis Colon Rectum, 32:1-8, 1989.

Chapter 12: Fiber

Glore SR, Van Treeck D, Knehans AW et al, Soluble fiber and serum lipids, A literature review, J Am Diet Assoc 94:425-436.

Holt S, Heading RC, Clement J. Effects of Dietary Fiber. Gastroenterology 80:1611, 1981.

Krotkiewski M., Effect of guar on body weight, hunger ratings and metabolism in obese subjects. Clin Sci 66:329-326, 1984.

National Research Council, Diet and Health, Implications for reducing chronic disease Risk, Washington DC: National Academy Press, 1989.

Ripsin CM, Keenan JM, Jacobs DR et al., Oat products and lipid lowering, a meta-analysis, JAMA 267: 3317-3325, 1992.

Rossner S., von Zweigbergk D, Ohlin A et al, Weight reduction with dietary fibre supplements. Results of two double-blind studies, Acta Med Scand, 222:83-88, 1987.

Royal D, Wolever TM, Jeejeebhoy KN et al. Clinical significance of colonic fermentations, AM J Gastroenterol 1990, 85: 1307-1312.

Solum TT, Ryttig KR, Solum E et al, The influence of a high-fibre diet on body weight, serum lipids and blood pressure in slightly overweight persons, A randomized, double-blind, placebo-controlled investigation with diet and fibre tablets (DumoVital), Int J Obesity 11(1):67-71, 1987.

Spiller GA, Dietary fiber in health and nutrition, Boca Raton, FL: CRC Press, 1994.

Temple N.J., and Burkitt, D.P., Western diseases, Humana Press, New Jersey, 1994.

Trowell H., Burkitt D, Western diseases: their emergence and prevention, Harvard University Press, 1981.

Trowell H., Burkitt D, Heaton K, Dietary fibre, fibre-depleted foods and disease, New York, NY: Academic Press, 1985.

Vahouny G, Kritchevsky D, Dietary fiber in health and disease, New York, NY: Plenum Press, 1982.

Chapter 13: Enzymes

Folkers K., Littaru G.P., Ho L et al., Evidence for a deficiency of coenzyme Q10 in human heart disease, Int J Vitam Nutr Res, 40: 380-390, 1970.

Folkers K., Wolaniuk J., Simonsen R. et al, Biochemical rationale and the cardiac response of patients with muscle disease to therapy with coenzyme Q10, Proc Natl Acad Sci, 82: 4513-4516, 1985.

Hanaki Y., Sugiyama S., Ozawa T, Ohno M., Ratio of low-density lipoprotein cholesterol to ubiquinone as a coronary risk factor, N Engl J Med, 325:814-815, 1991.

Lockwood K., Moesgaard S., Hanioka T., Folkers K., Apparent partial remission of breast cancer in "high risk" patients supplemented with nutritional antioxidants, essential fatty acids and coenzyme Q10, Molec Aspects Med, 15: S231-240, 1994.

Salim AS, Oxygen-derived free radicals and the prevention of duodenal ulcer relapse: a new approach, Am J Med Sci 300: 1-6, 1990.

Smith J.L., Scholler J., Moore H.W. et al, Studies on the mechanism of vitamin-like activity of coenzyme Q, Arch Biochem Biophys 116:129-137, 1966.

Steffen C. et al, Enzymtherapie im vergleich mit immunokomplex-bestimmungen bei chronischer polyarthritis, Z Rheumatol 44:51-56, 1985.

Stocker R., Bowry V.W., Frei B., Ubiquinol-10 protects human low density lipoprotein more efficiently against lipid peroxidation than does alpha-tocopherol, Proc Natl Acad Sci, 88:1646-1650, 1991.

Sugiyama S., Kitazawa M., Ozawa K. et al., Anti-oxidative effect of coenzyme Q10. Experientia 36:1002-1003, 1980.

Chapter 14: Coral Calcium

Barefoot R. Barefoot on Coral Calcium: An Elixir of Life. NEWARK, NJ: Wellness Publishing, 2001.

Halstead BW. Fossil Stony Coral Minerals and Their Nutritional Application. Cannon Beach, OR: Health Digest Publishing Company, 1999.

Hirota Y Ph. D. and Sugisaki T Ph.D. Effects of the coral calcium as an inhibitory substance against colon cancer and its metastasis in the lungs. Nutrition Research. Vol. 20, No. 11, pp 1557-1567, 2000

Holt S. Natures Benefit from Coral Calcium. Newark, NJ: Wellness Publishing, 2003.

Ishitani K, Itakura E, Goto S and Esashi T. Calcium Absorption from the Ingestion of Coral-Derived Calcium by Humans. J Nutr Sci Vitaminol 45:509-517, 1999.

Suzuki K, Uehara M, Masuyama R and Gotou S. Calcium utilization from natural coral calcium – A coral preparation with a calcium-magnesium content ratio of 2:1. Abstracts of papers presented at the 44th Japanese Society for Nutritional Betterment, Fukuoka, Japan, 1997. p 145.

Willcox BJ, Willcox DC, Suzuki M. The Okinawa Program: How the World's Longest-Lived People Achieve Everlasting Health--And How You Can Too. New York: Clarkson Potter Publishers, 2000.

Chapter 15: Weight Management

Anderson GH (1994) Regulation of food intake. In Shils ME, Olson JA, Shike M (eds), Modern nutrition in health and disease, 8th ed. Lea & Febiger, Malvern, pp 524-536.

Anderson GH (1995) Sugars, sweetness, and food intake. Am. J. Clin. Nutr. 62(suppl):

195S-202S.

Anderson GH, Li ETS, Glanville NT (1984) Brain mechanisms and the quantitative and qualitative aspects of food intake. Brain Res. Bull. 12:167-173.

Black R, Anderson GH (1994) Sweeteners, food intake and selection. In Fernstrom JD, Miller G (eds), Appetite and body weight regulation: sugar, fat and macronutrient substitutes. CRC Press, Boca Raton, pp 125-136.

Drewnowski A (1994) Human preferences for sugar and fat. In Fernstorm JD, Miller GD (eds), Appetite and body weight regulation. CRC Press, Boca Raton, pp 137-147.

Flatt J-P (1993) Dietary fat, carbohydrate balance and weight maintenance. Ann N Y Acad Sci 683:122-140.

Friedman MI (1990) Body fat and the metabolic control of food intake. Int J Obes 14(suppl) 3:53-67

Horton ES (1983) An overview of the assessment and regulation of energy balance in humans. Am. J. Clin. Nutr. 38:972-977.

Lissner L, Heitmann BL (1995) Dietary fat and obesity: evidence from epidemiology. Eur J Clin Nutr 49:79-90.

Mayer J, 1980 Physiology of hunger and satiety. In Goodhart RS, Schils ME eds, Modern nutrition and disease, 6th ed. Lea & Febiger, Philadelphia, pp 560-577

Chapter 16: Syndrome X

Bernstein R K, Dr. Bernstein's Diabetes Solution: A Complete Guide to Achieving Normal Blood Sugars, Little Brown and Company, Boston, 2000.

Blaylock R, Excitotoxins: The Taste That Kills, Health Press, Santa Fe, 1994.

Broadhurst C L, Diabetes: Prevention and Cure, Kensington, NY, NY, 1999.

Challem J, Berkson B, Smith M D, Syndrome X, John Wiley & Sons, Inc., 2000.

Corea G, The Hidden Malpractice, William Morrow and Company, Inc., NY, NY, 1977.

Cowett R M, Diabetes, Raven Press, NY, NY, 1995.

Daneman D, Marcia F, Kusiel P, When a Child Has Diabetes, Firefly, NY, NY, 1999.

Dufty W, Sugar Blues, Warner Books, NY, NY, 1976.

Eades M R, Eades M D, Protein Power, Bantam Books, NY, NY, 1996.

Ford ES, Giles WH, Dietz W. "The Prevalence of the Metabolic Syndrome Among U.S. Adults," JAMA, 297, 3, 356-359, 2002.

Gracey M, Kretchmer N, Rossi E, Sugars in Nutrition, Raven Press, NY, NY, 1991.

Greene B, Winfrey O, Make The Connection, Ten Steps To A Better Body – And A Better Life, Harpo Inc, NY, NY, 1996.

Gross M L, The Psychological Society, Random House, NY, NY, 1978.

Heller R, Heller R and Vagnini F, The Carbohydrate Addict's Healthy Heart Program, Ballantine Books, NY, 1999

Jarville-Taylor KJ, Anderson RA, Graves DJ. A hydroxychalcone derived from cinnamon functions as a mimetic for insulin in 3T3-L1 adipocytes. J Am Coll Nutr 2001; 20(4):327-336

Kelly GS. Insulin resistance: lifestyle and nutritional interventions. Altern Med Rev. 2000 Apr; 5(2): 109-32

Kowalski R E, Cholesterol & Children, Harper & Row, Publishers Inc., NY, NY, 1988.

Leeds A, Brand Miller J, Foster-Powell K, Colagiuri S, The Glucose Revolution, Hodder and Stoughton, London, UK, 1998.

Libov C, Beat Your Risk Factors, Plume, NY, NY, 1999.

McCool M H, Woodruff S, My Doctor Says I Have A Little Diabetes, Avery, Garden City Park, 1998.

Miller J B, Foster-Powell K, Colagiuri S, The G.I. Factor, Hodder Headline Australia PTY, Ltd., Rydalmere, Australia, 1996.

Norman JC (Editor), Medicine In The Ghetto, Meredith Corporation, NY, NY, 1969.

Pescatore F, Feed Your Kids Well: How to Help Your Child Lose Weight and Get Healthy, John Wiley and Sons, NY, NY, 2000.

Reaven G, Kristen Strom T, Fox B, Syndrome X, Overcoming the Silent Killer that can give you a Heart Attack, Simon & Schuster, NY, NY, 2000.

Romaine D S, Marks J B, Syndrome X, Managing Insulin Resistance, Harper Collins Publishers Inc., NY, NY, 2000.

Sale K, Human Scale, Coward McCann & Geoghegan, NY, 1980.

Sears B, Mastering the Zone, Harper Collins Publishers, NY, NY, 1997

Sears B, Lawren B, Enter The Zone, A Dietary Road Map, Harper Collins Publishers Inc., NY, NY, 1995.

Sentochnik DE, Elipoulos GM, Infection and diabetes, In: Kahn CR, Weir GC, eds. Joslin's Diabetes Mellitus, Malvern, PA: Lea & Febiger, 1994:867.

Sosin AE, Sobell S, The Doctor's Guide to Diabetes and Your Child, Kensington Publishing Corp, NY, NY, 2000.

Steward HL, Bethea MC, Andrews SS, Balart LA, Sugar Busters, The Ballantine Publishing Group, 1998.

Touchette N, The Diabetes Problem Solver, American Diabetes Association, Alexandria, VA, 1999.

Weir GC, Leahy JL, Pathogenesis of non-insulin-dependent diabetes mellitus, In: Kahn CR, Weir GC, eds. Joslin's Diabetes Mellitus, ed 13, Philadelphia: Lea Febiger, 1994:240.

Wright JV. Detect and prevent diabetes now – years, even decades in advance. Part 1: Are you at risk? Nutrition & Healing 2001; 8(7):1-3

Wright JV. Detect and prevent diabetes now – years, even decades in advance. Part 1: Are you at risk? Nutrition & Healing 2001; 8(8):1-4

Chapter 17: Blood Sugar

Bernstein R K, Dr. Bernstein's Diabetes Solution: A Complete Guide to Achieving Normal Blood Sugars, Little Brown and Company, Boston, 2000.

Blaylock R, Excitotoxins: The Taste That Kills, Health Press, Santa Fe, 1994.

Broadhurst C L, Diabetes: Prevention and Cure, Kensington, NY, NY, 1999.

Challem J, Berkson B, Smith M D, Syndrome X, John Wiley & Sons, Inc., 2000.

Corea G, The Hidden Malpractice, William Morrow and Company, Inc., NY, NY, 1977.

Cowett R M, Diabetes, Raven Press, NY, NY, 1995.

Daneman D, Marcia F, Kusiel P, When a Child Has Diabetes, Firefly, NY, NY, 1999.

Dufty W, Sugar Blues, Warner Books, NY, NY, 1976.

Eades M R, Eades M D, Protein Power, Bantam Books, NY, NY, 1996.

Ford ES, Giles WH, Dietz W. "The Prevalence of the Metabolic Syndrome Among U.S. Adults," JAMA, 297, 3, 356-359, 2002.

Gracey M, Kretchmer N, Rossi E, Sugars in Nutrition, Raven Press, NY, NY, 1991.

Greene B, Winfrey O, Make The Connection, Ten Steps To A Better Body – And A Better Life, Harpo Inc, NY, NY, 1996.

Gross M L, The Psychological Society, Random House, NY, NY, 1978.

Heller R, Heller R and Vagnini F, The Carbohydrate Addict's Healthy Heart Program, Ballantine Books, NY, 1999

Jarville-Taylor KJ, Anderson RA, Graves DJ. A hydroxychalcone derived from cinnamon functions as a mimetic for insulin in 3T3-L1 adipocytes. J Am Coll Nutr 2001; 20(4):327-336

Kelly GS. Insulin resistance: lifestyle and nutritional interventions. Altern Med Rev. 2000 Apr; 5(2): 109-32

Kowalski R E, Cholesterol & Children, Harper & Row, Publishers Inc., NY, NY, 1988.

Leeds A, Brand Miller J, Foster-Powell K, Colagiuri S, The Glucose Revolution, Hodder and Stoughton, London, UK, 1998.

Libov C, Beat Your Risk Factors, Plume, NY, NY, 1999.

McCool M H, Woodruff S, My Doctor Says I Have A Little Diabetes, Avery, Garden City Park, 1998.

Miller J B, Foster-Powell K, Colagiuri S, The G.I. Factor, Hodder Headline Australia PTY, Ltd., Rydalmere, Australia, 1996.

Norman JC (Editor), Medicine In The Ghetto, Meredith Corporation, NY, NY, 1969.

Pescatore F, Feed Your Kids Well: How to Help Your Child Lose Weight and Get Healthy, John Wiley and Sons, NY, NY, 2000.

Reaven G, Kristen Strom T, Fox B, Syndrome X, Overcoming the Silent Killer that can give you a Heart Attack, Simon & Schuster, NY, NY, 2000.

Romaine D S, Marks J B, Syndrome X, Managing Insulin Resistance, Harper Collins Publishers Inc., NY, NY, 2000.

Sale K, Human Scale, Coward McCann & Geoghegan, NY, 1980.

Sears B, Mastering the Zone, Harper Collins Publishers, NY, NY, 1997

Sears B, Lawren B, Enter The Zone, A Dietary Road Map, Harper Collins Publishers Inc., NY, NY, 1995.

Sentochnik DE, Elipoulos GM, Infection and diabetes, In: Kahn CR, Weir GC, eds. Joslin's Diabetes Mellitus, Malvern, PA: Lea & Febiger, 1994:867.

Sosin AE, Sobell S, The Doctor's Guide to Diabetes and Your Child, Kensington Publishing Corp, NY, NY, 2000.

Steward HL, Bethea MC, Andrews SS, Balart LA, Sugar Busters, The Ballantine Publishing Group, 1998.

Touchette N, The Diabetes Problem Solver, American Diabetes Association, Alexandria, VA, 1999.

Weir GC, Leahy JL, Pathogenesis of non-insulin-dependent diabetes mellitus, In: Kahn CR, Weir GC, eds. Joslin's Diabetes Mellitus, ed 13, Philadelphia: Lea Febiger, 1994:240.

Wright JV. Detect and prevent diabetes now – years, even decades in advance. Part 1: Are you at risk? Nutrition & Healing 2001; 8(7):1-3

Wright JV. Detect and prevent diabetes now – years, even decades in advance. Part 1: Are you at risk? Nutrition & Healing 2001; 8(8):1-4

Chapter 18: Fish Oil

Allard J.P., Kurian R., Aghdassi E., et al, Lipid peroxidation during n-3 fatty acid and vitamin E supplementation in humans, Lipids, 32: 535-541, 1997.

Billiyya G., Reddy K.K., Reddy G.P.R., et al, Lipid Profiles among fish-consuming coastal and non-fish-consuming inland populations, Eur J Clin Nutr, 44: 481-485, 1990.

Budiarso I.T., Fish oil versus olive oil, Lancet, ii 1313-1314, 1990.

Connor W.E., Do the n-3 fatty acids from fish oil prevent deaths from cardiovascular disease? Am J Clin Nutr, 66: 188-189, 1997.

Curb J.D., Reed D.M., Fish consumption and mortality from coronary heart disease, New Engl Med, 313:821, 1985.

Erasmus U., Fats and Oils, Vancouver, BC: Alive, p 248-249, 1986.

Harris W.S., Dietary fish oil and blood lipids, Curr Opin Lipidol, 7: 3-7, 1996.

Kinella J.E., Lokesh B., Stone R.A., Dietary n-3 polyunsaturated fatty acids and amelioration of cardiovascular disease: possible mechanisms, Am J Clin Nutr, 52: 1-28, 1990.

Riemersma R.A., Sargent C.A., Abraham R.A. et al, Fish and the heart, Lancet, ii: 1450, 1989.

Saynor R., Gillot T. Fish oil [Letter to editor], Lancet, ii: 810-812, 1989.

Sinclair H.M., The importance of fish in the prevention of chronic degenerative diseases, Nahr Meer (International Symposium), p 201-210, 1980.

Simopoulos A.P., Omega-3 fatty acids in the prevention-management of cardiovascular disease, Can J Physiol Pharmacol, 75: 234-239, 1997.

Stone N.J., Fish consumption, fish oil, lipids, and coronary heart disease, 65:1083-1086, 1997.

Vollset S.E., Heuch I., Bjelke E., Fish consumption and mortality from coronary heart disease, New Engl J Med, 313:821-821, 1985.

Weisburger J.H., Dietary fat and risk of chronic disease: mechanistic insights from experimental studies, J Am Diet Assoc 97(Suppl): S16-S23, 1997.

Yamori Y., Nara Y., Iritarri N., et al., Comparison of serum phospholipids fatty acids among fishing and farming Japanese populations and American inlanders, J Nutr Sci Vitaminol, 31:417-422, 1985.

Yetiv J.V., Clinical applications of fish oils, JAMA, 260:665-670, 1988.

Chapter 19: Cholesterol

Attwood C., Dr. Attwood's Low-Fat Prescription for Kids, Penguin, New York, 1995.

Booyens J, Van der Merwe C.F., Margarines and coronary artery disease, Med Hypothesis, 37: 241-244, 1992.

Cheraskin E., Orenstein N., Miner P., Lower Your Cholesterol in 30 Days, Perigree, 1986.

Erasmus U., Fats That Heal, Fats That Kill, 2nd ed., Alive Books, 1993.

Ford N., Eighteen Ways to Lower Your Cholesterol in 30 Days, Keats, 1992.

Holt S., The Natural Way to a Healthy Heart, M. Evans and Company, New York, NY, 1999.

Mensink R.P, Katan M.B., Effect of dietary trans fatty acids on high-density and low-density lipoprotein cholesterol levels in healthy subjects, New Engl J Med, 323:439-445, 1990.

Moyer E., Cholesterol & Triglycerides, People's Medical Pharmacy, 1995.

Verschuren W.M., Jacobs D.R., Bloemberg B.P., et al, Serum total cholesterol and long-term coronary heart disease mortality in different cultures, Twenty-five year follow-up of the Seven Countries Study, JAMA, 274: 131-136, 1995.

Willet W.C., Stampfer MJ., Manson J.E., Intake of trans fatty acids and risk of coronary heart disease among women, Lancet 341:581-585, 1993.

Chapter 20: Heart

Attwood C., Dr. Attwood's Low-Fat Prescription for Kids, Penguin, New York, 1995.

Cheraskin E., Orenstein N., Miner P., Lower Your Cholesterol in 30 Days, Perigree, 1986.

Erasmus U., Fats That Heal, Fats That Kill, 2nd ed., Alive Books, 1993.

Ford N., Eighteen Ways to Lower Your Cholesterol in 30 Days, Keats, 1992.

Goldstrich J., Healthy Heart, Longer Life, Ultimate Health Publishing, 1996.

Holt S., The Natural Way to a Healthy Heart, M. Evans and Company, New York, NY, 1999.

Moyer E., Cholesterol & Triglycerides, People's Medical Pharmacy, 1995.

Ornish D., Dr. Ornish's Program for Reversing Heart Disease, Ivy Books, 1996.

Shreeve C., A Healthy Heart for Life, City: Thorsens Publishing Group, 1988.

Shute E., The Heart and Vitamin E, Keats, 1977.

Sinatra S.T., Heartbreak and Heart Disease, Keats, 1996.

Verschuren W.M., Jacobs D.R., Bloemberg B.P., et al, Serum total cholesterol and long-term coronary heart disease mortality in different cultures, Twenty-five year follow-up of the Seven Countries Study, JAMA, 274: 131-136, 1995.

Chapter 21: Prostate

Belaiche P., Lievoux O., Clinical studies on the palliative treatment of prostatic adenoma with extract of Urtica root. Phytother Res 5: 267-269, 1991.

Buck A.C., Phytotherapy for the prostate, Br J Urol, 78:325-336, 1996.

Bush I.M., et al, Zinc and the prostate, Presented at the annual meeting of the AMA, 1974.

Chyou P.H., et al, A prospective study of alcohol, diet and other lifestyle factors in relation to obstructive uropathy, Prostate 22:253-264, 1993.

Farnsworth W.E., Slaunwhite W.R., Sharma M et al, Interaction of prolactin and testosterone in the human prostate, Urol Res 9: 79-88, 1981.

Habib F.K., Ross M., Lawenstein A., Identification of a prostate inhibitory substance in a pollen extract, The Prostate, 26: 133-139, 1995.

Morton M.S., Griffiths K., Blacklock N., The preventive role of diet in prostatic disease, Br J Urol, 77:481-493, 1996.

Scott W.W., The lipids of the prostatic fluid, seminal plasma and enlarged prostate gland of man, J Urol 53:712-718, 1945.

Wagner H., Search for the antiprostatic principle of stinging nettle (Urtica dioica) roots. Phytomedicine 1: 213-224, 1994.

Chapter 22: Sex

Boston Women's Health Book Collective, Our Bodies, Our Selves, Simon and Schuster, NY, 1979

Comfort A, The Joy of Sex, Simon and Schuster, NY, 1974

Diamond M, Sexwatching: Looking into the World of Sexual Behavior, Prion Books, London, 1992

Ford G, Listening to Your Hormones, Prima Lifestyles, Roseville, CA, 1997

Kodis M, Love Scents, E.P. Dutton, NY, 1998

Lawrence DH, Lady Chatterley's Lover, Penguin (reprint edition), NY, 1995

Love S, Dr. Love's Hormone Therapy, Random House, New York, 1999

Masters W, Johnson V, and Levin R, The Pleasure Bond, Bantam Books, NY, 1980

Mojay G, Aromatherapy for Healing the Spirit, Healing Arts Press, Rochester, VT, 2000

Morris D, The Naked Ape, Vintage/Random House, NY, 1994

Ornish D, Love and Survival: The Scientific Basis for the Healing Power of Intimacy, Perennial/HarperCollins, NY, 1999

Pearsall P, Sexual Healing, Random House, NY, 1995

Robert W and Fried M, Arginine Solution, Warner Books, NY, 1999

Chapter 23: Memory

Appa R.M.V.R., Srinivasan K., Koteswara R.T.L., The effect of Centella asiatica on the general mental ability of mentally retarded children, Ind J Psychiatry, 19: 54-59, 1977.

Gessner B., Voelp A, Klasser M., Study of the long-term action of a Gingko biloba extract on vigilance and mental performance as determined by means of quantitative pharmaco-EEG and psychometric measurements, Arzneim Forsćh, 35:1459-1465, 1985.

Kleijnen J., Knipschild P., Ginkgo biloba for cerebral insufficiency, Br J Clinical Pharmacol, 34:352-8, 1992.

Nerozzi D., Aceti F., Meila E., et al, Phosphatidylserine in age-related disturbance of memory, Clin Terapeutica, 120: 399-404, 1987.

Penland J.G., Dietary boron, brain function, and cognitive performance, Environ Health Perspect, 102: 65-72, 1994.

Petkov V.D., Kehayov R., Belcheva S., Konstantinova E., Petkov V.V., Getova D.,

Markovska V., Memory effects of standardized extracts of Panax ginseng (G 115), Ginkgo biloba (GK 501) and their combination Gincosan (PHL-00701), Planta Medica, 59: 106-114, 1993.

Chapter 24: Skin, Nail and Hair Support

Attar K., Abdel-Aal M.A., Debayle P., Distribution of trace elements in the lipid and non lipid matter of the hair, Clin Chem 36:477-480, 1990.

Clanet P, De Antonio S.M., Katz S.A., Schreiner D.M., Effects of some cosmetics on copper and zinc concentration in human scalp hair, Clin Chem, 28:2450, 1982.

Davis R.H., Kabbani J.M., Maro N.P., Aloe Vera and wound healing, J Am pod Med Assoc 77:165-169, 1987.

Klein A.D., Penneys N.S., Aloe Vera, J Am Acad Dermatol 18:714-719, 1988.

McKenzie J.M., Content of zinc in serum, hair and toenails of New Zealand adults, Am J Clin Nutr 32:570, 1979.

Mediros D., Sturniolo G.C., Martin A. et al, Trace elements in human hair, Lancet ii:608, 1982.

Passwater R.A., Cranton E.M, Trace elements, hair analysis and nutrition, New Canaan, C.T.: Heats Publ, p 291-303, 1983.

Saner G., Hair trace element concentration in patients with protein-energy malnutrition, Nutr Rep Int, 32:263-268, 1985.

Shelton R.W., Aloe Vera, its chemical and therapeutic properties. Int J Dermatol 30: 679-683, 1991.

Weber W., Nelson G., de Vaquera M.V., Pearson P.R., Trace elements in the hair of healthy and malnourished children, J Trop Peds, 36:230-234, 1990.

Chapter 25: Eye Care

Abel. R. Jr., The Eye Care Revolution, Prevent and Reverse Common Vision Problems, Kensington Publishing Corp, New York, NY, 1999.

Abel R. Jr., Stuart P.R., and Sardi B., The Case for Nutrition as Preventive Eye Care, Review of Optometry, August 15, 1995.

Absher K., Why Eye Problems Are Increasing, Journal of Longevity 4(6):7, 1998.

Duke J., The Green Pharmacy, Rodale Press, Emmaus, PA, 1997.

Goldberg J., et al, Factors Associated with Age-Related Macular Degeneration: An Analysis of Data from the First National Health and Nutrition Examination Survey, American Journal of Epidemiology, 128 (4):700-710, 1988.

Harkinson S.E., et al, Nutrient Intake and Cataract Extraction in Women: A Prospective Study, British Medical Journal 305:335-39, 1992.

Morgan B. L.G., Nutrition Prescription, Crown, NY, 1987.

Taylor A., Jacques P.F., and Epstein E.M., Relations Among Aging, Antioxidant Status, and Cataract, American Journal of Clinical Nutrition 62 (supppl): 1439S-47S, 1995.

Tabbara K.F., Nutritional Blindness: Vitamin A Deficiency, In Prevention of Eye Disease (ed. M.H. Friedlaender), Mary Ann Liebert, Publishers, New York, NY, 1988.

Wright J.V., Nutrition and Healing, Publisher's Management Corp, Phoenix, AZ, June 1998.

Chapter 26: High Energy

Briggs C., Peppermint, Medicinal herb and flavoring agent, Can Pharm J, March: 89-92, 1993.

Castellani C., Marai A., Vacchi P., The Centella asiatica, Boll Chim Farm, 120: 570-605, 1981.

Graham H.N., Green tea composition, consumption, and polyphenol chemistry, Prev Med 21: 334-350, 1992.

Hallstrom C., Fulder S., Carruthers M., Effect of ginseng on the performance of nurses on night duty, Comp Med East & West, 6: 277-282, 1982.

Hikino H., Traditional remedies and modern assessment: the case of ginseng, In: Wijeskera ROB, ed., The medical plant industry, Boca Raton, FL: CRC Press, p149-166, 1991.

Min Z., Peigen X., Quantitative analysis of the active constituents in green tea, Phytother Res, 5:239-240, 1991.

Chapter 27: Natures Calcium®

Arnaud D.C., Sanchez S.D., Calcium and phosphorus. Present knowledge in nutrition, 6th edn. Washington DC: Nutrition Foundation, p 212-221, 371-373, 1990.

Arnaud D.C., Sanchez S.D., The role of calcium in osteoporosis, Ann Rev Nutr 10:397-414, 1990.

Cook J., Dassenko S., Whittaker P., Calcium supplementation. Effect on iron absorption. Am J Clin Nutr 53: 106-111, 1991.

Chu J.Y., Margen S., Costa F.M., Studies in calcium metabolism, Am J Clin Nutr 28:1028-1035, 1975.

Fletcher M.P., at al, Nutrition and immunology. New York: Alan R. Liss, p 215-239, 1988.

Kanis J.A., Passmore R., Calcium supplementation of the diet – I, Br Med J, 298:137-140, 1989.

Kanis J.A., Passmore R., Calcium supplementation of the diet – II, Br Med J, 298:205-208, 1989.

Rivers J.M., Safety of high level vitamin C ingestion, Int J Vitamin Nutr Res, 30:95-102, 1989.

Chapter 28: Anti-Dependence

Chou T., Wake up and smell the coffee. Caffeine, coffee and the medical consequences, West J Med, 157:544-553, 1992.

Gilliand K., Bullick W., Caffeine: a potential drug of abuse, Adv Alcohol Subst Abuse, 3:53-73, 1984.

Holt S, Stewart IC, Dixon JM, Elton RA, Taylor RV, Little K. Alcohol and the emergency service patient. British Medical Journal 281:638-40, 1980.

Holt S, Skinner HA, Israel Y. Identification of alcohol abuse. II. Clinical and laboratory indicators. Canadian Medical Association Journal 124(10):1279-94, 1981.

Holt S., Skinner HA. Confronting alcoholism. Canadian Medical Association Journal 126:351-2, 1982.

Holt S. Tackling the alcohol problem: the case for secondary prevention. Journal of the South Carolina Medical Association 85(12):582-4, 1989.

Holt S. Identification and intervention for alcohol abuse. Journal of the South Carolina Medical Association 85(12):554-9, 1989.

Israel Y, Orrego H, Holt S, MacDonald DW, Meema HE. Identification of alcohol abuse: thoracic fractures on routine chest X-rays as indicators of alcoholism. Alcoholism: Clinical and Experimental Research 4:420-2, 1980.

Livshits O, Holt S, Skinner HA, Carlen P. Alcohol and male impotence. Substudy Publication, Addiction Research Foundation, Toronto, Canada 1980.

Skinner HA, Holt S, The Alcohol Clinical Index, Addiction Research Foundation, Toronto, 1993

Skinner HA, Holt S, Allen BA, Haakonson NH. Correlation between medical and behavioral data in the assessment of alcoholism. Alcohol Clinical and Experimental Research 4:371-7, 1980.

Skinner HA, Holt S, Israel Y. Identification of alcohol abuse. I. Critical issues and psychosocial indicators for a composite index. Canadian Medical Association Journal 124(9):1141-52, 1981.

Skinner HA, Holt S, Schuller R, Ray J, Israel Y. Identification of alcohol abuse using laboratory tests and a history of trauma. Annals of Internal Medicine 101(6):847-51, 1984.

Skinner HA, Holt S, Sheu WJ, Israel Y. Clinical versus laboratory detection of alcohol abuse: the alcohol clinical index. British Medical Journal 292(6537):1703-8, 1986.

Vasudeva R, Holt S. Observations on the management of alcohol withdrawal syndrome. The Journal of the South Carolina Medical Association. 86(1):24-6, 1990.

Chapter 29: Mood

Alpert J.E., Fava M., Nutrition and depression. The role of folate. Nutr Rev 55:145-149, 1997.

Byrne A., Byrne D.G., The effect of exercise on depression, anxiety and other mood states. A review, J Psychosom Res, 37:565-574, 1993.

Casper, R.C., Exercise and mood, World Rev Nutr Diet, 71:115-143, 1993.

De Smet P.A.G., Nolen W., St. John's wort as an antidepressant, BMJ, 313: 241-242, 1996.

Folkins C.H., Sime W.E., Physical fitness training and mental health, Am Psychologist, 36: 375-388, 1981.

Holzl J., Demisch L., Gollnik B., Investigations about antidepressive and mood changing effects of Hypericum perforatum, Planta Med, 55: 643, 1989.

Kreitsch K., Prevalence, presenting symptoms, and psychological characteristics of individuals experiencing a diet-related mood disturbance, Behav Ther, 19:593-594,

1985.

Reynolds E., Preece J., Bailey J. et al, Folate deficiency in depressive illness, Br J Psychiat 117:287-292, 1970.

Rosenthal N., Sack D., Gillin C. et al, Seasonal affective disorder: a description of the syndrome and preliminary findings with light treatment, Arch Gen Psychiat, 41: 72-80, 1984.

Russ C., Hendricks T., Chrisley B., et al, Vitamin B_6 status of depressed and obsessive-compulsive patients, Nutr Rep Intl, 27: 867-873, 1983.

Werbach M., Nutritional influences on mental illness: a sourcebook of clinical research. Tarzana, CA: Third Line Press, 1991.

Chapter 30: Allergy

Czap K, Alternative Medicine Review, Thorne Research, Dover, ID, 2002.

Gursche S, Encyclopedia of Natural Healing, Alive Publishing Group, Burnaby, Canada, 1997.

Hoffman RL, Intelligent Medicine, Simon & Schuster, NY, NY, 1997.

Pelletier KR, The Best Alternative Medicine, Simon & Schuster, NY, NY, 2000.

Tyler VE, The Honest Herbal, Haworth Press, Binghampton, NY, 1993.

Chapter 31: Specific Anti-Aging Factors for Natural Clinicians

Klatz, R., Kovarik, F., Goldman, R. Eds., Advances in Anti-Aging Medicine, Vol. 1, Mary Ann Liebert Inc., Larchmont, New York, 1996

Evans, W., Rosenberg, I., Thompson, J., Biomarkers: The 10 Keys to Prolonging Vitality, Simon & Schuster, New York, New York, 1992

West, S., Tyburn-Lombard, D., How to Live to be 100 and Enjoy It!, Aabbott McDonnell-Winchester, North Babylon, New York, 1977

Comfort, A., The Process of Aging, Signet Science Library, 1964

Walford, R., The 120 Year Diet: How to Double Your Vital Years, Simon & Schuster, New York, New York, 1986

Rabins, P., Lauber, L., Getting Old Without Getting Anxious, Penguin Group Inc., London, UK, 2005

Woodruff-Pak, D., The Neuropathy of Aging, Blackwell Publishers Inc., Malden, Massachusetts, 1997

Kyriazis, M., Anti-Aging Medicines, Watkins Publishing, London, UK , 2005

Smith, T., Renewal: The Anti-Aging Revolution, Rodale Press Inc., Emmaus, Pennsylvania, 1998

Hendler, S., The Complete Guide to Anti-Aging Nutrients, Simon & Schuster, New York, New York, 1985

Pesmen, C., How A Man Ages, Ballantine Books, a division of Random House Inc., New York 1984

Heinerman, J., Heinerman's Encyclopedia of Anti-Aging Remedies, Prentice Hall, Paramus, New Jersey, 1996

Willcox, B, Willcox, D., Suzuki, M., The Okinawa Program, Clarkson Potter, New

York, New York, 2001

Atkins, R., Buff, S., Dr. Atkins' Age-Defying Diet Revolution, St. Martin's Press, New York, New York, 2000

Holt, S., Combat Syndrome X, Y and Z…, Wellness Publishing, Little Falls, New Jersey, 2002

Holt, S., Wright, J.V., Holt, F.G.S., Nutritional Factors for Syndrome X, Wellness Publishing, Little Falls, New Jersey, 2003

Holt, S., A Certification Program for Dietary Supplement Counselors, Wellness Publishing, Little Falls, New Jersey, 2008

Ames, B.N., Shigenaga, M.K., Hagen, T.M., Oxidants, antioxidants and degenerative diseases of aging. Proc. Natl. Acad. Sci. USA, 1993 90: 7915-7922

Sohal, R.S., Sohal, B.H., Brunk, U.T., Relationship between antioxidant defenses and longevity in different mammalian species. Mech. Ageing Dev., 1990, 53: 217-227

Halliwell, B., Free Radicals, antioxidants and human disease. Curiosity, cause or consequence?, Lancet, 1994, 344: 721-724

Wang, H., Cao, G., Prior, R.L., Total antioxidant capacity of fruits, J. Agr. Food. Chem., 1996, 44: 701-705

Harman, D., Aging. A theory based on free radical and radiation chemistry, J. Gerontol., 1956, 11: 288-300

Gaby, A.R., Enzyme CoQ10, in Textbook of Natural Medicine, Pizzorno, J.E., Murray, M.T., Harcourt, Brace and Co Ltd, 1999, 2(1): 663-670

Brownlee, M., Vlassara, H., Cerami, A., Nonenzymatic glycosylation and the pathogenesis of diabetic complications. Ann. Int. Med. 1984, 101: 527-537

Miller, A.L., Kelly, G. S., Homocysteine metabolism: nutritional modulation and impact on health and disease, in Textbook of Natural Medicine, Pizzorno, J.E., Murray, M.T., Harcourt, Brace and Co Ltd, 1999, 2(1): 461-475

Mason, J., Miller, J., The effects of vitamins B12, B6, and folate on blood homocysteine levels, Ann. NY. Acad. Sci., 1992, 669: 197-203

Klatz, R., Kahn, C., Grow Young with HGH, HarperCollins, New York, New York, 1997

Horner, C., Waking the Warrior Goddess, Basic Health Publications Inc., Laguna Beach, California, 2005

Hau L., Bravata, D., Ingram, O., Smita, N., Roberts, B., Gerber, A., Hoffman, A., Systematic review: the safety and efficacy of growthe hormone in the healthy elderly, Annals of Internal Medicine, 2007 146(2): 104-115

Corpas, E., Blackman, M.R., Roberson, R. et al, Oral arginine-lysine does not increase growth hormone or insulin-like growth factor-I in old men, J. Gerontol., 1993, 48: M128-133

Hoffman, R., Endocrine aspects of aging, in Advances in Anti-Aging Medicine, Klatz, R., Ed., Mary Ann Liebert Inc., Larchmont, New York, 1996, 1: 43-49

Gaby, A.R., Dehydroepiandrosterone, in Textbook of Natural Medicine, Pizzorno, J.E., Murray, M.T., Harcourt, Brace and Co Ltd, 1999, 2(1): 695-699

Yen, S.C.C., Morales, A.J., Khorram, O., Replacement of DHEA in aging men and women. Potential remedial effects, Ann. NY, Acad. Sci., 1995, 774: 128-142

Regelson, W., Loria, R., Kalimi, M., Dehydroepiandrosterone (DHEA) – the "mother steroid." I. Immunologic action, Ann. NY Acad. Sci. 1994, 719: 553-563

Yu, H.S., Reiter, R.J., Eds., Melatonin Biosynthesis, Physiological Effects and Clinical Applications, CRC Press, Boca Raton, 1993

Pati, S., Bio-identical hormones: an update on the evidence, in Klatz, R., Goldman, R., Anti-Aging Therapeutics, A4M Publications, Chicago, Illinois, 2007, 9: 255-264

Humphries, K., Gill, S., Risks and benefits of hormone replacement therapy: the evidence speaks, Canadian Medical Association Journal, 2003, 168: 1001-1010

Writing group WHI Investigators, Risks and benefits of estrogen plus progestin in healthy postmenopausal women, JAMA, 2002, 288: 321-333

Chapter 32: Miscellaneous Topics

Bisset NG (Editor), Herbal Drugs and Phytopharmacueticals, CRC Press, Boca Raton, FL, 1994

Karch SB, The Consumers Guide to Herbal Medicine, Advanced Research Press, Hauppauge, NY, 1999

Mayell M, Off-The-Shelf Natural Health: How to Use Herbs and Nutrients to Stay Well, Bantam Books, New York, NY, 1995

Rakel D, Integrative Medicine, Saunders, Philadelphia, PA, 2003

Gursche S, Rona Z, Encyclopedia of Natural Healing, Alive Publishing Group, Burnaby, BC, 1997

Cupp MJ, Tracy TS, Dietary Supplements Toxicology and Clinical Pharmacology, Humana Press, Totowa, NJ, 2003

Blumenthal M, Busse WR, Goldberg A, Gruenwald J, Hall T., Riggins CW, Rister RS, The Complete German Commission E Monographs: Therapeutic Guide to Herbal Medicines, American Botanical Council, Austin, TX, 1998

Croft J, Health from the Seas: Freedom from Disease, Vital Health Publishing, Ridgefield, CT, 2003

Mowrey DB, The Scientific Validation of Herbal Medicine, Keats Publishing Inc., New Canaan, CT,1986

Wright JV, Gaby AR, Natural Medicine, Optimal Wellness: The Patient's Guide to Health and Healing, Vital Health Publishing, Ridgefield, CT, 2006

Griggs B, Green Pharmacy: The History and Evolution of Western Herbal Medicine, Healing Art Press, Rochester, VT 1981, 1991

Editorial, Anon. Nutrition and the metabolic response to Injury. Lancet. 1:995-97, 1989

Jacob, R.A. and Sotoudeh, G. Vitamin C function and status in chronic disease. Nutr. Clin Care. 5:66, 2002

Williams, J.Z. and Barbul, A. nutrition and wound healing. Surg. Clin. North Am. 89:571, 2003

Brown, Spencer A., Coimbra, Maria, Coberly, Dana M., Chao, James J., Rohrich, Rod J. Oral Nutritional supplementation accelerates skin wound healing: A randomized, placebo-controlled, double-arm, crossover study. Plastic and Reconstructive Surgery. 114:237, 2004

Shanmugasundaram, KR, Ramanujam S. and Shanmugasundaram, E.R. Amrita Bindu: A Salt-spice-herbal health food supplement for the prevention of nitrosamine induced depletion of antioxidants. J. Ethnopharmacol. 42:83, 1994

Shamosh, J.A., Herbal First Aid. J. Emerg. Nurs. 24: 553, 1998

Nguyen, DD., Nguyen, N.H., Nguyen, T.T. et.al. The Use of Water Extract from the bark of Choerospondias axillais in the treatment of second degree burns. Scand. J. Plastic and Reconstructive Surgery Hand Surg. 30:139, 1996

Werbach, M.R., Nutritional Influences on Illness. 2nd Ed. Third Line Press, Tarzana, CA, 1996

Dowling, R.J. Use of Fat Emulsion in Nutrition in Clinical Surgery. Edited by M. Dietel,. Williams and Wilkins, Baltimore, 1985

Holt, S. Combat Syndrome X, Y and Z. Wellness Publishing, Little Falls, NJ, 2003

Howat RCL., Lewis GD. The effect of bromelain therapy on epistomy wounds – a double blind controlled clinical trial. J Obstet Gynaecol BR Commonw. 79:951-3, 1972

Pollack, PJ. Oral administration of enzymes from Carica papaya: Report of a double-blind clinical study. Curr Ther Res. 4(5): 229-37, 1962

Kartnig T. Clinical applications of Centella asiatica (L.) Urb. Herbs Spices Med Plants. 3: 146-73, 1988

Klein, AD., Penneys NS. Aloe vera. J. Amer. Acad. Dermatology. 18:714-9, 1988)

Glowania HJ., Raulin, C., Swoboda M. Effect of Chamomile of wound healing – a clinical double-blind study. Z. Hautkr. 62(17): 1262, 1267-71, 1987, cited by Werbach MR., 1996

Baruch J. Effect of Endotelon in postoperative edema: Results of a double-blind study versus placebo in 32 female patients. Ann Chir Plast Esthet. 29(4): 393-5, 1984

Thomas, DR., Specific nutritional factors in wound healing. Adv. Wound Care. 10:40, 1997

Leipner, J., Iten F., and Saller R. Therapy with proteolytic enzymes in rheumatic disorders. Biodrugs 15:779, 2001

Desser. L., Holomanova D., Zavadova F., Pavelka K., Mohr T., and Herbacek I. Oral Therapy with proteolytic enzymes decreases excessive TGF-beta levels in human blood. Cancer Chemother, Pharmacol. 47:510, 2001

Taussig S., Batkin S. Bromelain, the enzyme complex of pineapple (Ananas comosus) and its clinical application. An update. J Ethnopharmacol. 22: 191-203, 1988

Cirelli MG. Five years of clinical experience with bromelains in therapy of edema and inflammation in postoperative tissue reaction, skin infections and trauma. Clin Med. 74(6): 55-59, 1967

Tassman G. et al. A double-blind crossover study of a plant proteolytic enzyme in oral surgery. J Dent Med. 20:51-4, 1965

Cowie DH. et al. A double-blind trial of bromelains as an adjunct of vaginal plastic repair operations. J Obstet Gynaecol BR Commonw. 77(4):365-68, 1970

Karch, SB. Herbal Medicine. Advance Research Press, 1999

Alonzo D, Lazarus MC, Baumann L. Effects of topical arnica gel on post-laser treatment bruises. Dermatol Surg. 2002 Aug; 28(8): 686-8

Ernst E, Pittler MH. Efficacy of homeopathic arnica: a systematic review of placebo-controlled clinical trials. Arch Surg. 1998;133:1187-1190

Hart O., Mullee MA., Lewith G., Miller J. Double-blind, placebo-controlled, randomized clinical trial of homeopathic arnica C30 (30X) for pain and infection after total abdominal hysterectomy. J R. Soc. Med. 1997: 90(2): 73-8

Conforti A, Bertani S, Metelmann H, Chirumbolo S, Lussignoli S, Bellavite P. Experimental Studies of the anti-inflammatory activity of a homeopathic preparation. Biol. Ther. 1997: 15(1):28-31

Tveiten D, Bruset S, Borchgrevink CF, Norseth J. Effects of the homeopathic remedy Arnica D30 on marathon runners: a randomized, double blind study during the 1995 Oslo marathon. Complement. Ther. Med. 1998: 6(2): 71-74

Vickers AJ., Fisher P., Smith C., Wyllie SE., Rees R. Homeopathic Arnica 30X is ineffective for muscle soreness after long distance running: a randomized, double-blind , placebo-controlled trial. Clin. J. Pain. 1998: 14(3): 227-231

Seeley, BM., Maas C. Effect of Homeopathic Arnica on Bruising in Face-Lifts, Archive of Facial Plastic Surgery. 8, 54-59, 2006

Kulich M. Proceedings of the American Society of Aesthetic Plastic Surgery (ASPAS), 2002

Chapter 32: Pets

Allport RB, Heal Your Cat the Natural Way, Reed International Books, NY, 1997.

Allport RB, Heal Your Dog the Natural Way, Reed International Books, NY, 1997.

Anderson N, and Peiper H, Are You Poisoning Your Pets? Garden City Park, NY, Avery Publishing Group, 1998.

Anderson N, and Peiper H, Super Nutrition for Animals, Garden City Park, NY, Avery Publishing Group, 1996.

Belfield, Wendell O, DVM and Zucker M, The Very Healthy Cat Book: A Vitamin and Mineral Program for Optimal Feline Health. New York, McGraw-Hill, 1988.

Castelman M, The Healing Herbs: The Ultimate Guide to the Curative Power of Nature's Medicines, Emmaus, Pa: Rodale Press, 1991.

Coulter AH, Alternative Veterinary Medicine Provides Relief for Pets, Alternative and Complementary Therapies, Vol. 2,4, 245-252, 1996.

DeBairacli Levy J, Cats Naturally: Natural Rearing for Healthier Domestic Cats, New York: Faber & Faber, 1991.

DeBairacli Levy J, The Complete Herbal Handbook for the Dog and Cat, New York, Faber & Faber, 1991.

Frazier A with Eckroate N, The New Natural Cat: A Complete Guide for Finicky Owners, New York: Penguin Books, 1990.

Gfeller RW, DVM and Messonier SR, DVM, Handbook of Small Animal Toxicology and Poisonings, Saint Louis, MO, Mosby, 1998.

Goldstein M, DVM, The Nature of Animal Healing: The Path to Your Pet's Healing, Happiness, and Longevity, New York: Knopf, New York, 1999.

Humphries J., Dr. Jim's Animal Clinic for Dogs, Howell Book House, NY, 1994.

Irlbeck NA, Nutrition and Care of Animals, Dubuque, Iowa: Kendall/Hunt Publishing, 1996.

Lazarus P, Keep Your Pet Healthy the Natural Way, Indianapolis: Macmillan, 1983.

Messonier S., The Arthritis Solution for Dogs. Prima Pets, Prima Publishing, Roseville,

Ca, 2000.

Monti DJ, Human and Animal Medicine Meet on the Bridge, News Section, Journal of the American Veterinary Medical Association, 217, No 12, pp. 1775 –8, 2000.

Norsworthy GD and Fooshee SK, Ask the Vet: Questions and Answers for Dog Owners, Guelph, Ontario, Canada: Lifelarn, 1997.

Patmore A and Couzens T, Your Natural Dog: A guide to Behavior and Health Care, New York: Carroll & Graf Publishers, 1998.

Pitcairn Rtl., Pitcairn Stl., Dr. Pitcairn's Complete Guide to Natural Health for Dogs and Cats, Rodale Press Inc., Emmaus, PA, 1995.

Puotinen CJ, The Encyclopedia of Natural Pet Care, Keats Publishing, New Canaan, CT. (McGraw Hill), 1998.

Schoen AM, DVM, Love, Miracles, and Animal Healing, New York: Simon & Schuster, 1997.

Self, HP, A Modern Horse Herbal. Addington, Buckingham, England: Kenilworth Press, 1996.

Siegal M and Cornell University. The Cornell Book of Cats, New York: Villard Books, 1989.

Siegal M and the School of Veterinary Medicine, University of California at Davis, UC Davis Books of Dogs, New York: HarperCollins Publishers, 1995.

Stein D, The Natural Remedy Book for Dogs and Cats, Freedom, Calif: Crossing Press, 1994.

Stein D., The Natural Remedy Book for Dogs and Cats, The Crossing Press, Freedom CA, 1994.

Volhard, W and Brown K, DVM, The Holistic Guide for a Healthy Dog, New York: Howell Book House, 1995.

Wolff HG, DVM, Your Healthy Cat: Homeopathic Medicines for Common Feline Ailments. Berkely, Calif.: North Atlantic Books, 1991.

Wulff-Tilford M and Tilford GL, Herbal Remedies for Dogs and Cats: A Pocket Guide to Selection and Use. Connor, Mont: Mountain Weed Publishing, 1997.

Wulff- Tilford ML, Tilford GL, All You Ever Wanted to Know About Herbs for Pets, Bowtie Press Inc., Irvine California, 1999.

Yamall, C, Cat Care Naturally. New York: Charles E. Tuttle, 1995.

CERTIFICATION EXAMINATION

INSTRUCTIONS

T HE following multiple choice examination is to be completed by the reader who wishes to become a Certified Dietary Supplement Counselor. Individuals who complete the certification examination should detach the answer page at the end of the certification examination. The certification candidate needs only to fill in the answer sheet as each question is answered. The completed answer sheet should be mailed to the following address: **Certification Program, Holt Institute of Medicine, 61 Stevens Avenue, Little Falls, NJ 07424.** Approximately two weeks after the exam questions are completed and mailed, the candidate for certification is requested to call 973-890-2378 and speak with Andrea Parris who will arrange for a short telephone interview to satisfy the academic staff of the Holt Institute of Medicine that the candidate has completed the requirements for certification in a satisfactory manner.

The examination is split into sections by chapter and the answers to most questions are found in the body of each chapter. Candidates are encouraged to try and complete the examination from memory, rather than from the book itself. However, when doubt arises, the candidate is permitted to revise the information during the examination. There may be an occasional question asked which requires a more in-depth knowledge than may be presented in the book. In the event that such a question is encountered the candidate is encouraged to research the question by referring to chapter references or other reliable sources of information. This certification program involves an honor system and the candidates are given the answers to the questions at the end of the book. The candidate is asked to report their score when they mail this answer sheet. It is expected that the candidate could score more than 85% because they have the book available to answer the questions. Furthermore, no candidate will be issued a certificate unless they have satisfied staff of the Holt Institute of Medicine that they have applied best efforts in the study program. The certification process is stringent because successful candidates are given credits toward a naturopathic degree from the Pan American School of Natural Medicine (call (973) 256-4660).

Please note that every question is answered by the simple response TRUE or FALSE. Read the questions carefully, some are tricky, in order to make you think!

Answer the questions by writing true (T) or false (F) on the question sheet. Then check your answers on the answer sheets on pages 367-369. Sign the declaration that you read the book and answered the questions in good faith. You will have an oral examination with a staff member of the Holt Institute of Medicine (call 973 256-4660 for details).

QUESTIONS

CHAPTER 1: MULTIVITAMINS

1. Fat soluble vitamins are toxic in high dosages
2. Vitamins A, C and E are examples of antioxidants
3. Vitamin D can be synthesized by the human body
4. Multivitamins pose no risk of adverse effects
5. Vitamin K can alter blood clotting
6. Dietary supplements can be recommended for the treatment and prevention of disease
7. Individuals on calorie controlled diets may be at special risk of vitamin and mineral deficiencies
8. Vitamin deficiencies are always obvious in their production of symptoms or signs
9. Recommended daily intakes (RDI) or recommended daily values (RDV) of vitamins and minerals are always sufficient to prevent diseases.
10. Most Americans manage to eat 5 servings of fruit or vegetables per day.
11. The elderly population seems to be at special risk for vitamin and mineral deficiency.
12. Some prescription drugs may deplete vitamin and mineral stores or their availability in the body.

CHAPTER 2: SLEEP

13. Sleep apnea should be evaluated by a medical practitioner
14. Simple sleep problems are best managed by drug prescriptions
15. Dietary supplements used to support the body function of sleep can be safely taken while operating machinery or driving
16. Behavioral therapies are quite valuable in common sleep problems
17. Alcohol consumption improves the quality and duration of sleep

18.   Drugs used to induce sleep often result in the development of tolerance
19.   Sleep is a complex cascade of body events
20.   Combining nutrients and botanicals can result in a synergistic approach to help combat sleeplessness
21.   Sleep deprivation can stimulate appetite and promote weight gain
22.   Over the counter sleeping drugs have not been associated with any serious adverse effects
23.   Mature men can have sleep patterns disturbed by prostatic enlargement

CHAPTER 3: MENOPAUSE AND PMS

24.   The risks of taking hormone replacement therapy (HRT) in uncomplicated menopause or peri-menopause may often outweigh any benefits.
25.   Uncertainty exists about the safety of bioidentical hormones in women with breast cancer.
26.   Menopause is due to a simple deficiency of estrogen.
27.   Conventional HRT, which combines animal estrogens with synthetic progestins, may cause breast cancer.
28.   Metabolic Syndrome X is associated with menstrual disorders.
29.   Menopause and Syndrome X combine to increase risks of chronic disease.
30.   Soy isoflavones are simple estrogens
31.   Black Cohosh is best used in a standardized extract in dietary supplements and is the form associated with an evidence base for symptom relief.
32.   Conventional HRT is always the treatment of choice for menopause
33.   Pre-menstrual syndrome occurs in women most commonly in the age range 30-40 years.
34.   After menopause women have a high risk of heart disease in comparison to pre-menopausal females.

CHAPTER 4: ANTIOXIDANTS

35.   Reactive forms of oxygen may damage tissue.

36. Inclusion of fruits and vegetables in the diet is the best source of antioxidants.
37. The body has no in-built defenses against oxidative tissue damage
38. High dosages of vitamin C when given by injection can sometimes cause an unwanted oxidative stress to tissues.
39. Ellagic acid has been shown to have potential benefits in breast cancer prevention in laboratory studies.
40. Oxidative stress can play a major role in the causation of complications in diabetes mellitus and Syndrome X.
41. Antioxidants are best used in combinations that reach fat and water loving tissue.
42. Antioxidants can play a valuable role in decreasing muscle pain and stiffness following aerobic exercise.

CHAPTER 5: ANTIAGING

43. The single most effective way of reversing aging is to take human growth hormone.
44. Anti-aging initiatives should focus on the prevention of chronic disease and disorders that cause premature death or disability.
45. Immune function often declines with age.
46. The thymus gland shrinks with age.
47. Osteoporosis is more frequent in elderly people.
48. Coral calcium is a holistic mineral supplement rich in calcium and other trace elements.
49. Diabetes mellitus can be considered to be a disease of premature aging.
50. Hormone replacement therapy has complete anti-aging benefits.
51. Poor people (underprivileged economics) tend to die young.
52. Loving relationships are associated with longevity.

CHAPTER 6: OSTEOPOROSIS: THIN BONES

53. Osteoporosis and osteomalacia are the same disease.
54. An indirect measure of the presence of osteoporosis in the population is the occurrence of hip fracture.
55. African-American women have a greater risk of osteoporosis than

Caucasian women.

56. Smoking and drinking alcohol are associated with an increased risk of osteoporosis.

57. Peak bone mass is reached in women in their early or mid-thirties age range.

58. Osteoporosis is often associated with osteoarthritis especially in the elderly.

59. Antigravity exercise is important in osteoporosis prevention.

60. Many mature adults may benefit from bone density assessment.

61. Nutritional support for bone structure and function is valuable in individuals taking bone building drugs e.g. bisphosphonates etc.

62. Calcium supplements alone are adequate to build bone strength.

63. Calcium intake in most American teenagers is most often at a level of recommended daily values.

64. Bone density often rapidly diminishes after the menopause.

CHAPTER 7: IMMUNE FUNCTION

65. Altered immune function with age is associated with auto-immunity.

66. Single nutritional or botanical supplements are preferred to combination supplements to support immune function.

67. Acquired Immuno Deficiency Syndrome (AIDS) often requires intensive nutritional support.

68. Several drugs are highly effective at preventing viral infections.

69. Altered immune function is associated with many diseases.

70. Immune function involves a complex cascade of events among body functions and structures which is more able to be supported by combination herbs, botanical or nutrients.

71. Oxidative stress damages immune function.

72. Supplements sold to support immune function are often supported by research on the specific supplement that carries the limited health claim.

73. Disorders of immune function are easily self managed.

74. Metabolic Syndrome X and diabetes mellitus are associated with impaired immune function.

CHAPTER 8: JOINT CARE

75. Dietary supplements can be used in a legally accepted manner to treat arthritis.
76. Pain, heat and swelling in a single joint is a medical emergency.
77. Chondroitin is well absorbed.
78. Certain herbs can inhibit cyclo-oxygenase type II (cox-2) enzymes.
79. High quality, low sodium glucosamine has an evidence base for the nutritional support of joint mobility and cartilage structure.
80. Glucosamine is a highly effective treatment for joint pain (analgesia).
81. Evidence suggests that certain types of collagen provide immune support for joint health.
82. Boswellia serrata may inhibit inflammatory compounds (leukotrienes) that promote inflammation in joints.
83. Non-steroidal anti-inflammatory drugs (NSAID) are the commonest class of drugs that involve adverse event reporting to the Food and Drug Administration in the U.S.
84. NSAID usage is often associated with significant bleeding from the upper and lower digestive tract.
85. NSAID may interfere with liver function.
86. NSAID may compromise renal function.
87. Cox-2 inhibitor types of NSAIDs have been associated with increased risk of heart attack and stroke.
88. Effective bone and joint rubs, such as those containing essential oils, emu oil and counter-irritants in combination, can reduce the need for NSAID or permit reduction in dosage of NSAID in individuals with joint pain or arthritis.

CHAPTER 9: DIGESTION

89. Probiotics are friendly bacteria that can implant themselves in the lower digestive tract and exert health benefits
90. Probiotics may be useful in preventing or managing travelers diarrhea
91. Probiotics of certain types may be valuable in patients with immune deficiency, e.g. AIDS
92. Digestive enzymes are considered to be most valuable in the presence of deficiency of these enzymes.
93. Digestive enzymes can sometimes be destroyed by stomach acid.

94.   Prebiotics are agents that promote the growth of healthy bacteria in the colon.

95.   Milk thistle (sylimarin) has valuable benefits in the support of liver function.

96.   Fava bean flour can neutralize stomach acid, with effects similar to regular mineral antacids.

97.   Gum mastica (mastic gum) has been used to help deal with Helicobacter pylori (H. pylori) infection, which is often associated with peptic ulcer.

98.   Antibiotic usage can promote yeast overgrowth.

99.   Reseeding the bowel with friendly bacteria (probiosis) is a valuable nutritional support following courses of broad spectrum, prescription antibiotics in both children and adults.

100.   Gentle colon cleansing with herbs and nutritionals may assist with body detoxification.

101.   Heartburn is most often caused by excessive backwash or reflux of acid from the stomach into the lower esophagus

102.   Apple cider vinegar is effective for most cases of heartburn.

CHAPTER 10: HEARTBURN

103.   Proton pump inhibitor drugs can completely abolish stomach acid for many hours.

104.   Some powerful antioxidants, such as ellagic acid may have an ability to block gastric proton pumps, which secrete acid.

105.   Immediate relief of the symptom of heartburn is possible by blocking stomach acid secretion with a proton pump inhibitor drug.

106.   The most effective and immediate way of relieving heartburn is to take a substance that neutralizes gastric acid.

107.   H. pylori infection causes much damage to the upper digestive tract by creating oxidative stress.

108.   Antioxidants may play an important role in preventing direct damage to the lining of the upper digestive tract in people with acid peptic disease.

109.   The first line approach to managing simple heartburn is lifestyle change.

110.   The symptoms of a peptic ulcer are always easily distinguished from cancer of the stomach or upper digestive tract.

111.   Magnesium containing antacids may cause diarrhea.

112.   Calcium containing antacids tend to cause diarrhea.

113.   High intake of calcium supplements should be avoided in individuals
       with failure of kidney function.

CHAPTER 11: COLON CLEANSING

114.   Soft, bulky stools that are easy to pass are present in individuals who
       take a high fiber diet and adequate fluid intake.

115.   Many individuals on a Standard American diet (SAD) do not consume
       enough dietary fiber.

116.   The administration of probiotics with dietary fiber may be more
       advantageous in health benefits than using either alone.

117.   Strong stimulant laxatives e.g. senna should never be taken on a long
       term basis.

118.   Some strong purgatives may damage the function of the colon.

119.   Taking adequate amounts of fluid with fiber is absolutely necessary to
       avoid digestive upset or complications.

120.   When a person increases fiber intake, they may go through a
       temporary phase of adjustment of bowel habit and flatulence.

121.   Adequate dietary fiber intake compliments body cleansing by
       enhancing or regulating bowel habits.

CHAPTER 12: FIBER

122.   Certain types of dietary fiber have a prebiotic effect.

123.   Insoluble fiber is the type of fiber that may generally have a laxative
       effect.

124.   Soluble fiber can be used to smooth out blood glucose elevations
       following meals.

125.   Enhancing dietary fiber intake in people with the Irritable Bowel
       Syndrome may reduce bowel spasms.

126.   Oat bran hydrocolloid (beta glucan) may reduce blood cholesterol by a
       factor of approximately 20%.

127.   Beta glucans from oat fiber are particularly valuable in regulating blood
       sugar in individuals with Metabolic Syndrome X or Diabetes.

128.   Oat beta glucans are soluble fiber that may decrease requirements for

diabetic drugs or insulin in people with Diabetes; and individuals with
Diabetes should be warned to avoid episodes of low blood sugar.

CHAPTER 13: ENZYMES

129.   Conventional medicine thinks that digestive enzyme supplementation
       is necessary to assist normal people with digestion of food and
       nutrients.
130.   Digestive enzymes are involved in driving chemical reactions inside the
       body.
131.   The body makes certain enzymes that operate to detoxify the body.
132.   Metabolic enzymes have just the same effects as digestive enzymes.
133.   Metabolic enzymes may go into the body when taken by mouth and
       provide nutritional support for many aspects of body chemistry.
134.   All metabolic enzymes are well absorbed into the body.
135.   Metabolic enzymes may assist in the support of immune function.
136.   Combination enzyme products should be examined in terms of the
       strength of the enzyme activity and the range of content of enzymes
       in the product.
137.   Some enzyme products are over priced in comparison to more
       complete formulas with a better range of ingredients.
138.   Nattokinase is a digestive enzyme.

CHAPTER 14: CORAL CALCIUM

139.   Coral calcium is not just a calcium supplement.
140.   Absurd and preposterous treatment claims have been made about
       coral calcium.
141.   There is a health precedent only for the use of coral calcium that
       originates in Okinawa, Japan.
142.   Much coral calcium sold in the dietary supplement market in the past
       few years did not originate in Okinawa, Japan.
143.   There are many testimonials concerning the health benefits of coral
       calcium use.
144.   Studies imply that coral calcium combined with exercise may be
       valuable in the management of Osteoporosis.
145.   The word "coral calcium" is misleading and it has led to ignorant

comparisons of coral calcium with regular calcium supplements.

146.   Human studies have shown that coral calcium treated water may help with relaxation responses.

CHAPTER 15: WEIGHT MANAGEMENT

147.   There is not a diet described in the history of medicine that can cause sustained weight loss or control in overweight individuals.

148.   Obesity is a significant cause of premature disability or death.

149.   As obesity rates increased in modern times, there has been a corresponding increase in the occurrence of Type II Diabetes and these phenomena appear to be closely related.

150.   Many people with obesity develop insulin resistance.

151.   Excess circulating insulin is often found in individuals with Syndrome X.

152.   Overcoming insulin resistance is often a key factor in the management of mature people with obesity.

153.   The most successful dieters are those who use dietary supplements or drugs alone to gain most weight loss.

154.   Every weight control program must involve a general health initiative.

155.   Treating obesity requires a holistic program with multiple interventions.

156.   Most people who lose weight by dieting regain their weight within a couple of years or so.

157.   Restriction of simple sugars in the diet is widely considered to be a useful dietary approach to weight control and the management of Syndrome X.

158.   Treating or managing obesity without considering the presence of Syndrome X will not result in good outcome for people involved in weight control programs.

159.   High dosages of stimulant appetite suppressant have been associated with cardiovascular risks.

CHAPTER 16: SYNDROME X

160.   Many people with Syndrome X may progress to develop Type II Diabetes.

161.   Syndrome X may affect up to 70 million American citizens.
162.   Syndrome X does not occur in children.
163.   Syndrome X is associated with many different diseases, disabilities and premature death.
164.   Syndrome X is the most common cause of liver disease.
165.   Obesity and Syndrome X are often associated with inflammatory responses in the body.
166.   EPA, found in fish oil, may assist in sensitizing the actions of insulin.
167.   Syndrome X is easily managed by drug treatments.
168.   There are many nutritional factors that can be combined to benefit the constellation of problems found in Syndrome X.
169.   Alpha lipoic acid may have both insulin sensitizing effects and benefits in the prevention of complications of oxidative stress in individuals with Syndrome X or Type II Diabetes.
170.   Special care is required with the use of supplements in children on weight control programs.

CHAPTER 17: BLOOD SUGAR

171.   The most highly educated person with Diabetes tends to have better clinical outcomes from their disease.
172.   About 20 million documented Americans have Diabetes, in some form.
173.   There may be several million people with Diabetes that is undiagnosed.
174.   Established Diabetes cannot be self managed.
175.   Several dietary supplements may reduce blood sugar in a potent manner and there is a significant risk of interaction between diabetic medications and dietary supplements.
176.   Type II Diabetes is the commonest type of Diabetes.
177.   High blood sugar can be present without obvious symptoms in some people.
178.   Type II Diabetes predisposes many people to significant risk of cardiovascular disease.
179.   Any suspicion of Diabetes should result in medical referral.
180.   No person should stop diabetic drug treatment or insulin administration without the advice of a medical practitioner.

CHAPTER 18: FISH OIL

181. Trans-fatty acids are healthy dietary fats.
182. There is a widespread deficiency of omega-3 fatty acids in many western diets.
183. Hydrogenated oils are best avoided.
184. Omega-6 types of essential fatty acids are quite common in western diets and they do not often require extra supplementation.
185. Omega-3 fatty acids have been reported to provide some protection against sudden death from heart attack.
186. In general, plant sources of omega-3 fatty acids are not reliable supplement sources of active omega-3 fatty acids.
187. People vary in their ability to convert omega-3 fatty acid precursors (found in plants or nuts) into active omega-3 type fatty acids, such as EPA or DHA.
188. Nutritional scientists have developed a general consensus that the ratio of dietary intake of omega-6 and omega-3 fatty acids is often out of balance with excessive intake of omega-6 fatty acids.
189. Medical literature suggests that it is very difficult for most people to get enough omega-3 fatty acids from regular fish oil liquids or regular fish oil capsules, without problems of compliance (sticking with the supplements).
190. Scientific studies show that targeted delivery, enteric coated, fish oil is absorbed much more efficiently and better tolerated than regular fish oil capsules or liquids.
191. Many physicians have stopped recommending fish oil liquids as supplements because these oils are likely to decompose rapidly when the container is opened.
192. Fish oil supplements are beginning to be preferred to increasing fish intake in the diet because of heavy metal contamination in certain fish.
193. Enteric coated fish oils may be more cost effective because of their better absorption and better tolerance by many individuals.
194. Fish oil usage must be monitored in people with bleeding tendencies.
195. EPA is a natural anti-inflammatory substance.
196. EPA is converted into DHA readily in the body.
197. DHA is converted to EPA readily in the body.
198. Fish oil supplementation may be very valuable in people with cardiovascular disease or Diabetes mellitus.
199. Conventional medicine has not universally accepted the benefits of

fish oil for disease management, despite a large body of scientific evidence showing health benefit.

CHAPTER 19: BLOOD CHOLESTEROL AND HOMOCYSTEINE

200.   Many individuals with Syndrome X take cholesterol lowering medication of the statin type.
201.   A significant number of individuals with high blood cholesterol have fatty liver (a component of Syndrome X), even though these people may be at risk of the known liver side effects of statin-type cholesterol lowering drugs.
202.   Elevated blood homocysteine levels are an independent risk factor for heart disease.
203.   High density Lipoprotein (HDL) is a good form of cholesterol and increases in its blood levels are associated with cardiovascular health potential.
204.   Taking blood cholesterol lowering drugs may sometimes give a person a false sense of security to lapse dietary control of blood cholesterol.
205.   The first line option to lower blood cholesterol is diet combined with exercise.
206.   Dietary supplements cannot be labeled with statements about lowering blood cholesterol in individuals with high blood cholesterol.
207.   Combining several nutritional or botanical substances that lower blood cholesterol may produce a synergistic or additive benefit in the promotion of a healthy blood cholesterol level.
208.   Individuals with high blood cholesterol are encouraged to lower blood homocysteine levels at the same time.
209.   One of the commonest reasons for discontinuation of statin-type cholesterol lowering drugs is disturbance of liver function tests.

CHAPTER 20: HEART

210.   There is no simple dietary supplements formula that can cover all aspects of the nutritional support of heart or cardiovascular health.
211.   Antioxidants are believed by most nutritional scientists to exert benefits in the promotion of cardiovascular health.
212.   Statin-type drugs deplete the body of co-enzyme Q10.

213.   Positive lifestyle is the most important approach to heart health

CHAPTER 21: PROSTATE

214.   Prostatic enlargement affects almost every man if he lives long
        enough.
215.   Soy based diets have been clearly linked to prostate health.
216.   Single item supplements for the nutritional support of prostate
        structure and function are often inadequate in their overall effects.
217.   Good scientific agreement exists that several nutrients, herbs or
        botanicals can benefit prostate structure and function.
218.   Some supplements used to support prostate function are prescription
        drugs in Europe.
219.   A comprehensive supplement approach for prostate health is
        advisable.

CHAPTER 22: SEX

220.   One of the commonest underlying problems in individuals with
        erectile dysfunction is poor cardiovascular health.
221.   Diabetes mellitus is commonly associated with erectile dysfunction.
222.   Drugs like Viagra®, Cialis® and Levitra® work to correct erectile
        dysfunction by enhancing the availability of nitric oxide in the body.
223.   A precursor to nitric oxide synthesis is L-Arginine.
224.   Nitric oxide is a powerful chemical messenger that regulates blood
        flow in several areas of the body.
225.   Drugs used to treat sexual dysfunction or erectile dysfunction should
        not be used in combination with dietary supplements that are used for
        sexual enhancement.
226.   Healthy sexual function has been associated with the reduction in
        occurrence of many diseases.

CHAPTER 23: MEMORY

227.   Sleep deprivation is a common cause of disturbance in memory.
228.   Exercising the brain with intellectual tasks assists in preventing
        declines in brain function.

229.   The principal fuel used by the brain during its function is glucose.

230.   Excessive stress may masquerade as poor brain function.

231.   Antioxidants are believed to play a major role in supporting brain function.

232.   Phospholipids have been shown in many studies to improve brain function in people with poor memory or decreased mental alertness.

233.   Acety-L-Carnitine complements the actions of phospholipids in supporting brain function.

234.   Acety-L-Carnitine may assist in increasing the neurotransmitter acetylcholine.

235.   Alpha-GPC may increase the availability of growth hormone in the body.

236.   The use of certain antioxidants in Alzheimer's disease seems quite promising.

CHAPTER 24: SKIN, NAILS AND HAIR

237.   Nutrients or beneficial dietary supplements for skin health may be more effective when taken by oral supplementation, compared with topical application.

238.   Much aging that appears in the skin is due to oxidative stress.

239.   There is a major move towards the use of more natural cosmetics because of the identification of potentially toxic, artificial ingredients in many cosmetics, moisturizers, shampoos, etc.

240.   All topical substances that contain potentially toxic artificial dyes should be avoided.

241.   The presence of some blue dyes (FDC) has been associated with serious toxic reactions when taken by mouth.

CHAPTER 25: EYE CARE

242.   Lutein is valuable in the support of the function of the retina.

243.   Eating bilberries has been associated with improvements in night vision.

244.   Vitamin C administration may be associated with cataract prevention.

245.   Combination antioxidant supplements are the preferred nutritional support for general eye health.

CHAPTER 26: HIGH ENERGY

246. Individuals who complain of lack of energy should define the cause of the problem.
247. Chronic Fatigue Syndrome may be associated with depressed immunity or chronic viral infection.
248. Green Tea is quite valuable as a healthy perk.
249. Sleeplessness drains energy.
250. Lack of energy is associated with the presence of body toxins.
251. Several simple botanicals may stimulate energy in a safe manner.
252. Strong stimulant supplements, e.g. ephedra are best avoided in mature adults.
253. All herbal stimulants should be avoided in childhood or pregnancy.

CHAPTER 27: NATURES CALCIUM

254. Eggshell calcium is the highest concentration of natural calcium known to the supplement industry on a weight for weight basis.
255. Eggshell calcium is more likely to be free of heavy metal contamination than marine sources of calcium.
256. Eggshell calcium has been associated with improvements in bone structure.
257. Eggshell calcium contains a desirable trace element profile, as well as calcium.
258. Calcium supplements are utilized by the body in a much more efficient manner when vitamin D is administered with the calcium.

CHAPTER 28: ANTI DEPENDENCE

259. Dietary supplements should not be used to treat serious forms of addiction.
260. Kudzu has been shown in human studies to reduce total alcohol intake in healthy volunteers.
261. Studies show that individuals taking Kudzu tend to drink less alcohol compared with people not taking Kudzu.
262. Dependence on substances is a tendency shed by almost every person.
263. Removal from substances of abuse e.g. alcohol or cigarettes creates stress.

264.　　Safe stress busting nutrients or herbs may be quite valuable in individuals who have problems with substance abuse or dependence.

CHAPTER 29: MOOD

265.　　Clear evidence of depression should always result in medical evaluation.

266.　　Individuals with depression have a greater risk of suicide.

267.　　Saint John's Wort may interfere with anti-viral drug treatments.

268.　　Allergies have been associated with mood disturbance.

269.　　Dietary supplements for mood support are best applied only in minor to moderate mood disturbance.

270.　　Supplements that alter mood should not be used in children or pregnancy.

CHAPTER 30: ALLERGY

271.　　True allergic responses involve the immune system.

272.　　Food intolerance should be distinguished from food allergy.

273.　　Individuals with general allergies may tend to have more allergies to botanicals or herbs.

274.　　Vitamin C has an effect somewhat similar to anti-histamines.

275.　　The key approach to allergic reactions is to remove the agent or substance that causes the allergy.

276.　　Allergy testing e.g. prick testing etc. is no substitute for a well taken medical history about offending allergens.

277.　　In cases of doubt substances that may cause allergy should not be administered.

CHAPTER 31: SPECIFIC ANTI-AGING FACTORS FOR NATURAL CLINICIANS

278.　　Hormonal supplementation is a stand alone intervention for anti aging.

279.　　Autoimmunity decreases with age.

280.　　Compounds that donate methyl groups in the body have a basis for rational use in anti aging medicine.

281.　　Calorie restriction has been associated with longevity in experimental animals.

282. Enhanced mineral intake has been linked to decreased life expectancies.

283. Coffee extracts and coffee drinking contribute to the development of Type 2 Diabetes.

284. Vitamins and phytochemicals contained in fruit, vegetable and berry powders are preferred baseline nutritional approaches for anti aging.

285. Advanced Glycation End Products (AGEs) can make cellular attachments and cause tissue damage.

286. Carnosine promotes the process of protein glycation.

287. Tri-methyl-glycine (TMG) is a methyl donor.

288. Individuals who have advanced exercise programs may benefit from methyl donors.

289. Some meta-analysis studies question the benefit of use of human growth hormone injections in anti aging medicine.

290. Compounds used as growth hormone secretagogues may lose their effectiveness over a period of time in some individuals.

291. Blood levels of DHEA often decline with age.

292. DHEA may cause depression in some individuals.

293. Melatonin is a powerful free radical that causes oxidative stress to tissues.

294. The term "adaptogen" strictly refers to assistance with adaptation of the body to stress.

295. Resveratrol has complex actions on the regulation of apoptosis.

296. Bioidentical hormone replacement therapy is without significant side effects.

297. Ecballium elaterium has been shown to benefit individuals with Hepatitis C infection.

298. All hormone replacement therapies must be supervised by a knowledgeable healthcare giver.

CHAPTER 32: MISCELLANEOUS

299. Fucoxanthin is found in several species of seaweed and it has been shown to have thermogenic properties that may assist in weight control

300. The value of seaweed in weight control may include many other factors than Fucoxanthin.

301. Polysaccharides in seaweed may stimulate immune function.
302. Seaweed has been extensively used in techniques for body cleansing.
303. Vitamin and mineral supplements used in children should be adjusted downwards in dosage.
304. Nutritional supplementation in children has been associated with improved measures of IQ.
305. Any substance used in health management that is natural is always safer than a drug.
306. New Zealand green-lipped mussel may be useful in the nutritional support of joint function.
307. The word apperient means gentle stimulation of bowel elimination.
308. Black cohosh has the same properties and actions as blue cohosh.
309. Curcumin is found in turmeric.
310. Chaparral (Larrea) has potential toxicity and is best avoided.
311. Fennel has soothing effects on upper digestive function.
312. Valerian is a sedative herb.
313. Goldenseal can be taken to help an individual disguise their use of illicit drugs.
314. Licorice may cause fluid retention and is to be avoided in high dosage in people with high blood pressure.

CHAPTER 33: PETS

315. It is always advisable to take the advice of a vet before treating any illness in companion animals.
316. Separation anxiety experienced by companion animals is a common reason for placing pets into animal shelters for adoption.
317. Hip arthritis or dysplasia is a very common problem in mature dogs.
318. Several nutrients can support vibrant, coat appearance in dogs or cats.
319. Supplements or strange food should not be given to exotic animals.
320. Cats may suffer from altered immune function more than dogs.
321. The administration of food supplements to animals is regulated by the Dietary Supplement Health and Education Act (1994).

BONUS QUESTIONS

322. Third party literature about dietary supplements can be located in the same area as dietary supplements in a retail setting.

323. A very common cause of heartburn is absence of stomach acid.

324. Colloidal silver is an effective anti-microbial.

325. Colloidal silver has versatile effects on stimulating immune function.

326. Additions of essential oils, e.g. peppermint oil and Polysorbates can enhance the anti-microbial killing action of colloidal silver (augmentation).

327. Particle dispersion and orderliness in photographs of silver colloids are not in any way representative of the effectiveness of silver colloid as an antimicrobial.

328. Human exposure to several herbicides or pesticides are associated with weight gain in scientific studies.

329. Body cleansing or detoxification is best approached by using substances or maneuvers that work on all organs of detoxification.

330. Individuals with severe addiction often have underlying psychological disorders.

331. Curcuminoids found in turmeric have analgesic actions (pain killing).

332. The regularity of taking probiotics may be more important than the actual amount taken on a single or short term basis.

333. Lipase and pancreatic enzymes are often destroyed by gastric acid.

334. Popular combined enzyme supplements are often deficient in their range of content of enzymes.

335. Liquid fish oil products are obsolete or disadvantageous because they decompose rapidly when the bottle is opened and stored.

336. Most natural agents that stimulate sexual function work quickly, within one hour of taking them.

337. The Federal Trade Commission regulates truth in labeling of dietary supplements.

338. Plant sources of omega-3 fatty acids are reliable ways of obtaining the active omega-3 fatty acids EPA and DHA.

339. Modern nutraceutical technology provides complex formulations of natural substances to meet the complexity of cascades of body structures and functions.

340. More than 80% of all dietary supplements sold in the U.S. are formulated by sales or marketing staff without any biomedical training.

341. Homeopathic Arnica montana is an evidence-based natural agent

that may diminish pain and swelling following medical procedures or trauma.

Questions: Appendix C

342.   Metabolic Syndrome X has been associated with an increased occurrence of Alzheimer's disease.

343.   Soluble fiber is metabolized in the colon to yield saturated fats.

344.   A high glycemic index property of foods is related often to the rate at which glucose is absorbed into the body.

345.   Diets proposed for the management of Syndrome X should be enriched with omega-6 fatty acids in most individuals.

346.   Reductions in inflammatory cytokines have been noted to occur with weight loss.

347.   Significant amounts of inflammatory cytokines are elaborated by adipose tissue.

348.   Sleep deprivation may increase appetite promoting hormones.

349.   Many diets used alone are successful in producing sustained weight loss.

350.   Carbohydrate restriction does not consistently overcome insulin resistance.

ANSWER SHEET

To be detached and mailed with your score and signature

1. T	29. T	57. T	85. T
2. T	30. F	58. T	86. T
3. T	31. T	59. T	87. T
4. F	32. F	60. T	88. T
5. T	33. T	61. T	89. T
6. F	34. T	62. F	90. T
7. T	35. T	63. F	91. T
8. F	36. T	64. T	92. T
9. F	37. F	65. T	93. T
10. F	38. T	66. F	94. T
11. T	39. T	67. T	95. T
12. T	40. T	68. F	96. T
13. T	41. T	69. T	97. T
14. F	42. T	70. T	98. T
15. F	43. F	71. T	99. T
16. T	44. T	72. F	100. T
17. F	45. T	73. F	101. T
18. T	46. T	74. T	102. F
19. T	47. T	75. F	103. T
20. T	48. T	76. T	104. T
21. T	49. T	77. F	105. F
22. F	50. F	78. T	106. T
23. T	51. T	79. T	107. T
24. T	52. T	80. F	108. T
25. T	53. F	81. T	109. T
26. F	54. T	82. T	110. F
27. T	55. F	83. T	111. T
28. T	56. T	84. T	112. F

detach and mail

113. T	152. T	191. T	230. T
114. T	153. F	192. T	231. T
115. T	154. T	193. T	232. T
116. T	155. T	194. T	233. T
117. T	156. T	195. T	234. T
118. T	157. T	196. T	235. T
119. T	158. T	197. F	236. T
120. T	159. T	198. T	237. T
121. T	160. T	199. T	238. T
122. T	161. T	200. T	239. T
123. T	162. F	201. T	240. T
124. T	163. T	202. T	241. T
125. T	164. T	203. T	242. T
126. T	165. T	204. T	243. T
127. T	166. T	205. T	244. T
128. T	167. F	206. T	245. T
129. F	168. T	207. T	246. T
130. F	169. T	208. T	247. T
131. T	170. T	209. T	248. T
132. F	171. T	210. T	249. T
133. T	172. T	211. T	250. T
134. F	173. T	212. T	251. T
135. T	174. T	213. T	252. T
136. T	175. T	214. T	253. T
137. T	176. T	215. T	254. T
138. F	177. T	216. T	255. T
139. T	178. T	217. T	256. T
140. T	179. T	218. T	257. T
141. T	180. T	219. T	258. T
142. T	181. F	220. T	259. T
143. T	182. T	221. T	260. T
144. T	183. T	222. T	261. T
145. T	184. T	223. T	262. T
146. T	185. T	224. T	263. T
147. T	186. T	225. T	264. T
148. T	187. T	226. T	265. T
149. T	188. T	227. T	266. T
150. T	189. T	228. T	267. T
151. T	190. T	229. T	268. T

detach and mail

269. T	290. T	311. T	332. T
270. T	291. T	312. T	333. T
271. T	292. T	313. F	334. T
272. T	293. F	314. T	335. T
273. T	294. T	315. T	336. F
274. T	295. T	316. T	337. T
275. T	296. F	317. T	338. F
276. T	297. T	318. T	339. T
277. T	298. T	319. T	340. T
278. F	299. T	320. T	341. T
279. F	300. T	321. F	342. T
280. T	301. T	322. F	343. F
281. T	302. T	323. F	344. T
282. F	303. T	324. T	345. F
283. F	304. T	325. F	346. T
284. T	305. F	326. T	347. T
285. T	306. T	327. T	348. T
286. F	307. T	328. T	349. F
287. T	308. F	329. T	350. T
288. T	309. T	330. T	
289. T	310. T	331. T	

_____Your self score on the exam, number of questions
answered correctly out of 350 questions.

I certify that I have read this book and
answered the questions in good faith.

_____

Sign Here

detach and mail

INDEX

Absorption, 22, 24-25, 76, 78, 100, 106, 128, 133, 139, 147, 151-153, 155, 162, 199-200, 215, 243, 267, 271, 308-309, 317

Acid, 23, 29, 40, 43-45, 58-59, 80, 82-84, 86-92, 106, 110, 129-131, 133, 141-143, 145, 147-154, 159, 164, 172, 177, 182, 188, 191, 210, 219-220, 226, 239, 242-243, 245, 247, 255, 258, 262, 277, 279-280, 287-289, 292, 308-309

Addiction, 28, 201, 204, 319

Adrenal, 184, 289

Aging, 15, 25, 27, 31, 39, 44, 46-49, 51-54, 129, 137, 184, 191, 205, 217-224, 226-227, 229, 312

Alcohol, 29-30, 57, 89-90, 129, 131, 171, 173, 195, 201-206, 209, 219, 272, 319

Alfalfa, 235-236

Allergic, 109, 209, 211-216, 252-253, 255, 283

Aloe, 63, 72-73, 96, 191, 228, 234, 236-237, 280

Alternative Medicine, 4, 33, 79, 96, 187, 224, 237, 269, 295

Alzheimer's, 39, 125, 132, 180-181, 183-187, 221, 223, 234, 245, 249, 304, 310

Analgesic, 72, 231

Angelica, 35, 237

Animals, 88, 113, 139, 191, 216, 226, 238-239, 241, 255, 258, 264, 279, 290-293

Anti-Aging, 5-6, 16, 23, 37, 39, 44, 47-49, 51-55, 178, 183, 185-187, 190-191, 217-219, 221-227, 229-230, 245, 253, 262

Antibody, 62, 286

Antidepressant, 153, 209-210, 253

Antioxidant, 21, 23-24, 37-39, 42-44, 46-48, 51, 54, 63, 66, 70, 79, 82, 88, 91-92, 105, 129, 133, 141, 143, 145, 151, 157, 164, 171, 177, 179, 186, 190, 193, 197, 205, 215-216, 220, 224, 226, 228, 243-245,

253, 255-256, 258, 262, 266, 276, 281, 287, 311

Anxiety, 27, 172, 180, 206-207, 233, 241, 289

Apricot Pits, 237

Arnica, 235, 240, 282-285

Arthritis, 15, 39, 46, 61, 68, 70, 72, 74, 107, 151, 191, 212, 234, 239-240, 243-244, 256, 272, 291-292, 310

Autoimmune, 61, 105, 107, 222, 236, 272

A to Z Guide to Commonly Used Herbs, 235

Bacteria, 23, 62, 76-78, 81, 83-84, 94, 99-100, 102-103, 243, 265-269, 273, 291-292

Barberry, 69, 71, 82, 237, 245

Bayberry, 237-238

Beauty, 48, 189-191, 257

Berries, 38-40, 42, 46, 79, 131, 145, 171-172, 195, 205, 220, 259, 277, 279, 287

Betony, 238

Bilberry, 39-40, 192-193, 238

Biorhythm, 27, 32, 120, 196, 224

Black Cohosh, 35-37, 238-239

Bleeding, 68, 83-84, 109, 153, 233, 244, 270

Blood , 5, 15, 23, 35-36, 51, 58, 62, 64, 99, 101-102, 107, 109, 113, 117-119, 121-123, 125-130, 132-145, 150-151, 153, 155-171, 176-179, 182, 185-186, 188, 194, 197, 203-204, 212-213, 222-223, 225-226, 231, 233-234, 236, 240-241, 247-250, 257, 259, 265, 269, 275, 282-283, 307-308, 310-311, 317

Blood Cholesterol, 15, 36, 64, 99, 101-102, 113, 117-118, 125-127, 129-130, 132-133, 137-141, 144-145, 151, 156-171, 182, 185, 225-226, 240, 250, 257, 275, 307, 310, 317

Blood Clotting, 23, 107, 109, 130, 150, 159, 163, 171

Blood Flow, 35, 171, 176-179, 186, 204, 248-249

Blood Homocysteine, 58, 156, 159-160, 164, 166-168, 170, 182, 188

Blood Lipid, 156-157

Blood Pressure, 15, 36, 101, 109, 113, 117-119, 121, 125-126, 132, 145, 150-151, 161, 164, 169, 171, 177, 197, 212, 222, 225, 233-234, 247, 250, 275, 282, 310

Blood Sugar, 5, 99, 102, 109, 113, 133-143, 145, 161, 182, 194, 248, 308

Blood Vessels, 107, 125, 155, 163-164, 177, 186, 212, 233, 241

Body Chemistry, 23, 57, 95, 104, 119, 129-130, 136, 149, 154, 189, 231, 259

Body Structure and Function, 87

Bone, 22, 52, 56-60, 62, 68-69, 71-74, 89, 113, 198-199, 239, 259, 291

Borage, 149, 239

Boswellia, 69-70, 191, 235, 239-240, 245, 250, 291

Botanicals, 7, 12, 28, 33, 44, 56, 61-63, 66, 70-71, 84-85, 88, 96, 138, 140, 142-143, 156, 160, 163-164, 170-175, 178, 184, 188, 190-193, 195-197, 210, 215-216, 224, 227, 231, 234, 256, 259, 268, 274, 277, 280, 288, 292, 299, 307

Bowel, 75-77, 83-84, 91, 93-99, 155, 208, 232-233, 241, 248, 254, 257, 265-267, 270-271, 308

Brain, 6, 34, 39, 45, 79, 93, 104, 112, 125, 155, 159, 177, 180-188, 195, 203-204, 210, 221, 225, 277, 312

Breast, 34-35, 43, 89, 220, 247, 261, 263, 286-288

Caffeine, 30, 195, 209, 241-242, 247

Calcium, 5-6, 22, 52, 56, 58-60, 76, 87-88, 91, 100, 111-114, 144, 191, 194, 198-200, 219, 236, 258, 281, 288, 319

Calendula, 73, 242

Calorie, 20, 102, 117, 119-122, 184, 225-226, 262-263, 275-277

Cancer, 22-23, 34, 39, 45, 61, 65-66, 75-76, 80, 82-83, 90, 94, 101, 104-105, 108, 113, 125-126, 132, 145-146, 149, 173, 190-191, 194, 199, 205, 208, 219-221, 223, 236-238, 240, 242, 246, 250, 259, 261-263, 266, 271-272, 286-288, 310

Capsicum, 235, 242

Carbohydrate, 98, 116, 119, 130, 154, 182, 304, 315-316

Cardiovascular Disease, 34, 36, 105, 125-127, 131-132, 136, 141, 145-147, 155-156, 158-159, 165-166, 168, 170-171, 180, 182, 219-220, 222, 261-262, 276, 303, 310

Cartilage, 69-70, 239, 259, 291, 319

Cat, 291

Cellular Function, 45

Chaparral, 242

Children, 29, 109, 115, 119-120, 124, 127, 132-133, 136, 147, 149, 151, 197, 214, 275-277, 301

Cholesterol, 6, 15, 36, 64, 77, 94, 99, 101-102, 113, 117-118, 121, 125-127, 129-130, 132-133, 137-145, 151, 155-171, 182, 185, 225-226, 234-235, 240-241, 250, 257, 275, 305, 307-308, 310, 317

Chondrus crispus, 257

Chromium, 121, 131, 139, 141, 144-145, 164, 198, 259

Cognitive Decline, 159, 181-182, 187, 220, 261

Colon, 5, 23, 76-78, 83-85, 93-97, 99-100, 102, 113, 199, 232, 240-241, 254, 261, 264-270, 308

Comfrey, 73, 234, 242

Constipation, 77, 87, 93, 95, 109, 234, 267

Coral Calcium, 5, 52, 111-114, 194, 219, 319

Cosmetics, 72-73, 189-190

COX-2, 69-71, 238, 244-245

Cranberry, 39-40, 235, 243, 292

Curcumin, 43-45, 243-245

Curcuminoids, 24, 191, 243-245

Dandelion, 245

Dementia, 180-182, 184, 186-188, 222, 249

Dependence, 201-202, 204-206, 276

Depression, 27, 145, 155, 171-172, 188, 195, 207-209, 224, 228, 234, 239, 253

Detoxification, 23, 78, 81, 84, 94, 97, 122, 143, 195-196, 213-214, 264, 267-271

Devil's Claw, 69, 71, 215-216, 245

Diabetes Mellitus, 15, 20, 25, 27, 44-45, 49-50, 64, 101-102, 117, 123-124, 126-130, 132-141, 143-145, 151, 162, 168, 186, 192-194, 201, 221-222, 236, 303, 307, 310-311, 318

Diet, 10, 17, 19-21, 23, 25, 27, 30, 35, 38-39, 42, 45-46, 57-60, 64, 78-80, 91, 94-95, 98-100, 102, 109, 116-117, 119-122, 126, 131-132, 136-137, 144-149, 151, 155-156, 158-159, 162, 172-173, 182, 184, 188, 190, 195, 199, 202, 205, 207, 209, 219, 241-242, 257, 262, 265, 267, 270, 276-277, 280, 286-288, 292, 313, 315-317

Digestion, 5, 75-76, 78-79, 81, 84-85, 92, 98, 100, 104, 208, 232, 240, 248, 280, 296, 320

Digestive Tract, 68, 75-76, 78, 80, 82-85, 88, 90-92, 95, 99, 102, 155, 162, 181, 244, 265, 270

Dog , 291

Dong Quai, 35, 37, 246

Dyspepsia, 76, 82-83, 86, 89-91, 101, 234, 244, 270

Echinacea, 63-64, 66, 228, 234-235, 246, 250, 274, 280

Education, 6-7, 10-11, 14, 53, 58, 60, 76, 132, 134, 142, 157, 169, 171, 276, 292, 294-295, 298-300, 302

Egg, 199

Energy, 6, 46, 100, 117, 120, 123, 136, 154, 185, 194-197, 208, 226, 258

Enzyme, 71, 78-80, 82, 105-110, 203, 216, 238, 245, 251, 262, 270, 281-283, 308

Ephedra, 121, 197, 246-247, 316

Erectile Dysfunction, 176, 178-179

Evening Primrose, 35, 37, 149, 247, 288

Exercise, 30, 39, 46, 58-59, 94, 105, 113, 117-118, 120, 122, 126, 131-132, 135, 137, 144, 156, 158, 160, 165, 171, 183, 185, 195-196, 207, 209, 214, 219, 222, 254, 258, 267, 270, 275, 277, 292, 304

Eye, 6, 22, 127, 136, 143, 192-193

Fat, 21, 25, 43, 46, 73, 80, 116-117, 119-120, 122, 125, 131-132, 136, 146-148, 150, 156, 173, 184, 189, 219, 257-258, 264, 275, 284, 310-311

Fatigue, 109, 123, 136, 194-195, 197, 208, 220, 234

Fennel, 96, 215-216, 234, 248

Feverfew, 71, 234, 245, 248

Fiber, 5, 21, 38, 46, 51, 78, 80, 84, 94-95, 98-103, 119, 121-122, 128-129, 133, 141, 161-162, 184, 219, 236, 240-241, 257, 267, 270-271, 275-276, 287, 307-309, 317

Fish Oil, 5, 21, 80-82, 97, 119, 130-131, 144-155, 166, 170, 172, 182, 188, 191, 209, 219, 247, 263, 277, 279-280, 287, 309

Fo-Ti, 248

Free Radicals, 38-39, 46, 105, 129, 205, 220, 265, 311

Fucose, 257-258

Fucoxanthins, 122, 258

Garlic, 63, 82, 141, 164, 171-172, 228, 234-235, 248, 287, 292

Ginger, 69, 71, 97, 234, 245, 248-249

Gingko Biloba, 36, 171-172, 179

Ginseng, 63, 143, 178-179, 197, 228, 249, 288-289

Glucose, 51, 64, 101-102, 122-123, 125-126, 128-130, 135-136, 138-144, 182, 220, 225, 241, 307-308, 312, 317

Glycemic Index, 99, 128, 131, 144, 308

Goldenseal, 63, 228, 250

Green Tea, 24, 35, 40, 44-46, 51, 62-63, 66, 69, 71, 82, 88, 91, 105, 121, 188, 191, 197, 210, 220, 227, 241, 245, 259, 287, 292

Guggulupid, 250

Hair, 6, 57, 189-190, 211, 253

Hawthorne, 172, 250

Heart, 6, 21, 31, 34, 36, 39, 68, 98, 107, 130-131, 137, 149-151, 155-164, 166, 168-172, 176-177, 179, 197, 204-205, 231-233, 235, 240-241, 244, 247, 250, 270, 276, 282, 295, 319

Heartburn, 5, 86, 89-92, 113

Heavy Metal, 113, 198-199, 214, 269, 273

Herb, 59, 63-64, 66, 70-71, 80, 140, 142, 191,

206, 210, 215-216, 231, 233, 238-239, 241-242, 245-246, 248-250, 253-256, 274, 282

Homeopathic, 223, 235, 240, 277, 282-285, 301

Homocysteine, 6, 58, 156, 159-160, 164-168, 170-171, 182, 188, 221-222

Hormone, 15, 29, 33-34, 37, 48, 104, 113, 117, 120, 122, 126, 139, 182, 187, 222-224, 226-227, 230, 233, 255, 259-263, 275, 286, 288-289, 312

Hypertension, 127, 129-130, 137-138, 221, 303-304, 316

Immune Function, 5, 22, 27, 44, 61-67, 77, 101-102, 133, 155, 168, 181, 185, 215-216, 222, 227-228, 236, 257-259, 274, 292

Immunity, 45, 47, 61-66, 107, 145, 177, 227-228, 246, 258, 274, 277

Infection, 76-77, 82, 91, 101, 195, 232, 243, 271-272, 274

Infertility, 125, 132, 145

Inflammation, 70, 75-76, 83, 90-91, 104, 107-108, 125-126, 129-130, 132, 138, 145, 149-150, 155, 164, 166, 194, 208, 212, 217, 221-223, 225, 228, 232, 239-240, 244-245, 266, 271, 281-282, 310, 318

Insomnia, 27-28, 208, 235, 241, 247, 255, 264, 312, 319

Insulin, 15, 22, 36, 64, 102, 113, 116-123, 125-126, 128-130, 132, 135-141, 144-145, 151, 154, 164, 166, 223, 225, 275, 280, 303-304, 308-311, 316-318

Insulin Resistance, 36, 116-120, 122-123, 125, 129-130, 132, 136-139, 145, 151, 154, 166, 223, 275, 280, 303-304, 308-311, 316-318

Iodine, 198, 257-258, 288-289

Joint, 5, 60, 68-74, 234, 239-240, 244-245, 259, 291

Kidney, 68, 127, 136, 233, 243, 247

Kudzu, 202-206

Leaky Gut, 266, 271-272

Licorice, 45, 82, 234-235, 250-251, 289

Lifestyle Change, 9, 15-16, 31, 33, 37, 49, 57, 60, 89, 117-118, 131, 156, 160-161, 165, 169, 182, 226, 228-230, 286, 313, 316

Lipid, 51, 150, 154, 156-157, 245, 309

Liver, 23, 68, 78, 85, 118, 125-126, 129, 132, 139, 143, 161, 163-166, 185, 233, 239, 242, 244, 250-251, 254, 269-271, 308, 310, 318

Magnesium, 20, 29, 59, 87-88, 91, 111-113, 144, 171-172, 198, 200, 215, 254, 257, 262-263, 289

Marine Nutraceuticals, 256

Memory, 6, 23, 177, 180-184, 186-188, 195, 210, 249

Menopause, 5, 15, 32-37, 57, 170, 180-182, 194, 209, 227, 249, 260-263, 296, 313, 320

Metabolic Enzyme, 105, 108-110

Metabolic Syndrome, 6, 15, 36, 44, 49-50, 64, 101, 116-121, 123-127, 129-133, 138, 141, 143, 151, 154, 165-166, 168-170, 172, 182, 193-194, 201, 221, 275, 278, 280, 303-305, 307-310, 312, 316-318

Milk Thistle, 78, 80, 82, 143, 215-216, 251, 271

Minerals, 4, 19-22, 25, 29, 52, 91, 105-106, 111-112, 140, 144-145, 157, 191, 195, 200, 219, 257-258, 261-262, 275-276, 279, 288

Mistletoe, 234, 251, 259

Mood, 6, 30, 153, 155, 207-210, 228

Mushrooms, 64, 66, 102

Myrrh, 251

Nervous System, 23, 35, 72, 130, 148, 154-155, 183-188, 203, 209, 233, 241, 247, 254, 277

Nettles, 235, 251

Oat Bran, 101-102, 119, 133, 141, 145

Obesity, 15, 19, 27, 50, 109, 115-119, 122, 125-127, 129-130, 132-133, 136-138, 141, 145, 168, 201, 217, 240, 245, 263-264, 275, 278, 303-305, 307, 310-313, 315-319

Oil, 5, 21, 35, 37, 72-73, 80-82, 84, 97, 119, 130-131, 144-155, 166, 170, 172, 182, 188, 191, 209, 219, 234-235, 239,

247-248, 252, 255, 263, 277, 279-280, 283, 287-288, 292, 309

Okinawa , 52, 111-114, 219

Omega 3 Fatty Acids, 21, 82, 119, 130, 147-148, 150, 152-153, 155, 157, 184, 188, 276-277, 279-280, 291, 308-310

Omega 6 Fatty Acids, 147, 149, 279

Osteoarthritis, 68, 239-240, 244, 291

Osteoporosis, 5, 34, 39, 52, 54, 56-60, 113, 159, 200, 222, 261

Overweight, 15, 20, 31, 36, 115-120, 125, 127, 132, 275, 278, 280, 306, 311-313

Oxidative Stress, 38-39, 43-44, 46-47, 54, 63, 66, 70, 91, 129, 136, 141, 145, 168, 185, 205, 213, 217, 225-226, 311

Pain, 46, 57, 70-74, 76, 83, 86, 90, 95, 105, 151, 195, 231, 241-245, 248, 278, 282

Pain Control, 242-245

Papaya, 251-252, 280

Parsley, 252, 288

Peptic Ulcer, 39, 68, 76-77, 82, 90-91, 100-101, 242, 244, 250

Perimenopause, 33-36, 58-59, 261-262, 313

Pet, 213, 290-293

PMS, 5, 33-37, 170, 180-181, 194, 260, 262, 296, 320

Pollen, 197, 211, 213, 252

Postmenopause, 33, 180

Prebiosis, 77, 81, 84, 99, 271

Pre-diabetes, 15, 50, 64, 117, 123, 126-127, 129, 132, 136, 138, 141, 145, 154, 171, 186, 193-194

Premature Aging, 27, 31, 44, 48-49, 54, 129, 137, 191, 205, 217, 221, 226, 312

Probiosis, 77, 81, 99

Propolis, 252

Prostate, 6, 44, 162, 173-175, 220, 224, 251, 254

Protein, 21, 119, 129, 131, 140, 144, 162, 164, 168, 173, 185, 219-222, 225-226, 236, 251, 258, 262, 275-276, 309-311

Pycnogenol, 220, 253

Relaxation, 35, 76, 99, 112, 177, 183, 194, 207

Royal Jelly, 197, 253

Sargassum muticum, 257-258

Saturated Fat, 21, 119, 131, 146-147, 173, 184, 219

Saw Palmetto, 235, 253-254

Seaweed, 256-259, 287-288

Senna, 254

Sex, 6, 30, 57, 122, 173, 176, 178-179, 208, 222-223, 227, 256, 259-262, 286, 320

Sexual function, 173, 176-179, 207, 249

Skin, 6, 46, 48, 72-73, 109, 165, 189-191, 211-213, 220-221, 224, 232-233, 236-237, 242, 255, 257, 269, 272-273, 278, 283, 285, 291

Skullcap, 29, 69, 71, 245, 254

Sleep, 5, 27-32, 120, 180-183, 194-197, 208-209, 217, 224, 228, 255, 296, 312-313, 318, 320

Smoking, 30, 57, 89, 131, 173, 195, 204-205, 209

Soy, 35-37, 59, 119, 129, 131, 144, 148, 162, 173, 186, 191, 203, 255, 259, 261, 267, 286-287, 308, 317, 319

Soy Isoflavones, 35-36, 59, 144, 191, 203, 255, 259, 267, 286-287

Spirulina, 40, 197, 255-256

St. John's Wort, 234, 253

Statin, 158, 163-166

Steroid, 289

Stomach, 68, 82-84, 86-92, 102, 106, 122, 152, 186, 203, 233, 235, 239, 241, 244, 257-258

Stool, 23, 94-97, 99, 264-265, 267, 270

Stress, 21, 27, 30, 32, 38-39, 43-44, 46-47, 54, 57, 63, 65-66, 68, 70, 75, 82, 86, 88, 91, 96, 129, 136, 138, 141, 145, 153, 156, 168, 170, 172, 182-183, 185, 194, 205, 210, 213, 217, 224-226, 228, 233, 244, 269, 276-277, 283, 289, 291, 311, 313, 318

Stroke, 36, 68, 121, 125, 159, 163, 165-166, 182, 244, 270

Sugar, 5, 21, 45, 64, 99, 102, 109, 113, 120-121, 126, 128-129, 131-145, 161, 163, 182, 185, 194, 201, 204, 248, 275-276, 304, 308

Syndrome X, 5-6, 15, 27, 36, 44, 49-50, 54,

64, 98, 101, 116-127, 129-133, 136-138, 141-143, 151, 154-155, 161, 163, 165-166, 168-170, 172, 181-182, 186, 193-195, 201, 221, 223, 228, 247, 275, 278, 280, 295-296, 303-313, 315-320

Synergy, 10, 29, 31, 62, 69, 74, 78, 81, 91, 99, 102, 108, 159, 161, 185, 193, 216, 291

Tea Tree Oil, 255

Teeth, 20, 22, 113, 199

Thalassotherapy, 257

Thyroid, 224, 257, 288-289

Toxin, 213-214, 268-270

Trace Mineral, 219

Trans-Fatty Acids, 146-147, 157

Trauma Recovery, 240, 277-278, 284-285

Triglycerides, 36, 125, 129-130, 137, 151, 155-157

Turmeric, 24, 43-45, 59, 62-63, 66, 69, 71, 82, 88, 91, 188, 220, 227, 234, 243-245, 288-289

Unsaturated Fat, 146

Valerian, 29, 234-235, 255

Veterinary, 290, 292

Virus, 66, 195, 274

Vision, 136, 192-193

Vitamin A, 20-23, 25, 214-215

Vitamin B, 215

Vitamin C, 20, 23, 43, 59, 62-63, 66, 88, 191, 193, 210, 215, 228, 232, 250, 253, 258, 262-263, 277, 281-282, 289, 291-292

Vitamin D, 19-20, 22, 73, 191

Vitamin E, 20-23, 43, 73, 88, 171, 191, 193, 220, 262-263, 291

Vitamins, 4, 19-25, 29, 36, 58, 76, 91, 100-101, 105-106, 114, 129, 131, 140-141, 144-145, 147, 157, 159, 171, 173, 215-216, 219-220, 224, 236, 257, 261-263, 275-276, 279, 288

Weight, 5, 15, 19, 28, 30-32, 45, 50, 94, 101-102, 113, 115-122, 127, 132-133, 135-137, 142, 154, 169-171, 182, 195, 199-200, 208, 214, 226, 228, 255-259, 262-264, 266, 275-276, 278, 304, 306-307, 310, 312-317

Weight Loss, 101, 116-117, 119-121, 136-137, 142, 208, 255-256, 258, 276, 310, 312, 315-316

Wound healing, 23, 72, 221, 240, 242, 246, 255, 277-281, 283-284

Yeast, 64, 77, 83, 101-102, 151, 163, 223, 234, 246, 272

Yohimbe, 255-256

Zinc, 20, 44, 58-59, 62-63, 66, 88, 91, 145, 193, 198, 228, 262, 279, 288-289